D0838063

Aphasia Treatment
World Perspectives

Edited by

Audrey L. Holland, Ph.D.
University of Arizona

Margaret M. Forbes, Ph.D.
University of Pittsburgh

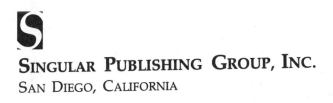

SINGULAR PUBLISHING GROUP, INC.
SAN DIEGO, CALIFORNIA

RC
425
.A6714
1993
27726124

Singular Publishing Group, Inc.
4284 41st Street
San Diego, CA 92105-1197

Copyright © 1993 by Singular Publishing Group, Inc.

Typeset in 10/12 Palatino by CFW Graphics
Printed in the United States of America by BookCrafters

All rights, including that of translation, reserved. No part of this publication may be reproduced, stored in a retrieval system, or transmitted in any form or by any means, electronic, mechanical, recording, or otherwise, without the prior written permission of the publisher.

Library of Congress Cataloging-in-Publication Data

Aphasia treatment : world perspectives / Audrey L. Holland, Margaret
  M. Forbes, editors.
    p.   cm.
  Includes bibliographical references and index.
  ISBN 1-879105-64-0
  1. Aphasia—Treatment   I. Holland, Audrey L.   II. Forbes
Margaret M.
  [DNLM: 1. Aphasia—therapy.   WL 340.5 A641645 1993]
RC425.A6714 1993
616.85'5206—dc20
DNLM/DLC
for Library of Congress   93-18644
                                                                   CIP

Augustana College Library
Rock Island, Illinois 6120

Contents

List of Contributors

Elizabeth Armstrong, Ph.D.
Department of English and
  Linguistics
Macquarie University
North Ryde
New South Wales, Australia

Anna Basso, Ph.D.
Associate Professor in Clinical
  Neuropsychology
Milan University
Neurological Clinic
Milano, Italy

Brigitte Bertoni, Ph.D.
Speech Pathologist
Department of Neurology
University of Zurich
Zurich, Switzerland

Sally Byng, Ph.D.
Reader in Clinical Aphasiology
Department of Clinical
  Communication Studies
City University
London, England

Claire Croteau, Ph.D.
École d'orthophonie et
  d'audiologie, Faculté de
  Médecine
Université de Montréal
Montréal, Quebec, Canada

Marie-Pierre de Partz, Ph.D.
Cognitive Neuropsychology
  Research Unit (NECO)
Faculty of Psychology
Universite of Louvain
Louvain-la-Neuve, Belgium

Matthias Fünfgeld
Neurologische Universitatsklinik
Freiburg, Germany

Gillian Gailey, Ph.D.
Executive Director
Aphasia Centre of Ottawa-Carleton
Ottawa, Ontario, Canada

Manfred Herrmann
Neurologische Universitatsklinik
Freiburg, Germany

Walter Huber, Ph.D.
Professor of Neurolinguistics
Department of Neurology and
  School of Logopedics
Medical Faculty,
Rheinisch-Westäflische
  Technische Hochschule
Aachen, Germany

Yves Joanette, Ph.D.
Professeur titulaire de recherche
École d'orthophonie et
  d'audiologie, Faculté
  de Médecine
Université de Montréal and
  Laboratoire Théophile-
  Alajouanine
Montréal, Québec, Canada

Helga Johannsen-Horbach
Director, School of Speech
  Therapy
Neurologische Universitatsklinik
Freiburg, Germany

Aura Kagan, Ph.D.
Director, Communication
  Program
The Aphasia Centre-North York
North York, Ontario, Canada

Guylaine Le Dorze, Ph.D.
Assistant Professor
École d'orthophonie et
  d'audiologie, Faculté de
  Médecine
Universife de Montréal
Montréal, Quebec, Canada

Maria M. Pachalska, Ph.D.
Professor
Institute and Clinic of
  Rehabilitation
Academy of Physical Education
Kraków, Poland

Richard Peach, Ph.D.
Rush-Presbyterian-St. Luke's
  Medical Center
Rush University
Department of Communication
  Sciences and Disorders
Chicago, Illinois, U.S.A.

Claire Penn, Ph.D.
Professor and Chair
Department of Speech Pathology
  and Audiology
University of the Witwatersrand
Johannesburg, South Africa

Sumiko Sasanuma, Ph.D.
Tokyo Metropolitan Institute of
  Gerontology
Itabashi-ku
Tokyo, Japan

Xavier Seron, Ph.D.
Cognitive Neuropsychology
  Research Unit (NECO)
Faculty of Psychology
Université of Louvain
Louvain-la-Neuve, Belgium

Luise Springer, Ph.D.
Chief Speech Therapist
Department of Neurology and
  School of Logopedics
Medical Faculty,
Rheinisch-Westäflische
  Technische Hochschule
Aachen, Germany

Claus-W. Wallesch, Ph.D.
Neurologische Universitatsklinik
Freiburg, Germany

Klaus Willmes, Ph.D.
Department of Neurology and
  School of Logopedics
Klinikum, Rheinisch-Westäflische
  Technische Hochschule
Aachen, Germany

Sandra M. Weilaert
Speech Therapist
Rotterdam Aphasia Foundation
Erasmus University Rotterdam
Rotterdam, The Netherlands

Dorothea Weniger, Ph.D.
Department of Neurology
University of Zurich
Zurich, Switzerland

Conny Wenz
Neurologische Universitatsklinik
Freiburg, Germany

Nel M. van Amerongen
Neuropsychologist
Department of Internal Medicine
  I and Geriatric Medicine
Erasmus University Rotterdam
Rotterdam Aphasia Foundation
Rotterdam, The Netherlands

**Mieke E. van de
  Sandt-Koenderman**
Clinical Linguist
Rotterdam Aphasia Foundation
Erasmus University Rotterdam
Rotterdam, The Netherlands

Frans van Harskamp
Behavioral Neurologist
Department of Neurology
University Hospital
  Rotterdam-Dijkzigt
Erasmus University Rotterdam
Rotterdam, The Netherlands

Evy G. Visch-Brink
Clinical Linguist
Department of Neurology
University Hospital
  Rotterdam-Dijkzigt
Erasmus University Rotterdam
Rotterdam, The Netherlands

Preface

During the past 10 years of my life, I have begun to satisfy a lifelong ambition. I started to see the world. I have been lucky enough to have been invited by colleagues to participate in their meetings and conferences. Thus, some of this travel has been professional. Some has been just for personal delight, but even then, I have sought out my fellow aphasiologists: Perhaps the most obvious professional fallout from my travel is that I have developed an intense awareness of how truly little I really knew about the work of my colleagues in other parts of the world. I don't think I am alone with this problem, and it seems to me that many of my fellow American clinical aphasiologists share my limited world view. Finally, I have developed a growing awareness that our colleagues around the world are more aware of what is going on in the United States than we Americans expect.

It is clear that a major barrier to freer communication about treating aphasic patients is language; we represent a uniquely English-speaking perspective on aphasia treatment even though our own country is becoming more multilingual with every passing year. But the problem is probably deeper than that; our geographic vastness and our relative professional isolation from other continents of the planet take their toll as well. As a profession, we have been able to remain myopic rather easily. But, as my vision has been stretched by my contact with what is still a smattering of the world's aphasia experts, I have become truly excited about sharing these experiences with my American colleagues. This is the motivation from which this volume initially developed.

Margaret Forbes and I began to develop the notion of editing a volume in which a group of international experts describe their approaches to aphasia rehabilitation for an American audience when we attended the International Aphasia Rehabilitation Congress in Edinburgh, Scotland in 1990. There, our own insularity finally became overwhelming, and we decided to do something about it.

First, we identified a number of individuals who were recognized as experts in aphasia treatment in their respective countries. However, because we, like many of our American colleagues, are not facile with other languages, we felt it necessary to limit our invitations to individuals who could write in English. Therefore, one of the first surprises of this book is that, although sometimes a fairly large amount of editing was required, all of the authors included were not daunted by our requirements to produce a chapter in English. Can you imagine a similar response if a group of English-speaking clinical aphasiologists was asked to write in German, or in French?

The second surprise, I suspect, is that you will be amazed at the extent of the English-language references throughout these chapters. This in no way means that the literature in aphasia treatment is limited to English. A careful study of the respective bibliographies will disabuse a reader of that idea. Great international cross-pollination of ideas is practiced in most parts of the world. This international interaction should suggest that access by non-American professionals to what we can read is not nearly as limited as access by American professionals to what else is afoot in the world of aphasia treatment.

The third surprise is that, regardless of the languages in which the therapies described are conducted, the methods have cross-linguistic application. The formal cross-linguistic study of aphasia has prepared us for understanding differences and similarities in sentence processing cross-linguistically, and to be alert for cross-cultural differences when we provide treatment for aphasia. However, many of the clinical principles and approaches to helping patients to cope with aphasia rise above these extremely important concerns. As you read these approaches, be aware of how many of them can be adapted to our own work, regardless of the language and culture in which they are being described.

As you read this book, you will detect a number of common themes concerning the process of therapy. Most notably, the interest in Cognitive Neuropsychology and its application to treatment is a thread that runs through many of these chapters. Concern with pragmatic issues is almost equally strong. A surprising number of chapters also refer to the World Health Organization's distinctions between disability, impairment, and handicap, and invoke this three-pronged concept as cardinal to notions of functionalism in treatment for aphasia.

Differences also appear, most notably in terms of the backgrounds of the clinicians represented here and the settings and service delivery models that prevail in some places. Although these authors represent an international collection of stars of aphasia therapy, they have diverse backgrounds. Some of them have been trained as speech-language pathologists in ways that are not dissimilar from training in the United States. Included here would be Aura Kagan and Guylaine Le Dorze of Canada, Claire Penn of South Africa, Sally Byng of England, Luisa Springer and Helga Johansen-Horbach of Germany, and Dorothea Weniger of Switzerland. In fact, at least one author, Sumiko Sasanuma of Japan, received her doctoral degree from the University of Iowa. Others are from other disciplines, including Psychology (e.g., Xavier Seron of Belgium) and Neuropsychology (e.g., Anna Basso of Italy and Maria Pachalska of Poland), Linguistics (e.g., Walter Huber of Germany), Neurology (e.g., Claus Wallesch of Germany and Franz van Harskamp of The Netherlands). Some represent disciplines that are not familiar to Americans, such as Clinical Linguistics (e.g., Marie-Pierre de Partz of Belgium and Evy Visch-Brink of The Netherlands). Finally a number of the chapters in this book represent an interdisciplinary collaboration among professionals to an extent that is unusual in the United States. In most of the world, the American definition of the speech-language pathologist as the professional who provides clinicial services to aphasic adults does not strictly apply.

In a related vein, work settings and clinical time frames for service delivery vary. Some of the authors describe their circumstances. We suspect that American readers will be jealous of some of them and see familiarity in far fewer of them. But, regardless of work setting, many of the authors' ideas have direct applications to American clinical service.

Margie and I began this work with a naive (possibly even stupid) idea that we could produce a "World Perspective" on aphasia treatment for colleagues in the United States. As this book has developed, we have changed this stance, thinking that practitioners in other countries might benefit from this book as well. Therefore, an American summary chapter was added. Richard Peach took on the enormous burden of explaining the prevailing American Zeitgeist in a context in which most of the book's readers already know that Zeitgeist. He deserves special thanks for his difficult contribution.

We also recognized that there is no way to do a "World Perspective." Some of our authors were not able, for personal reasons, to meet the deadlines. Our own horizons were not broad enough to have sampled the (even English-fluent) world.

We solved the first problem by the simple expedient of changing the title to "World Perspectives." But we are more pleased with our alternative solution. This book will be followed in a few years by another volume, representing countries not included here, such as some Scandinavian, South American, and Far-Eastern contributions.

We had a wonderful time creating this book. We are pleased and excited by its contents, and we expect you will be as fascinated by what our colleagues around the world are doing as we are. We thank Singular Publishing Group, Inc., for agreeing to support this rather unusual publishing venture. We also thank Pamela Adams for her typing and for her good cheer in helping us, and Pelagie Beeson and Laura Murray and Scott Jackson (bless his compulsive heart) for their careful reading and relentless editing of each chapter. Finally, we are ever grateful to our international colleagues for making this project a reality.

We dedicate this volume to those students of aphasiology and their patients whose mutual work will help us to increase our understanding of aphasia, across international boundaries and across languages.

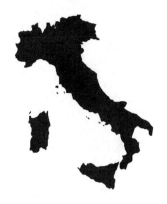

CHAPTER 1

Therapy for Aphasia in Italy

ANNA BASSO
Institute for Neurological Clinic
University of Milan
Milan, Italy

The Aphasia Rehabilitation Service of the Neurological Clinic of Milan University started on a voluntary basis in 1962. For many years it remained the only Aphasia Rehabilitation Service in Italy, and aphasic patients living outside Milan had no chance of being rehabilitated. This state of affairs persuaded us in the late 1960s to organize specialization courses for aphasia therapy, since neurological disorders were not taught in logopaedics schools. This, in turn, directly affected the kinds of patients who came to the Service. Initially, all of our patients had been admitted to the neurological wards, generally because of vascular disease. However, soon thereafter speech therapists who had attended the specialization courses on aphasia therapy began to send us patients for counseling and supervision.

We have now seen 4,500 left-brain-damaged patients, some acute and some chronic. Acute patients are inpatients referred to the Aphasia Service for diagnosis, and may or may not be aphasic. Chronic patients come from various parts of Italy, and all are aphasic. They come either for

1

diagnosis or for a decision about whether therapy is in order for them. A few patients settle down in Milan for 6 months of rehabilitation. All of the patients examined in our Aphasia Service are invited to return. If therapy is provided, either directly in our Service or elsewhere, they are asked to come back for a reevaluation every 3 to 6 months, depending on how far they live from Milan. If they had language disorders, but for various reasons had not been enrolled in therapy, they are invited for control examinations approximately every 2 years.

Our experience with this population is the subject of this chapter. What I have written does not pretend to be anything other than the expression of my thoughts at this moment. Therapy for aphasia is relatively new. It started on a large scale basis some 50 years ago, with only pedagogic principles for theoretical support. Since then it has incorporated new knowledge from various interdependent areas, such as linguistics, clinical neuropsychology, and cognitive psychology. What appears correct in the field of aphasia therapy today will soon be considered outdated. Having often written on aphasia therapy, I always find myself rejecting what I had asserted only a few years before, and I hope that this chapter too will soon be outdated.

People in the field are currently making an effort to base aphasia therapy on scientifically sound procedures, but for the moment it still depends heavily on the therapist's expertise. To detail a coherent and rational therapeutic program is a difficult (perhaps an impossible) task. In the absence of a common cultural background, it requires a long and meticulous exposition, which I will try to make clearer and shorter by discussing some patients we have treated and describing the basis of our treatments.

ASSESSMENT

Before describing the procedures used in our Aphasia Unit to assess whether a patient is aphasic and, if so, to identify his language and other neuropsychological impairments, let me consider some practical issues related to the selection of suitable candidates for aphasia therapy and duration of treatment. I must state beforehand that, from this point of view, Italy is a happy island. The Italian National Health Service pays all expenses; decisions about who, when, for how long, and so forth, to treat are decided entirely by the person prescribing.

Both data from the literature and practical constraints are taken into account in selecting patients for rehabilitation. The effectiveness of aphasia therapy has not been established beyond doubt. In general terms it never will be, because not all patients benefit from therapy. However, a number of clinical studies have established with *reasonable* certainty that an unselected group of treated patients fares better than an unselected group of untreated patients, if the period of aphasia therapy is not too short. Unfortunately, we cannot be more precise about which patients will benefit from aphasia therapy. Some factors are known to have a negative effect on prognosis (the most important being severity of aphasia, time post-onset, and extent of lesion). The effects of other factors, such as age, handedness, and etiology, are less clearly established (see Basso, 1992, for a review). There are, however, indications that these factors have a negative effect only on spontaneous recovery and do not influence the effects of rehabilitation. Wertz et al. (1986), for instance, did not find a negative effect of deferred rehabilitation; and Basso, Capitani, and Vignolo (1979) found no significant interaction between improvement, severity of aphasia, and rehabilitation. Although it is highly probable that the joint effects of many negative factors will prevent recovery, we are not entitled a priori to exclude a patient from therapy.

We have seen that therapy can begin a long time post-onset without diminishing the chances of recovery. Once it has started, though, how long should it be continued? A careful reading of the literature on the effectiveness of aphasia therapy indicates that when patients are treated for rather short periods of time, no difference can be found between them and others who received no therapy (Levita, 1978; Sarno, Silverman, & Sands, 1970; Vignolo, 1964); however, when treatment lasts longer, patients fare better (Basso et al., 1979; Hagen, 1973; Marshall, Tompkins, & Phillips, 1982; Sarno & Levita, 1981). Thus duration of treatment has proved to be a significant factor in recovery (Basso, 1987). Therefore, when we engage a patient in the rehabilitation adventure, we program a minimum of 6 months of daily therapy. If a control examination after this period does not disclose any progress, we usually give up. When amelioration is evident, we proceed for another 3 months, and this is repeated for as long as the patient continues to progress.

Finally, adequate assessment is necessary before starting rehabilitation. A standard assessment battery must concentrate on language, as well as on the cognitive functions that also are frequently impaired in aphasic patients (probably for anatomical reasons). We routinely use such a battery for all our patients, because approximately 90% of them suffer from cerebrovascular disease, mostly in the left hemisphere. Praxis, calculation, abstract thinking, and language are all evaluated. Specifically, language is assessed using the Token Test (DeRenzi & Vignolo, 1962) and à standard language examination. All the tests are standardized, with a cut-off score calculated on normal controls, and they allow us to say whether the subject's performance falls within the normal range and how impaired he is relative to a control group.

The Token Test, probably the most widely used test for evaluation of auditory comprehension, discriminates fairly well between patients with and without language comprehension disorders. However, comprehension is not a unitary process, and it can be impaired because of a lexical disorder, a syntactic deficit, or even a short-term memory impairment, among other things. The Token Test does not identify the cause of the failure; it simply states whether the patient falls within the normal range.

Our standard language examination provides an orderly and standardized description of the patient's behavior in gross language functions. It is detailed enough to permit classification into one of the classical aphasia syndromes that are based on an analysis of speech production (fluent vs. nonfluent) and on comparison of the patient's behavior in different language functions, such as repetition, oral comprehension, naming, reading, writing, verbal production, and so on. The selection of the items and of the different subtests is not, however, informed by any theory of normal language processing, but rather by the observation that lesions in different parts of the language area give rise to different patterns of impairment. To take a simple example, lesions in the perisylvian region generally cause disruption of repetition with frequent phonetic/phonemic errors; lesions outside this area leave repetition unaltered at the phonetic/phonemic level, although paraphasias can occur (Cappa, Cavallotti, & Vignolo, 1981).

For many years treatments have been framed according to the classical syndromes (Broca, Wernicke, Conduction, etc.) or to the symptoms (naming disorders, jargon, agrammatism, etc.) (see, for example, Albert, Goodglass, Helm, Rubens, & Alexander, 1981; Lecours, Lhermitte, & Bryans, 1983). Our original routine evaluation was sufficiently detailed for such needs, and I still believe that for many severely impaired patients there is no need for further examination.

However, the nature of the subjacent disorders responsible for the impaired processing was neither looked for nor captured by the sort of evaluation based on the classical syndromes. Pretherapeutic assessment might have the additional goal of disclosing the possible cause of the impaired behavior. This is particularly true if one believes that therapy must be coherent with some hypotheses of the nature of the processing deficits. Then, patients' disorders should be interpreted by reference to a model of what is currently known about the normal language processing system.

Whenever we consider a patient a possible candidate for therapy and he is not too severely impaired, we submit him to the "Screening Battery for Aphasia" (Miceli, Laudanna, & Burani, 1991). Information derived from results of the various subtests of the battery can be used for a clinical diagnosis, but because this battery is based on the theories of the organization of language developed by cognitive neuropsychology, it also allows us to make a first hypothesis about the functional deficit with reference to normal language processing. This hypothesis should be substantiated, whenever necessary, by more specific and in-depth examinations.

The battery is divided into four sections. Part One explores the patient's capacity to process a sublexical phonological, or orthographic input, presented either auditorily or visually, and to produce an oral or written response to a sublexical input. Part Two is devoted to the study of the lexical-semantic system. This is explored by lexical decision tasks with auditory and visual input, transcodification tasks (repetition, reading aloud, writing to dictation, and delayed copying), lexical comprehension with auditory and visual naming, written and oral confrontation naming, and naming to verbal description.

Part Three explores the processing of grammatical structures. The choice of grammatical subtests is not based on theories, as we do not have at the moment sufficiently detailed theories of production and comprehension of grammatical structures. Practical considerations of what happens in aphasic individuals have guided the choice. First, patients can perform well on a grammatical judgment task but not on the comprehension of grammatical structures. Tasks of oral and written grammaticality judgment are therefore included. Second, processing of grammar can be impaired separately for comprehension and production, and separate tasks of comprehension and production of sentences are included. Third, in both comprehension and production, all sentences are not equally difficult; active sentences, for instance, are generally easier to process than passive sentences. Different types of sentences are therefore included. The final section of the battery is devoted to verbal memory. However, relationships between language processing and verbal memory are unclear, and thus we do not consider the test's results in treatment planning, except for very exceptional cases who have a highly specific and severe verbal short-term memory impairment.

None of the tests listed here is designed for rehabilitation planning. Their main objective is diagnosis, but this can be more or less precise and more or less motivated by a theoretical view of the nature of the disorder. A precise and theoretically motivated diagnosis can be a good starting point for rehabilitation. The more refined the diagnosis, the more precisely therapeutic intervention can be directed toward the functional damage. The assessment battery is a first step toward such an end.

TREATMENT

Based on the results of these language and neuropsychological tests, we recognize two groups of aphasic patients. The first group consists of all

patients for whom we have been unable to arrive at a precise diagnosis
of the specific locus (or loci) of impairment. Most of the patients in this
group are severely impaired and often present with other neuropsychological deficits in addition to aphasia. Some less severely impaired patients whose deficits are about the same in all language functions also
belong to this group. The therapeutic approach to these patients is underspecified. We cannot immediately attempt to restore previous language abilities because we do not know exactly what language abilities
are compromised. Therefore, therapy is initially directed toward recovery of functional communication which, in any case, is the goal of therapy. Patients with more specific and restricted deficits make up the second group. Treatment of these patients is directed toward restoration of
the impaired abilities. We will briefly expound the underlying principles for each group, and then describe two treated patients.

REHABILITATION AIMED AT RESTORING COMMUNICATION

Patients in this group generally are severely impaired, with equivalent
impairment in all language modalities. The group, however, is not homo-
geneous; global, Broca, Wernicke, and transcortical sensory aphasics can
be found in it. In some patients impairment is so severe that test results
are all nil; for other less severely impaired patients, the communicative
use of language appears to be the predominant impairment. Common to
all patients is a severe impairment in functional communication, sometimes more severe than would be expected from their test results.

   As noted earlier, treatment for these patients is determined by our failure to find the functional loci of impairment rather than by a rational
choice of what to do. In effect, there is no greater reason to treat, say, the
lexicon instead of reading, or comprehension instead of confrontation naming. However, because any successful treatment is supposed to restore
the communicative function of language, we endeavor to enable the patient to make the most effective use of whatever language he has.

Turn-taking

The most common situation in which language is used to communicate
is conversation, and the easiest conversation is that which takes place between two persons. This is the situation in aphasia therapy, and we try to
turn the rehabilitation session into a conversation.

   In addition to the content of the exchange between listener and speaker, a conversation has a formal structure, with turn-taking its main aspect. Some patients seem to think the interlocutor is there only to listen;
others never try to say anything although they are willing to listen. For

both types of patients, the first step in aphasia therapy is to re-accustom them to being speaker and listener in turn. Even though this may not be a simple task, it is usually accomplished rather quickly, and the therapist then pays more attention to the content of the exchange.

Comprehension

If the patient's comprehension is good and he is willing to interact verbally, even a severe production impairment will not severely disrupt communication. The interlocutor does not depend on the patient to introduce a new argument; as long as he is able to shape the questions in such a way that the answers do not require much production, as in yes/no questions, the interlocutor can talk with the patient about various matters. However, when comprehension is severely disrupted, verbal exchanges are not possible. For that reason, we initially pay more attention to comprehension than to production.

Classical comprehension exercises generally considered only the level of impairment. Typically, these started by asking the patient to point to one of an array of 4 to 6 semantically unrelated pictures, then to complex pictures, and eventually to understand a narrative. In normal language use, however, it is not enough to associate the word *cat*, for example, with the picture of a cat, or *The boy is eating* with the picture of a boy eating. The process of comprehension cannot stop at this point. It is equally important to understand the purposes of the speaker. In classical aphasia therapy, by asking the patient only to point to the correct picture, the therapist verified whether he or she was able to understand the linguistic content of the sentence, but this is not enough. If a patient is able to point to the correct picture when hearing the sentence *Dinner is ready* (among a choice of, say, a woman cooking in the kitchen, a man reading the newspaper in a dining room with a partly laid table, a laid table with a bowl of steaming spaghetti on it), but does not come and sit down on hearing the same sentence at home, he has not understood the sentence. In classical aphasia therapy no attention was paid to understanding the intent of an utterance or to understanding the inferences that generally are drawn by the listener. Much of what a speaker intends is, in fact, omitted; it is the hearer's job to reconstruct these intentions from what the speaker does say.

A speaker who says "John is tired" may want to convey more than the simple statement that John is tired. For example, he may wish to explain that John has gone to bed, or that John is in a bad mood, or that he will not go to the party. The hearer must discover what information the speaker wants to convey, based on his knowledge of John, the current situation, and, more generally, his knowledge of the world. A patient who reads in a newspaper that Mr. X murdered his wife and does not make the necessary inference that Mrs. X is dead, has not understood the news. In our everyday life, we draw hundreds of inferences each day, some necessary and some optional. Inferences can, in fact, be wrong, causing a disruption of communication that must then be repaired. There are indications that aphasic patients understand indirect speech acts pretty well (Green & Boller, 1974; Kadzielawa, Dabrowska, Nowakowska, & Seniow, 1981; Wilcox, Davis, & Leonard, 1978), but I do not know of any experimental study on other important aspects of comprehension, such as inferences or conversational implications.

After this brief excursion into the area of pragmatics, let us return to the aphasia therapy session. We have a patient with severe aphasia, no chance to locate his functional deficits precisely and we have decided to concentrate on auditory comprehension in a conversational setting. Each day, 5 days a week for months, we must find new topics and create conversational situations in which the burden is carried mainly by the therapist. This can be achieved with a vivid imagination or with some external support such as pictures or short stories. My personal preference is for the short story, which must be read, explained, re-read, and so on, to the patient as many times as necessary for the patient to understand and remember it. Patient and therapist are now ready to engage in a conversation about the content of the story that has become part of the patient's knowledge.

The goal of the therapist is to simulate, as far as possible, a real conversation. To do this, he must use whatever means he has at his disposal (prosody, facial expressions, gestures, etc.) to enable the patient to understand his questions. These questions should, of course, be worded in such a way as to require much attention from the patient and sometimes in a way he cannot understand and thus must ask for repetition. This is because the goal of this exercise is to improve comprehension. The answers required, however, must be easy and short, and the therapist should behave as if he does not know them.

Production

For patients who seem unable to produce language (although speech is not impaired) but have relatively preserved comprehension, the main goal is to have them speak. The situation may be the same as the one just described, but the questions should be shorter and easier. This time, however, the questions must require varied and heterogeneous answers, which initially can consist of a noun, a yes or no, an adverb, or even a gesture, and which become longer and more complex as the patient recovers.

Answering a question never is a simple task. One must determine what part of the question is already known and what part is new, that is, what exactly is asked. Even an apparently simple question like "Has Mary gone out?" can be about either *who* has gone out or *what* Mary has done. Prosody, knowledge of what has been said before, and the actual situation disambiguate the question. Second, one must determine the bit of information requested, and third, one must answer in such a way that the listener comprehends. We must remember to whom we are talking and phrase our speech according to what the interlocutor knows or does not know. This can be very difficult for aphasic patients, and it is our first goal in remediation of production. I once asked an agrammatic patient with severe apraxia of speech who spoke very little, using single words, how he had spent the previous Sunday. The patient said "Peter." The answer was correct, and the patient gave me the information requested, since he had spent the day with Peter (his brother). However, this wording was not very efficient, because I had no idea who Peter was. A more informative answer in this case would have been "brother."

Summarizing what we have said so far, for some severely aphasic patients, it is not possible to identify the functional disorder nor is it very informative to do so because all language processes appear to be equally impaired. For these patients, rehabilitation is focused on restoring efficient use of language, mainly in a conversational setting. Either comprehension or production can be the main focus, but the patient is always asked to alternately be the listener and speaker. Each day the therapist must provide a new topic for conversation and weigh his or her interventions so that the patient must either make an effort to understand, or can understand easily but must strive for the correct answer.

A patient who progresses may reach a stage at which it is possible to identify one or two specific disorders that appear to be the most devastating. When this is achieved, the therapeutic approach changes totally. It is no longer undifferentiated and directed only toward functional communication. To the contrary, therapy strives to be as specific as the individuation of the locus(i) of impairment and knowledge about language processing allow it to be.

A Case of Rehabilitation of Production

MT is a 46-year-old right-handed housewife with 5 years of education. She is married, with two children. In 1981 she had a first ischemic attack with right hemiparesis from which she recovered in a few days. In May 1990, she manifested a right-sided weakness and an inability to speak. A computed tomography (CT) scan performed on the same day showed multiple ischemic lesions in the periventricular white matter and the deep nuclei in both hemispheres. A control CT scan 2 months later showed three small left cortical temporal lesions, in addition to the deep lesions already mentioned.

MT was first examined at the Aphasia Service 45 days post-onset. Speech was nearly absent; she could name 6 of 20 pictures of common objects and repeat and read aloud a few single words, but apraxia of speech was clearly present. She could not write spontaneously or to dictation. She could only trace a few letters and write her surname but not her first name. Comprehension for words was good, mildly impaired for simple sentences, and she scored 16/36 on the Token Test. MT had severe oral apraxia (she scored 2/20; cut-off score, 16/20), mild ideomotor apraxia (48/72; cut-off score, 53/72), and a severe calculation disorder, scoring 18/101 (cut-off score, 74/101). On the Raven's Colored Progressive Matrices (RCPM) (Raven, 1962), she scored 19/36.

MT left for the summer but returned to attend the Aphasia Service regularly at the end of September 1990. The battery performed at that time showed that the patient failed all subtests except for the phonemic discrimination tasks and the oral and written comprehension of nouns. The impairment was about the same in all subtests. Notwithstanding a score of 21 out of 36 on the Token Test, the patient never spoke spontaneously. Further, she spoke only when urgently requested and even then with a great effort unexplained by her mild apraxia of speech. We decided that our first goal in rehabilitation was to have the patient speak more, paying special attention to verbs, which were even rarer than nouns, in a confrontation-naming task and in spontaneous speech. We therefore engaged MT in conversations, using a complex picture as a starting point but always trying to go beyond what was represented in the picture. If, for instance, the picture represented a family lunch, we used it to ask MT questions about her family lunch (what time they had lunch, what they liked to eat, who cooked, etc.). If the picture represented a train station, we used it to ask about her journeys and so on. Very soon we abandoned pictures in favor of short stories. MT's responses slowly became easier and more varied although she spoke slowly and used very few words. Despite her improvement, she reported that she did not speak at home, and this was confirmed by her daughter.

Word-finding difficulties did not seem a sufficient explanation; she could correctly name 80–90% of the pictures of nouns and nearly as many verbs in a confrontation-naming task. In sentences some verbs were omitted and prepositions were occasionally incorrect; but most of her sentences were correct, although simple and short. Phonological errors apparently were due only to her low educational level. The impression was that she *could* have spoken more and we were at a loss to find out why she did not, despite continuous slow progress in the rehabilitation setting.

We finally concluded that MT did not speak mainly because she did not know what to say. Therefore, we sought a way to help her to clarify and sharpen her thoughts so that they could be expressed more easily in words. As before, we read a short story with the patient in order to have something to talk about, but now we asked MT to form a mental image of what was happening in the story. The image had to be as clear and detailed as possible. She could no longer talk about "a man," for example; the man had to be a specific man that she could see in her mind in every detail: how tall he was, what he looked like, how he was dressed, and so forth. In the beginning, MT had great difficulty comprehending what we wanted her to do, but later she started to conjure up progressively more detailed scenes, and she could tell us more and more about what was happening in her mental picture. Such transposition of a story into a series of pictures has another advantage: Events that were not expressed in the story must be made explicit in the pictures. One of Aesop's fables, for example, concerns a dog with meat in its mouth seeing its image in the river. Retelling the story, one can say that the dog wanted to seize the other's dog meat and jumped in the river where, however, it found nothing. One need not consciously realize what happened to the meat in the dog's mouth. However, if the patient *sees* the event, he must see that, when the dog opens its mouth to seize the other dog's meat, its own falls in the river. A control examination performed in May 1991, after 8 months of rehabilitation, showed moderate general amelioration, which was confirmed by MT and her relatives. At the same time, it was now possible to isolate two areas of more severe damage: Writing (via sublexical and lexical routines) and grammatical comprehension. Recovery of these functions will be the next goal in rehabilitation.

A Case of Rehabilitation of Comprehension

AB is a 56-year-old right-handed male construction worker with 8 years of education. Following the rupture of an aneurysm of the left middle cerebral artery he underwent surgery in July 1990. A neurological examination showed a right hemianopia and severe fluent aphasia. The patient was first examined at the Aphasia Service in January 1991, when a control CT scan was also performed. There was a large cortico-subcortical fronto-temporo-parietal hypodense area in the left hemisphere with enlargement of the left ventricle. The patient appeared depressed. His speech was fluent but rather sparse and devoid of meaningful information. Although errors (mainly nonwords) were relatively rare, the patient frequently uttered recurring automatic phrases ("I don't know, what is it?," "I can't speak"). AB performed poorly on all subtests of the assessment battery, with no indication of relatively more preserved or more severely damaged areas. He scored 8/36 on the Token Test and 14/36 on the RCPM. Oral apraxia (13/20) and acalculia (48/101) were also present.

AB's comprehension scores were just above chance level (66% correct in the picture-word matching task with two choices, and 57% correct in the sentence-picture matching task, also with two choices). However, in speaking with him, one had the impression that his comprehension was even more severely impaired than would be expected from the test results, primarily because he appeared to pay no attention to the interlocutor.

We decided that AB should listen and recover some useful comprehension first. This was attempted by engaging him in simple conversations, starting with a picture. The therapist tried to make himself understood by using short sentences accompanied by unambiguous prosody, facial expressions, and gestures. Most of the time, AB did not seem to have the slightest idea what he was being asked. Sometimes, however, he gave an answer apparently related to the question. If the answer was correct, the therapist explicitly noted that it was the requested answer and rephrased the same question, making it clear to the patient that the question was the same. This was done for two reasons: To determine whether AB's answer was correct only by chance; and because we hoped that rephrasing the same question would improve his understanding. If the answer was wrong, this also was demonstrated to AB (sometimes with difficulty), and the therapist tried to explain his question better. Despite our efforts, a control examination 3 months later showed no improvement.

We felt relatively sure that our failure was due to AB's depression and withdrawal rather than the choice of exercises. Rehabilitation continued along the same lines but we used short stories instead of pictures, in hope of motivating the patient.

Six months after starting rehabilitation, AB scored 14 on the Token Test, and slight amelioration was evident in the battery. All of the subtests remained uniformly impaired. At this writing, rehabilitation had been interrupted for the summer.

REHABILITATION AIMED AT A SPECIFIC IMPAIRMENT

In the last few years major changes have occurred in neuropsychology, especially in the study of aphasia. Semiology of language disorders is much more refined, due mainly to the contributions of cognitive neuropsychology. Cognitive neuropsychology extends the principles developed by cognitive psychology to study normal processing to the study of brain-damaged patients. This work is based on the assumption that brain

damage cannot produce new functions, but causes the loss of some previously acquired capacities.

Highly complex and detailed models of normal cognitive functions,
such as the lexical-semantic model, have been developed. Despite some
differences, the functional architecture of the lexical-semantic system is
generally conceptualized as consisting of a set of autonomous, interconnected components. Components involved in the comprehension of
words are distinct from those involved in the production of words. Modality of input and output, phonological or graphemic, defines a second
major distinction between components. These four lexical components
are interconnected through a semantic system that is the repository of
the meanings of words. Any of the components of the model can be
damaged, alone or in combination with others, giving rise to a large number of different disorders.

A cognitive model is only a series of hypotheses about the structure
and the functioning of a mental process. It can serve as a guide for the
analysis of the patient's language. Identification of the lesion in the cognitive system is more or less difficult according to the structural complexity of the reference model. Integrity of any particular component can only
be examined indirectly, by observing the patient's performance on different tasks. This is because each component has a certain function and
will be utilized in all tasks that require that function; further, any one task
involves many components of the cognitive system.

To arrive at a correct diagnosis, much attention must be paid to the
types of errors that the patient makes because they may be highly informative. A patient described by Miceli and Caramazza (1988), for example,
made frequent morphological errors in spontaneous sentence production and repetition of single words. Careful analysis of his errors showed
that most of them were substitutions of inflectional affixes. Derivational
errors were rare. This finding was interpreted by the authors to support
the thesis that inflectional and derivational processes are represented
separately in the lexicon. The consequence for rehabilitation is that for
this patient only the inflectional component must be retrained, not morphology as a whole, as a more superficial analysis would have suggested.

First, using performance on the battery to diagnose a patient's disorder, we consider whether the impairment is in phonology, lexicon, or
grammar. Rehabilitation will always be directed toward the impaired
process and not the *symptom*. We will not treat impaired repetition, for
instance, but either the phonological input or output, depending on our
test results.

At the phonological level, processing of the input phonological stimulus or the phonological output can be investigated separately. Damage to
the processing of phonological input will affect repetition, writing to dictation, and phonemic discrimination. In the case of damage to phonolo-

gical output, reading aloud must be impaired in a similar way. An impairment of sublexical phonology or orthography prevents processing of nonwords, not a particularly important aspect of communication. There may be, however, many reasons for rehabilitation for impairment of sublexical routines. First, severe damage of phonemic discrimination disrupts oral verbal comprehension; second, when there is damage to the lexicon, reading and writing of regular words (and in Italian most words are spelled regularly) can still be performed through the (undamaged) sublexical routines; and finally, there is some evidence that lexical and sublexical routines interact (Miceli, Giustolisi, & Caramazza, 1991).

Retraining of sublexical processes is, however, monotonous and repetitive, and direct intervention by the therapist is needed only for supervision; drilling can usefully be done at home with someone's help.

As we have just seen, the lexical-semantic system has a complex structure, and identification of the functional lesion is not an easy task. Frequently patients have several coexisting deficits. The patient's performance on all lexical (and sublexical) subtests must be analyzed together with reference to a model of normal lexical processing. Analysis of the type of errors is helpful, but one must take care to compare errors from different tasks. If a patient makes semantic errors in comprehension and production, both oral and written, as well as in reading, writing to dictation, and repetition, damage to the semantic system may well be present. However, if sublexical processing is intact, it can be sufficient to partially compensate, resulting in correct repetition, reading, and writing to dictation for most Italian words. Lexical semantic errors in transposition tasks, therefore, are not necessary for a diagnosis of damage to the semantic system.

A post-semantic lexical impairment can be restricted to the phonological or orthographic lexicon, although in clinical practice it is much more common to find similar impairments in oral and written naming. This occurs either for a fortuitous anatomical reason or because of a functional relationship.

It is difficult to summarize rehabilitation of lexical-semantic deficits in a few pages because intervention should be specific for each of the numerous functional impairments. Therefore, we will describe the rehabilitation of two patients: One with damage to the semantic system and the other with damage to the output lexicons.

As mentioned earlier, Part Three of our assessment battery is of limited value because of the lack of a detailed model of normal grammatical processing. This lack also has direct consequences for rehabilitation. Rehabilitation of structures longer than single words has not changed much, at least in our Service, in part because of this lack of a detailed and shared model of normal processing of grammatical structures. Moreover, in Milan, we have not developed any great interest in rehabilitation of grammatical impairments, partly because, strange as it may appear, clinically agrammatic patients are extremely rare in our series. We do try to incorporate in the therapy all the information derived from the patient's test results and from other more specific tasks, but I must admit that our therapeutic intervention is not as specific as would be desirable. However, even thorough investigation of the patient's disorder and application of an apparently rational therapeutic method do not guarantee success.

Two recent studies (Byng, 1988; Jones, 1986) described the treatment of three patients who were clinically agrammatic in both speech production and comprehension. In all patients a specific difficulty with "thematic roles" (i.e., in the mapping between syntactic roles, subject, object, etc., and semantic roles, agent, patient, etc.) was considered the origin of their difficulties. Jones' patient was trained to identify different semantic roles in sentences of increasing syntactic complexity. Byng taught her patients about thematic roles in prepositional phrases. Jones' patient and one of Byng's patients improved in speech comprehension and production. Byng's first patient showed considerable improvement after only 2 weeks of therapy specifically devised for this mapping disorder, whereas her second patient showed no improvement after 6 weeks of the same therapy. After a complete change of the therapeutic regime, the second patient also improved. In summary, the same therapy technique which worked quite well with one patient was clearly unsuccessful with another who had the same functional impairment, and three different techniques helped recovery in three patients with the same disorder.

What can we conclude about therapy from this background? I believe the major change that has taken place in aphasia therapy in recent years lies in the attitude of the therapist, who no longer approaches the patient with a pre-established therapeutic program based on the clinical diagnosis. We know that groups with the same diagnostic label contain highly different patients, and we are much more aware that we have to carry out detailed analyses of the patient's performance if we want to understand the underlying causes of the disorder. However, identification of the underlying impairment, while necessary, does not define therapy.

As for the content of therapy, it has changed more or less for the different functional disorders. Rehabilitation of lexical deficits has probably taken most advantage of recent research in neuropsychology; rehabilitation of sublexical routines is now more frequently taken into consideration. Finally, rehabilitation of grammatical structures has not changed much, at least in our Service.

A Case of Damage to the Semantic System

BA is a 42-year-old right-handed draftsman with 13 years of education. On September 29, 1988 he was shot during a holdup. The bullet entered through his right cheek and came out in the left fronto-temporal region. BA underwent surgery on the same day and remained comatose for 10 days. A neurological examination 2 weeks later disclosed a confusional state, with right hemiparesis, blindness of the left eye due to retinal hemorrhage, and severe fluent aphasia. A CT scan performed in April 1989, 7 months after the shooting, showed three lesions in the left hemisphere: fronto-temporal, lenticular, and occipital parasagittal; a small bone fragment was visible in the right thalamus.

In May 1989, BA's speech therapist referred him to our Service for advice. The patient's speech was fluent and abundant, with rare content words and little communicative value. Repetition and reading aloud were correct for nonwords, words, and sentences, and writing to dictation was generally correct, with only occasional errors. BA could name 8 of 20 pictures despite severe perseverations (he correctly named an envelope, for instance, and then went on saying "envelope" for the subsequent 7 pictures) but, strangely, could point only to 4 of the same 20 pictures. The same was true for written confrontation naming (7 of 20 correct) and written word-picture matching (5 of 20 correct). He could perform oral and written simple commands and scored 10/36 on the Token Test. He had no apraxia and he scored 24/36 on the RCPM. In the written calculation test he scored 42/101.

Semantic processing ability was examined further. The patient was asked to name and point to 10 objects in each of six semantic categories: animals, musical instruments, fruits and vegetables, objects, body parts, and means of transportation. All categories were severely impaired except for the body parts (he correctly named all 10 pictures and pointed to 7). In three categories (means of transportation, objects, and body parts) naming was better than pointing. He was also shown 20 pictures of real and 20 of nonexistent animals and 20 pictures of real and 20 of nonexistent objects and was asked to differentiate between real and unreal animals and objects. He correctly sorted 36 animals and 26 objects, rejecting 11 real objects. BA was also asked to say for the animals and objects whether or not a series of perceptual and functional characteristics were real, but the test could not be administered because BA reported that he had no idea of what the words meant. When asked to draw an object from memory he usually refused, saying that he did not know what it was. The rare times when he acknowledged that he knew the object, his drawings were unrecognizable. BA could copy a model — he had no constructional apraxia — but immediately afterward he could not reproduce it if it was no longer in sight. (Remember that BA was a draftsman.)

From our analysis we concluded that sublexical routines were grossly spared as were grammatical structures. His main deficit was semantic-lexical. The patient could not correctly point to or name pictures, producing semantic errors and frequent perseverations. In drawing, too, he sometimes drew a semantically related object or perseverated on previously presented objects. In judging whether objects were real or unreal, he made frequent errors and a semantic category effect was present (the category of body parts was selectively preserved). We concluded that the main deficit was damage to the semantic system and decided that therapy should be directed toward its restoration. The main obstacle to any therapy was the fact that perseverations disrupted all behavior; he perseverated in naming, pointing, drawing, demonstrating objects' use, and so on. Even when the task was changed for a short time, on returning to the previous task he resumed his perseveration.

The therapy was performed in his hometown and consisted of categorization tasks and odd-one-out tasks. BA was presented 73 with pictures from two semantic categories, drawn from the categories of clothing, toys, jewelry, food, animals, and furniture, and asked first to show how an object was handled and used and then to put it in the correct category (one item from each category was in front of the subject). BA could sometimes correctly mime the use of an object, but more often he could not or he perseverated on a previous gesture. Even when he correctly demonstrated the use of the object, he was totally inconsistent in categorization, the only exception being jewelry. In the odd-one-out task, BA was given five pictures, four of which belonged to the same semantic category. Again he could not sort the odd one out.

After 5 months of rehabilitation, in November 1989, no hint of recovery was evident, and rehabilitation was interrupted. In April 1990, BA again came to our Aphasia Service for advice. He perseverated a bit less and could correctly point to 42 of 72 pictures and name 24 of 70. The total number of correct responses was approximately the same from day to day, but he was inconsistent about which pictures he could correctly name or point to, and often appeared puzzled about his own answers. At that time a series of tests was performed using the same 56 objects: of these he could name 24, spell 23, and recognizably draw 18. He never failed in repeating and reading, but he misspelled two of the words written to dictation.

We decided to take a second chance, and rehabilitation was resumed. Our main goal was still recovery of the semantic system, but this time we decided not to work on semantic fields in general but to concentrate on single concepts, one at a time, asking the patient to draw objects. An object was first shown to him and he was asked to copy it; every part of the object was discussed to make clear why it should be as it was. The handle of the hammer, for instance, is used to hold it; the blunt end of the head to beat nails, and the flat end to pull nails out. The category of tools was chosen first and BA started to draw a hammer. It took approximately a month before BA could reliably draw a hammer without seeing it. From May 1990 to April 1991, work was done in three categories: tools, kitchen implements, and clothing.

A control examination performed in September 1991 disclosed general improvement. The first important result was a drastic reduction of perseveration in all behavior; he also was more consistent and more confident in his answers. Results on the battery confirmed good phonological processing (all the scores were in the normal range) and moderate-to-severe lexical damage. In a lexical decision task, he made errors on 8 of the 80 items and could name 23 of 30 nouns and 21 of 28 verbs. Written naming was better preserved than oral naming (22/22 nouns and 18/22 verbs). Because lexical comprehension had improved, the errors in grammatical comprehension tasks could be safely attributed to a deficit in grammatical processing. In an auditory grammaticality judgment task, BA scored 12 out of 48, and 11 of 24 in a written form, rejecting nearly all the correct sentences; in a sentence-picture matching task with two choices he scored 55 of 60.

Rehabilitation is being continued without much change. Grammar will be considered after the lexical-semantic impairment is further reduced.

A Case of Damage to the Output Lexicons

GH, a 46-year-old right-handed university professor of biochemistry, was admitted to a hospital in April 1990 for a prolonged myocardial ischemic crisis. In the following days right hemiparesis and aphasia appeared. A CT scan showed an ischemic hypodense area in the left temporo-parietal region with a hemorrhagic hyperdense zone inside. The right hemiparesis resolved in the following days; the aphasia persisted unchanged. The patient was examined at the Aphasia Service 40 days post-onset. His speech was fluent, but GH only produced a few comments that were adequate ("this is new," "I don't know," "one two three," "I can't," "this is this"). He never produced a content word but was able to make himself understood through the intelligent use of gestures, mimes, and so forth. He could correctly point to some pictures given the word, but looked amazed and did not understand what to do when confronted by the tokens of the Token Test. However, comprehension outside the test situation was good unless the interlocutor used a content word that sounded totally incomprehensible to the patient. In a picture-word matching task, he could correctly point to 10 of 20 pictures, but in 10 cases he was totally unable to grasp the meaning of the word. He could not repeat, read aloud, or write anything but his signature. Oral apraxia (10/20) and acalculia (24/101) were also present. On the RCPM he scored 32/36.

Rehabilitation with the following goals was immediately started: To have GH understand as many content words as possible and to restore repetition, since, despite GH's efforts, all attempts to repeat even a CV syllable failed. We considered repetition important because the patient *never* produced a content word on any occasion, and we had no means to help him because repetition and reading aloud were totally absent.

Three months later he could repeat, read, and spell some syllables and a few, very easy words, and he scored 10/36 on the Token Test. Output phonology was severely impaired. At the lexical level, oral lexical decision and oral and visual comprehension tasks were nearly in the normal range; all transposition tasks, except for delayed coping, were very severely impaired. GH could name to confrontation only 3 of 30 nouns and no actions and he gave 4 correct responses of a possible 22 nouns and named 1 of 29 actions in a written naming-to-confrontation task. Auditory grammatical judgments and grammatical comprehension were only mildly impaired. However, GH correctly understood only 1 of 45 written sentences. GH could easily draw from memory and frequently used drawing and correct circumlocutions to circumvent his word-finding difficulties.

Based on these results, post-semantic damage to the output lexicons seemed highly probable. Reading and writing lexical and sublexical routines also appeared to be severely damaged. We decided to work on the output lexicons and asked GH to work on phonology at home. GH's son was asked to have the patient repeat, write, and read simple CV syllables for 1 to 2 hours per day. As this task became easier, CVCV nonwords could be utilized. In confrontation naming, it was now becoming evident that damage to the phonological and graphemic output lexicons were totally independent. GH could sometimes correctly name a picture but was totally unable to write it; more frequently he could write (although sometimes some of the letters were missing) the name of the picture but this never helped him to say the word. As written naming was slightly less impaired and the patient could sometimes write the first letter(s), we concentrated on written naming-to-confrontation. Frequent and orthographically easy words were chosen, and GH was given as much time as he felt necessary to write the word. When he did not succeed or the word was incomplete, the therapist wrote the word letter-by-letter, leaving enough time for the patient to complete the word after each letter. When the word was correctly spelled, the therapist asked GH to repeat it, but he was frequently unsuccessful. However, as sublexical reading improved, he could with effort read some of the words he had correctly spelled.

In addition to daily rehabilitation, from December 1990 to March 1991, GH underwent a series of tests specifically designed to investigate the functional locus of his word-finding difficulties and the factors that influenced his naming. Results indicated that GH was impaired in naming nouns and actions independent of modality of input (visual, tactile, definition) or output (oral or written). Low frequency words were more impaired than high frequency words. There was no hint of any damage to the semantic system as GH performed correctly and without hesitation all tasks that evaluated processing by the semantic system (verifying categorical relation, discrimination between real and unreal animals and objects, completing drawings of animals and objects, choosing the correct attribute, etc.).

Rehabilitation continued along the same lines, and in July 1991 a final control examination was performed. As expected, major gains were evident in repeating, reading and writing nonwords, and in oral and written naming, although naming of actions was still moderately impaired. GH could, in fact, now name 27 of 30 pictures of nouns and 20 of 28 of verbs orally, and 21 of 22 written nouns and 16 of 22 written verbs. A very mild grammatical impairment was still present; in a 48-item grammaticality-judgment task, he made 3 errors and in a 60-item sentence-comprehension task, 4 errors; 3 involved reversible sentences and 1 was a morphological error. However, except for a series of adequate sentences that he produces easily, it is still always an effort for GH to find a specific word or to read or write. He always begins by saying that he does not know the word; if the interlocutor insists, he generally eventually comes up with the correct word.

Therapy continues with two goals: To restore the output lexicons and to make GH's use of sublexical routines for reading, writing, and repeating easier and more automatic.

CONCLUSIONS

Did aphasia therapy help our patients? It is a difficult question, but we can venture some opinions.

MT started rehabilitation 4 months post-onset with moderate-to-severe impairment of all language functions and severe reduction of spontaneous language. After 8 months of daily therapy, she had better scores on all subtests and reported speaking more at home. Rehabilitation had no effect in the first 3 months and only after she was taught to "see" events in her mind did she start getting better. At this point it was possible to identify two areas of major impairment: Grammatical comprehension and sublexical and lexical writing. I am confident that whatever results were obtained are due to therapeutic intervention, but they are of little value to the patient unless we overcome her reluctance to speak.

AB started rehabilitation 5 months post-onset and had therapy daily for 6 months. In his case, too, it was not possible to detect a specific area for intervention, because like MT, he presented with an across-the-board impairment, although he was more severely impaired. In his case, rehabilitation has been a nearly total failure. His major improvement has been in the Token Test (from 8 to 14/36), but no changes are evident in his language behavior in daily life.

Things were more complicated for BA. After 5 months of apparently useless aphasia treatment, therapy was changed, and some very slow recovery became apparent. After such a delayed and slow start, however, recovery now seems to be proceeding slightly faster, and it is a reasonable guess that recovery is due to treatment.

Finally, GH is something like a miracle. He started rehabilitation 1½ months post-onset and has been treated daily for 15 months, with a 2-month break during the summer. His gains are astonishing. When he started he could say a few words, such as "I do not know" or "this is new," and understand very few commonly used nouns, but otherwise language was totally abolished. He can now read, write, and follow a conversation, although nothing is accomplished easily. He reads and writes using a letter-by-letter strategy, and finding a content word always takes some time. However, one must be cautious about concluding that GH's recovery is due to therapy. He started therapy soon after onset, when he was still in the spontaneous recovery period, and above all, he is a very intelligent and motivated person who is able to take advantage of any clue. For example, he was once asked to find the names of means of water transportation. Most of them are compound words made up of something like water, engine, wings, hull, and so forth. By reasoning, GH first found these words and then tried different combinations looking for something that sounded right. I am personally convinced that rehabilitation has helped GH, if in no other way than accelerating recovery. (He would not have worked on sublexical routines had we not asked him to, for example.) However, I do not dare to say what is due to aphasia therapy, to spontaneous recovery, or specifically to GH's intelligence and perseverance.

Finally, for patients MT and AB we started rehabilitation without having a clear idea of the nature of the disorder. For BA and GH, on the contrary, we were convinced that we had localized the disorder and that we had devised appropriate therapeutic strategies. However, results for BA and GH, for whom we had a specific hypothesis about treatment, have not been markedly different from results for MT and AB who were treated in a global way. Unfortunately, even when we can be confident that we have correctly localized the functional lesion in a patient (and few people would deny that this is the only sound basis for guiding therapeutic intervention), we still are at a loss about what to do. Identification of the functional damage specifies what *not* to do (e.g., it would be useless to do exercises for something that is not damaged), and the more precise the identification the larger the number of things that are presumably useless. Even precise identification of the deficit does not tell us what to do. This is because we do not have a theory of rehabilitation that specifies the modification that a damaged system undergoes as a function of the different types of exercises that a patient is requested to do.

All we can say is that therapy cannot ignore possible guidance from theory, but at the same time it cannot wait for it, since patients have a right to rehabilitation.

REFERENCES

Albert, M. L., Goodglass, H., Helm, N. A., Rubens, A. B., & Alexander, M. P. (1981). *Clinical aspects of dysphasia.* Wien: Springer Verlag.

Basso, A. (1987). Approaches to neuropsychological rehabilitation: Language disorders. In M. Meier, A. Benton, & L. Diller (Eds.), *Neuropsychological rehabilitation* (pp. 294–314). London: Churchill Livingstone.

Basso, A. (1992). Prognostic factors in aphasia. *Aphasiology, 6,* 337–348.

Basso, A., Capitani, E., & Vignolo, L. A. (1979). Influence of rehabilitation on language skills in aphasic patients: A controlled study. *Archives of Neurology, 36,* 190–196.

Byng, S. (1988). Sentence processing deficits: Theory and therapy. *Cognitive Neuropsychology, 5,* 629–676.

Cappa, S., Cavallotti, G., & Vignolo, L. A. (1981). Phonemic and lexical errors in fluent aphasics: Correlation with lesion site. *Neuropsychologia, 19,* 171–177.

DeRenzi, E., & Vignolo, L. (1962). The Token Test: A sensitive test to detect receptive disturbances in aphasics. *Brain, 85,* 665–678.

Green, E., & Boller, F. (1974). Features of auditory comprehension in severely impaired aphasics. *Cortex, 10,* 133–145.

Hagen, C. (1973). Communication abilities in hemiplegics: Effect of speech therapy. *Archives of Physical Medicine and Rehabilitation, 54,* 454–463.

Kadzielawa, D., Dabrowska, A., Nowakowska, M. T., & Seniow, J. (1981). Literal and conveyed meaning as interpreted by aphasics and non-aphasics. *Polish Psychological Bulletin, 12,* 57–62.

Jones, E. (1986). Building the foundations for sentence production in a non-fluent aphasic. *British Journal of Disorders of Communication, 21,* 63–82.

Lecours, A. R., Lhermitte, F., & Bryans, B. (1983). *Aphasiology.* Eastbourne: Bailliere Tindall.

Levita E. (1978). Effects of speech therapy on aphasics' responses to the functional communication profile. *Perceptual and Motor Skills, 47,* 151–154.

Marshall, R. C., Tompkins, C. A., & Phillips, D. S. (1982). Improvement in treated aphasia: Examination of selected prognostic factors. *Folia Phoniatrica, 34,* 305–315.

Miceli, G., & Caramazza, A. (1988). Dissociation of inflectional and derivational morphology. *Brain and Language, 35,* 24–65.

Miceli, G., Giustolisi, L., & Caramazza, A. (1991). The interaction of lexical and non-lexical processing mechanisms: Evidence from anomia. *Cortex, 27,* 57–80.

Miceli, G., Laudanna, A., & Burani, C. (1991). Batteria per l'analisi dei deficit afasici. Milan: Associazione Sviluppo Ricerche Neuropsicologiche.

Raven, J. C. (1962). *The Coloured Progressive Matrices Test.* London: H. K. Lewis.

Sarno, M. T., & Levita, E. (1981). Some observations on the nature of recovery in severe aphasia. *Brain & Language, 13,* 1–12.

Sarno, M. T., Silverman, M., & Sands, E. (1970). Speech therapy and language recovery in severe aphasia. *Journal of Speech & Hearing Research, 13,* 607–623.

Vignolo, L. A. (1964). Evolution of aphasia and language rehabilitation: A retropective exploratory study. *Cortex, 1,* 344–367.

Wertz, R. T., Weiss, D., Aten, J. L., Brookshire, R. H., Garcia-Bunuel, L., Holland, A. L., Kurtzke, J. F., LaPointe, L. L., Milianti, F. J., Brannegan, R., Greenbaum, H., Marshall, R. C., Vogel, D., Carter, J., Barnes, N. S., & Goodman, R. (1986). Comparison of clinic, home, and deferred language treatment for aphasia. *Archives of Neurology, 43,* 653–658.

Wilcox, J. J., Davis, G. A., & Leonard, L. B. (1978). Aphasics' comprehension of contextually conveyed meaning. *Brain and Language, 6,* 362–377.

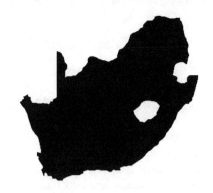

CHAPTER 2

Aphasia Therapy in South Africa: Some Pragmatic and Personal Perspectives

CLAIRE PENN
Department of Speech and Audiology
University of the Witwatersrand
Johannesburg, South Africa

This chapter provides a perspective on aphasia therapy that is centered on the pragmatic approach. It is based on my own personal beliefs about aphasia and on my growing impatience with the fact that many assessment procedures prove an end-point rather than a beginning point for therapy. Much of this frustration may stem from the context in which I have worked since graduation and the type of patient population that I have had to assess and treat. The South African aphasic population is a unique one from many perspectives, and it has become clear to me that to be accountable in this context, some changes of directions are essential. In this chapter I discuss certain of these changes, making reference to a few of the specific challenges, both theoretical and practical, and to their potential solution.

APHASIA IN SOUTH AFRICA

Certain characteristics of the South African aphasic population may be identified as unique. These characteristics present challenges to the clinician and researcher and make it difficult or inappropriate to adapt the more Western-style and traditional approaches to aphasia work that we are trained in and familiar with.

The first characteristic is multilingualism. The majority of aphasic patients in South Africa are multilingual or bilingual. Varying throughout the country, the number of languages acquired by an individual is dependent on social, economic, and geographic circumstance. Nine African languages have been raised to literary and educational status, although many more exist informally (Lanham, 1978; Wilkes, 1978). In addition, the educative norm for most South Africans has until now required the coordinate acquisition of the official languages of the country, English and Afrikaans. Proficiency in these languages largely defines success in further education and employment.[1] The complexity of the situation is compounded by the fact that most speech-language pathologists are English- or Afrikaans-speaking with little or no competence in African languages. Thus, most aphasic patients, while bilingual, are tested in their second or third languages. Further, despite several informal attempts (e.g., Epstein, 1976; Semela, 1978; Tughendaft, 1972), no properly standardized versions of tests have been developed for local aphasic patients. Probably of more importance is the fact that aphasia tests are not culture-free. Even for English-speaking aphasic patients, many of the items on tests currently in use are not appropriate.

The next group of problems lies with the facilities available for the treatment of aphasia. Despite the fact that in South Africa the incidence rates for most disorders that result in aphasia are among the highest in the world, facilities for treatment and rehabilitation are very inadequate (Fritz & Penn, 1992). Time spent in an acute care hospital is much shorter than in other countries. In addition, almost no rehabilitation hospitals or facilities are available to patients following discharge. In the hospital setting, few patients, except in urban areas, have access to a range of rehabilitative therapies. Because there are so few filled posts (particularly in rural settings), it is rare that aphasic patients in any setting other than an urban one are seen by a speech-language therapist. Finally, unrealistic medical insurance limits exacerbate the problem, with the result that most patients cannot afford private treatment after discharge.

---

[1] For a detailed and current perspective on the complexities of language and language change in Southern Africa, the reader is referred to Herbert (1992).

Certain sociopolitical factors also have had a substantial impact on aphasia rehabilitation. Due to a long history of inequality and educational disadvantage, the majority of aphasic patients in South Africa are further disadvantaged in relation to receiving treatment by a lack of transportation and income. Many patients reside far from available facilities. Many patients are poorly educated, often functionally illiterate or barely literate, making the application of formal testing inappropriate. Finally, high levels of unemployment and the breakup of traditional family structure make for a mobile and inaccessible aphasic population.

The aphasia clinician working in a large hospital normally can expect to see a patient only during the acute phase. After discharge, unless the patient lives near the hospital or clinic and is mobile, it is unlikely that there will be follow up. The burden of rehabilitation thus often falls on the caregivers and those working in the community.

For these reasons, as an aphasia clinician, I have been both challenged and frustrated in this complex land. The field of pragmatics has provided some solutions to some of these challenges.

PRAGMATICS

What exactly is meant by a pragmatic way of characterizing and treating aphasia? During the last decade, pragmatic language models have had a profound effect on our thinking about adult language disorders. In effect, the development of the field of pragmatics has reflected a shift away from structural models toward models with a more functional perspective. In considering these effects, I will first provide a definition and some theoretical underpinnings to the topic and then discuss some lines of current pragmatic research in aphasia. On the clinical side, I will attempt to show how a pragmatic perspective enhances our clinical approaches to patients, while simultaneously providing insight into the nature of the underlying linguistic and cognitive deficits.

DEFINITION

The main goal of pragmatic language models is to characterize communicative competence. In general, this reflects complex interrelationships among three types of knowledge (see Figure 2–1), all of which become necessary prerequisites for appropriate communication in context:

1. *Knowledge of language and its structure.* This includes knowledge about phonology, syntax, and semantics and their interrelationships.

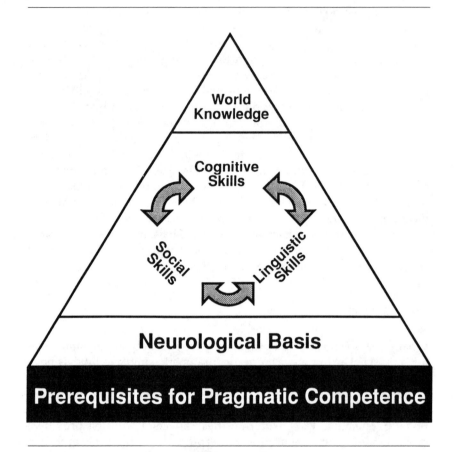

Figure 2–1. Prerequisites for Pragmatic Competence

2. *Knowledge of the world,* that is, knowledge about objects, events, and relations among objects, events, and actions. This is the cognitive domain and includes what Gallagher (1990) refers to as presuppositional knowledge, or the ability to make appropriate judgments about the form an utterance must take to communicate the speaker's intent adequately.
3. *Social knowledge,* that is, knowledge of the discourse rules governing conversation in the speaker's society. This view was highlighted beautifully by the late Carol Prutting (1982), who wrote with clarity and vision about the field.

I think that aphasiologists, possibly more than any other group, have welcomed the shift in direction from structural to functional with open arms. A pragmatic viewpoint tends to be compatible with their intuitions about the nature of aphasia and its crippling social consequences, as well as with the acknowledged often limited success of traditional structural aphasia therapy methods.

Briefly, the effect of this revision of approach has been to change many aspects of our management of patients. Not only have our assessment activities changed, but also our analysis methods, our goals of intervention, and our tasks, agents, and contexts of intervention. An examination of language in context demanded a move toward the elicitation and analysis of discourse. We have seen the development of a variety of pragmatic tools ranging from taxonomies to more formal tests such as Communicative Activities in Daily Living (CADL) (Holland, 1980) and more recently the Amsterdam Nijmegan Everyday Language Test (ANELT) (Blomert, 1990) and the Communicative Effectiveness Index (CETI) developed in Canada by Lomas et al. (1989). Similarly, a variety of new therapy techniques such as the PACE method of Davis and Wilcox (1985) and Holland's Conversational Coaching method (Holland, 1990) have emerged. Particularly for patients at either end of the severity continuum, pragmatic therapy approaches have provided the therapist with a number of useful options.

It seems surprising then that some reservations are now being expressed about the field. What are these reservations and how do we explain them? The first problem seems to be related to a lack of clarity with regard to the central constructs of pragmatics. For example, the very definition of the term "context" has been an issue of endless debate. In part because the field of pragmatics has such a mixed academic heritage, there is a terminological confusion and profusion which tends to frighten even the most avid researcher. This relates to the second point commented on by authors such as McTear (1985), who noted a lack of theoretical cohesiveness in the area. This lack is evident, for example, in disagreement as to the role of speech act theory and the relative independence of the pragmatic level of language from the other levels. Third, there has been increasing acknowledgment of the infinite complexity inherent in a description of language in context. Hence, surprisingly few published assessment protocols have emerged, relative to the number of years that pragmatic aspects of aphasia have been studied.

In response to these concerns, there appears to have been a resurgence of interest in more modular syntactic models of language, such as the government-binding theory of language discussed by Connell (1987) and Leonard and Loeb (1988).

I would suggest that the reason for these reservations may be that people have not effectively embraced the linguistic component in their definitions of pragmatics. Despite the fact that there may be a seemingly infinite extralinguistic side to pragmatics, there is undoubtedly a strongly structural component as well. I do not believe that it is necessary to abandon the framework altogether; rather an expansion of framework seems necessary to alleviate some of this unease.

ASSESSMENT

THE PROFILE OF COMMUNICATIVE APPROPRIATENESS

Viewing pragmatics as I do, as having both linguistic and extralinguistic characteristics, and dissatisfied with the sensitivity of traditional tests and purely syntactic measures, I devised a profile which attempts to formalize our intuitions about the communicative abilities of aphasic patients. This protocol focuses on aspects of aphasia that are not highlighted by traditional testing or by analysis of structural language alone. The protocol, the Profile of Communicative Appropriateness (PCA), is illustrated in Figure 2–2, and comprises six scales described in detail elsewhere (Penn, 1983a; Penn, 1988).

Scale A: Response to Interlocutor

This scale is concerned with the interactional component of conversation in that it measures the appropriateness of the patient's response to the interlocutor's input. It thus indirectly examines the patient's comprehension and knowledge of the turn-taking or cooperative aspect of conversation.

Scale B: Control of Semantic Content

This is basically a measure of semantic coherence. It is concerned with the linking together and organization of content units in the text. The categories for analysis of this component will depend on the task at hand. For example, in narrative structure, there is a well-defined set of rules for coherence, whereas in spontaneous discourse, there is another set of rules. Coherence is a reflection of knowledge about the world as well as the cognitive side of language. What is ignored in some of the published studies is that there is a strong linguistic overtone to this notion of coherence. For example, take the notion of successive verbs (i.e., verbs that are related in meaning to the previous verb). Contrast these two sentence pairs:

Bill punched George.	George called the doctor.
Bill punched George.	George liked the doctor.

Profile of Communicative Appropriateness (Penn, 1983)

Name _____   Features of sampling _____

Date _____   Unit of analysis _____

Person eliciting sample _____

		I	II	III	IV	V	VI	COMMENTS
Response to interlocutor	Request							
	Reply							
	Clarification request							
	Acknowledgement							
	Teaching probe							
	Others							
Control of semantic content	Topic initiation							
	Topic adherence							
	Topic shift							
	Lexical choice							
	Idea completion							
	Idea sequencing							
	Others							
Cohesion	Ellipsis							
	Tense use							
	Reference							
	Lexical substitution forms							
	Relative clauses							
	Prenominal adjectives							
	Conjunctions							
	Others							
Fluency	Interjections							
	Repetitions							
	Revisions							
	Incomplete phrases							
	False starts							
	Pauses							
	Word-finding difficulties							
	Others							
Sociolinguistic sensitivity	Polite forms							
	Reference to interlocutor							
	Placeholders, fillers, stereotypes							
	Acknowledgements							
	Self correction							
	Comment clauses							
	Sarcasm/humour							
	Control of direct speech							
	Indirect speech acts							
	Others							
Non-verbal communication	Vocal aspects: Intensity							
	Pitch							
	Rate							
	Intonation							
	Quality							
	Non-verbal aspects: Facial expression							
	Head movement							
	Body posture							
	Breathing							
	Social distance							
	Gesture and pantomime							
	Others							
	TOTALS							

Key:
I = Inappropriate; II = Mostly inappropriate; III = Some appropriate. IV = Mostly appropriate; V = Appropriate; VI = Could not evaluate

Figure 2–2. The Profile of Communicative Appropriateness

Much more inference is required in the second pair of sentences than in the first pair. Our knowledge of the inter-sentence features of verbs makes it easy for us to link the first two and to recognize them as being linked. This example demonstrates that there is a direct correlation between linguistic features and pragmatic features. For example, Sinoff (1992) found that factoring out linguistic elements that correlated with overall ratings of coherence in the narratives of a large group of adolescent children isolated successive verbs and their use as one of the most powerful predictors of coherence.

Scale C: Cohesion

Cohesion refers to the way in which sentences are linked within discourse via a variety of syntactic or lexical devices. This includes aspects such as reference, substitution, ellipsis, and conjunction. All of these aspects have been discussed at length by authors such as Halliday and Hasan (1976).

Scale D: Fluency

Although fluency is a term frequently used to describe and differentiate aphasic expressive output, it is often so loosely defined that it is of limited usefulness. When I refer to fluency in a pragmatic context, I refer to a broad definition, which incorporates temporal and sequential aspects of speech and includes factors such as pauses, repetitions, and interruptions. These elements have been found to relate closely to cognitive and linguistic factors in both normal and pathological language and provide a useful window into the patency of the communicative system (Penn, 1983b).

Scale E: Sociolinguistic Sensitivity

This scale measures the speaker's awareness of and sensitivity to the contextual features of his utterance and his ability to modify his message in terms of this context. Some of the manifestations of sociolinguistic sensitivity are listed here and include, for example, the phenomenon of self-correction — a strong prognostic indicator in aphasia.

Scale F: Nonverbal Communication

The area of nonverbal communication is divided into its vocal aspects and nonverbal aspects. Nonverbal communication has been fairly well researched, and a number of suitable taxonomies exist.

These six scales were the basis of my research concerning the interactive conversational discourse of aphasic patients. Their abilities were rated on a five-point scale of appropriateness and compared with their performance on standard tests of aphasia and on a structural syntactic analysis. Before discussing the results, it might be useful to consider research evidence from that which supports the validity of these divisions of the Profile of Communicative Appropriateness (PCA).

RESEARCH EVIDENCE

Table 2–1 attempts to draw together research evidence concerning levels of pragmatic competence in aphasia. As Table 2–1 indicates, some published evidence exists for noting relative retention of certain communicative competencies in aphasia. For example, in terms of the behaviors measured on Scale A many studies have noted a relatively well preserved response to the interlocutor and an ability to participate in the conversation.

Similarly for Scale B, the main content units in narrative tasks seem to be retained. The same can be said for Scales E and F where research evidence suggests strengths in these areas which reflect a sensitivity to contextual features, as well as an ability to adapt and compensate for communication difficulties. However, for Scales C and D, which rely very strongly on linguistic factors for their realization, aphasic patients have been judged to be less appropriate.

These observations were confirmed with a group of 18 aphasic patients of differing severity and type. A cluster analysis of their pragmatic profiles revealed a grouping that did not correlate with their structural language performance, nor with type of aphasia, but did correlate overall with severity (Penn, 1987).

This group of patients demonstrated separate cluster outcomes for each of the six scales. This confirms that, in some areas, pragmatic competence is relatively well preserved in the majority of aphasia patients. Specifically, these patients preserve the ability to communicate as measured by those skills which do not require linguistic fine-tuning. Scales A, E, and F and certain elements of Scale B are well preserved, reflecting relatively intact cognitive and social skills. Elements that are highly dependent on the linguistic component of the message are more likely to be judged inappropriate.

Some support for the linking of these constructs was found statistically when performance of the patients was correlated on the Scales. For example, Scales A and B and Scales A and E correlated highly, suggesting not only an element of overlap but also a possible common

Table 2-1. Research evidence for abilities of aphasic patients on scales of the Profile of Communicative Appropriateness

Scale	Aspects	Supporting Research
A: Response to Interlocutor	Turn-taking well preserved Good comprehension of stated main ideas Near normal repertoire of speech acts Able to benefit from prior contextual narratives	Brookshire & Nicholas (1984); Schienberg & Holland (1980); Silvast (1990); Klippi (1990).
B: Control of Semantic Content	Overall preservation of narrative structure Main content units retained	Ulatowska et al. (1981); Armus et al. (1989); Yorkston & Beukelmann (1980); Ernest-Baron et al. (1987); Hough & Pierce (1989).
C: Cohesion	Problems with reference Conjunction errors Errors in tense use and ellipses	Berko-Gleason et al. (1980); Armstrong (1991); Chapman & Ulatowska (1989).
D: Fluency	Lexical retrieval strategies involving temporal delay	Brown & Cullinan (1981); Penn (1983).
E: Sociolinguistic Sensitivity	Well preserved social conventions Ability to repair conversational failure Able to demonstrate difficulty in understanding Responsive to feedback Compensatory stereotypes	Busch et al. (1988); Panzeri et al. (1987); Whitney & Goldstein (1989).
F: Nonverbal Communication	Well retained co-verbal behavior Able to substitute nonverbal for verbal behavior Able to indicate range of needs and emotions through varied speed and pitch	Glosser et al. (1986); Behrmann & Penn (1984); Katz et al. (1988); Hermann et al. (1988, 1989); Ahlsen (1991).

underlying basis, that of relatively intact cognitive processes in aphasia, despite linguistic deficits.

Although text management depends on both cognitive and linguistic competence, it nevertheless becomes clear that the reasons for breakdown of text are different in purely aphasic patients than in persons with more widespread brain damage. In the former, identifiable and predictable breakdown occurs linked to lexical and syntactic factors. A wide variety of compensatory strategies may be developed to overcome these deficits. By and large, we agree with Weisenberg and McBride (1935, as cited in Schuell, Jenkins, & Jiminez-Pabon, 1964) who declared:

> The typical aphasic patient is a sensible fellow who is able to cope with the routine of everyday life in so far as it does not involve language. (p. 43)

By definition, the lesion in the aphasic patient tends to be more localized to the language areas, whereas the lesion in closed head injury, for example, is much more widespread, often tending to focus in the frontal lobe. When there is frontal involvement in aphasic patients, we can expect a different pragmatic profile. We see this in older aphasic patients and in patients with proven frontal lobe lesions (Glosser, Wiener, & Kaplan, 1990; Kascmarek, 1984). Higher order cognitive processes which are disrupted with lesions in frontal and prefrontal regions include focusing sustained attention, fluency and flexibility for novel responses, and planning and execution of sequential goal-directed activities. All of these are very important components of adequate pragmatic competence, a point I return to later.

THERAPY IMPLICATIONS

The framework of analysis just described has informed my approach to therapy with the aphasic patient. To illustrate this point, I will present two case studies, which illustrate some of the important aspects of what I have alluded to above:

1. The linguistic, social, and cognitive sides that characterize pragmatic assessment and therapy.
2. The flexibility of the pragmatic approach, particularly in a cross-cultural context of assessment and remediation.
3. Its relevance, particularly for the mildly aphasic patient, to the social and employment context of the patient.
4. The mutual roles of therapist and patient in devising the tasks, materials, and procedures of therapy.

5. The value of discourse as a method of analysis and a basis
for therapy.

CASE A: CROSS-LINGUISTIC DISCOURSE THERAPY

BACKGROUND

The first case was a multilingual aphasic patient, who was 38 years of
age. He was premorbidly right-handed and was a defense attorney with
19 years of formal education. In 1986, he suffered a left-sided posterior
embolic thrombosis. A computed tomography (CT) scan revealed a low
density lesion in the left posterior parietal region. In May 1989, 9 months
prior to testing, during a court case, TG reported a sudden loss of
expressive and receptive ability in Afrikaans and some impairment in
receptive function in his other languages. A small embolic thrombosis to
the same area of the brain as before was diagnosed. He was seen for a
period of speech and language therapy, during which time formal non-
standard and standard testing was conducted. At the time of intake, he
had a mild aphasia with relatively intact receptive abilities, fluent output,
and marked word-finding difficulty.

The language history of this patient is particularly interesting. He
knew and used no fewer than 10 languages in various contexts, namely:
Ndebele, Pedi, Zulu, English, Afrikaans, South Sotho, Siswati, Tswana,
Tsonga, and Xhosa. He was born of Ndebele-speaking parents who were
both equally fluent in Pedi. Raised in an African township in Pretoria, he
acquired several languages in his preschool and primary years, including English (which was the medium of instruction at school), Afrikaans,
Zulu and Xhosa, and Siswati. His most frequently used language in a
work setting was Afrikaans in a job which demanded interaction with
government officials. His reported order of language proficiency before
the strokes was as follows: Pedi and Ndebele (equal proficiency), South
Sotho, Afrikaans, Zulu, English and Xhosa, Tswana, Siswati, and Tsonga.
Following his stroke, Pedi and Ndebele continued to be the languages in
which he felt least impaired, followed by English, South Sotho, Xhosa,
and Zulu. Afrikaans, which had previously been easy for him, had become very difficult, and his main reason for coming to speech therapy
was his fear of losing his position. He was still practicing law with a reduced emphasis on court work.

ASSESSMENT

TG was tested in some of his languages to confirm his subjective impression of differential breakdown. The languages tested were English and

Afrikaans (which are largely inflectional languages) and two languages from the Southern Eastern family of Bantu languages (Zulu, from the Nguni group of languages, and Pedi from the Sotho group).[2] The decision to test these two languages was based on the availability of linguistically and culturally matched examiners.

Testing involved the administration of both formal tests of aphasia and devised narrative discourse tasks across four languages. Trained judges were then asked to rate the subject according to appropriateness on the PCA.

The details of the methods used and the subject's performance on the testing are reported elsewhere (Penn & Beecham, 1992) but may be summarized as follows: on the test of aphasia used (the Western Aphasia Battery [WAB], Kertesz, 1980), TG performed differentially across the four languages tested, with his test profiles deriving a diagnosis of Conduction aphasia in Afrikaans and Zulu (with aphasia quotients of 58.2 and 69.2, respectively), whereas in English and in Zulu, the WAB classification was Anomic aphasia (with aphasia quotients of 77.1 and 81.4, respectively).

A variety of narrative and procedural discourse tasks were analyzed using the PCA. This analysis revealed that TG experienced a considerable pragmatic breakdown in certain areas, regardless of the languages in which he was tested. Analysis was undertaken by two monolingual English examiners who independently rated TG's discourse samples in collaboration with first language speakers (depending on the language). High agreement (93%) was reached between the two raters. Table 2–2 summarizes these results.

TG's main difficulties lay in Scales B, C, D, and E of the PCA. Although he was able to respond appropriately to the initial input of the interlocutor, his topic management was judged to be inappropriate in all languages. He showed poor control of topic shift and maintenance as well as sequencing. This was exacerbated by excessive circumlocution and poor lexical choice and a lack of cohesion which was reflected in Scale C. Particularly for pronouns, there was a lack of reference frequently judged as inappropriate. For example (from a Zulu translation):

> She (nurse) phoned Pretoria and told that there was someone here, he can't talk. She said he lives in Daveyton . . . But now he's in Maritzburg. They came here.

Fluency was judged to be a particular problem, with excessive use of placeholders and stereotypes (Scale D); and on Scale E, he was judged to be insensitive to the rules of turn-taking. Although the degree of severity

[2] Further details regarding the structure of these languages may be found in the classic text of Doke (1954) and the more recent work of Gregorson (1977).

Table 2-2. Pragmatic abilities of patient TG on the Profile of Communicative Appropriateness

Scale	Overall Judgment	Specific Behaviors
A: Response to Interlocutor	Mostly appropriate	Initial response appropriate, but turn-taking impaired
B: Control of Semantic Content	Mostly inappropriate	Poor topic adherence Inappropriate turn length Unclear topic shift Unspecific lexical choice
C: Cohesion	Some appropriate	Poor text cohesion evidenced in lack of reference and inappropriate use of ellipsis
D: Fluency	Some appropriate	Excessive use of repetitions and revisions and pauses
E: Sociolinguistic Sensitivity	Mostly inappropriate	Poor turn-taking Excessive use of placeholders, stereotypes, and comment clauses
F: Nonverbal Communication	Mostly appropriate	Nonverbal behaviors congruent with verbal abilities

appeared to differ among languages, there was good agreement among the judges as to which behaviors appeared to be the most penalizing and as to the general level of disorganization manifest within the narrative discourse of the patient.

THERAPY

On the basis of the pre-therapy testing, a short-term discourse-based therapy program was implemented with a focus on some of the communicative behaviors identified as being inappropriate.

Therapy took place in English and was conducted by a monolingual clinician over a 14-week period. Nine therapy sessions were conducted, focused on specific targeted structures identified by the analysis. Materials were selected to minimize cultural and linguistic differences between TG and the therapist. Extensive use was made of audio- and videorecordings to develop self-monitoring skills. Therapy was focused at two main levels. The first was the macro level of discourse, with the goal of increasing the organizational structure of narrative discourse. The second level of therapy was aimed at a finer tuned (micro) level in which a detailed analysis of specific communicative behaviors was undertaken and self-monitoring skills were developed. Each therapy session combined both levels.

Activities at the first (macro) level included:

1. Analysis of written and spoken narratives, conversations, and picture descriptions (including single pictures and sequence cards) in terms of elements of story grammar identified by writers such as Mandler and Johnson (1977). These elements included topic, sequence, actors, complicating event, conclusion, and so forth. This material was graded for complexity, starting with simple texts (accompanied by visual support) and moving to more complex dyadic interaction. A written hierarchy was used, and each text was analyzed using this framework.
2. Self-monitoring of audiotaped conversations along these same dimensions (graded for complexity).

At the micro level, the following activities were included:

1. Certain specific aspects were targeted during the therapy period. The pragmatic behaviors targeted were pronominalization and specific fluency behaviors, chosen because of their large contribution to inappropriateness in all the discourse samples judged.
2. Clarification was sought on the specific behavior targeted for the session. For example, in targeting his inept pronominalization, multiple actor sequence stories were used and the therapist would probe with a statement such as, "When you say 'he' is that the policeman or the man who was arrested?"
3. At the natural end of TG's narration, the tape was replayed and the self-monitoring encouraged, based on the clarifications needed by the therapist. For example:

   T: Why did I need to ask you that?

   TG: Because I had not told you that the car was stolen.

4. Analysis of number, type, and position of inappropriate placeholders, moving from reading tasks to picture description, sequence story, and narrative tasks. Although TG used many dif-

ferent strategies that affected fluency (such as pausing, coughing and so forth), the judges agreed that his use of the tag question *ne* (an Afrikaans word) was used with unacceptable frequency,. and it was agreed to monitor the word specifically
(using tape-recorded samples of TG's own discourse).

(cough) Now it's like (pause) (laugh) you heard me say now ne?
(laugh) When it still comes to that (pause) what a person is going to
say, ne? (pause) So nearly but still we can't ne?

Well (pause) a plate as well as (pause) meat (pause, cough) inside.
And there's a (pause) dog when has been leashed, ne? To a tree. We
notice that this cat has been moving around the tree to (pause) dici
(pause, cough) divitiate, ne?

The judges agreed that *"ne?"* should be used less frequently and in
more appropriate contexts rather than being eliminated altogether in
TG's speech. Using recordings, development of self-monitoring began
with a criterion of 80% correct identification of the targeted dysfluency.
Progression to the next level of narrative complexity was determined not
by percentage of achieving criterion, but by mutually determined judgments of successful communication of the message.

THERAPY RESULTS

After therapy the same discourse tasks were elicited and analyzed and
the following results were obtained: Relative to the pre-therapy performance, improvement in the target areas was noted in all languages
despite the fact that therapy was conducted only in English (cf. the results of Fredman, 1975); the specific targeted behaviors (pronominalization, placeholders, and fluency) were assessed as being markedly more
appropriate across the tested languages.
    An extract from a post-therapy sample illustrates this:

I can say it in short, ne? that the cat was enjoying his meat right at the end.
But from the story we can see that (pause) the dog and the cat was very
close and there's a board — and there's some meat inside. Then we notice
that the dog was being held by a leash. Then the cat noticed that the best
thing is dis . . . distract ne. Your attention on this dog so that he must continue running around this tree, that gradually the dog notice that the cat
wants to eat his meat . . .

Interestingly, some of the untreated behaviors also showed improvement. For example the turn-taking behavior, which was judged as inap-

propriate prior to therapy, showed improvement across all languages. This is probably directly attributable to the nature of the therapy activities which involved a great deal of interaction and therapist intervention.

The rate of TG's speech was noted to slow down after therapy. Although this aspect had not been identified as inappropriate, either before or after therapy, and was not specifically targeted during intervention, it seemed to be particularly sensitive to the procedures adopted. A post-hoc analysis of the spontaneous discourse samples was undertaken to confirm this subjective impression. Rate in syllables per minute was measured on three narrative tasks in the four languages. A slowing in rate occurred in English, Afrikaans, and Zulu (by 15, 6, and 8 syllables per minute, respectively) but not in Pedi. Although not statistically significant, the trend toward a slower rate with increased monitoring was clinically interesting and confirms the results of Whitney and Goldstein (1989), who suggested that slowing is an adaptive delay strategy that serves to facilitate more fluent and organized discourse.

In interpreting these results, it should be noted that TG himself reported a decrease in functional handicap across languages. By the seventh session he attempted to return to active court work, negotiating with court officials and conducting a trial in a mixture of English and Afrikaans. The court transcript of this trial was used as a basis for the following session. TG spontaneously evaluated his narrative performance and identified areas that could be further improved (predominantly at the organizational level). This evidence of increasing self-reliance corresponds with his report that the therapy program furnished him with methods to continue autonomous improvement in his language performance.

CASE B: HIERARCHICAL DISCOURSE THERAPY

To further illustrate some of these points, the process of therapy with another patient will be reported. His therapy, like TG's, was specifically designed around a number of linguistic and cognitive pragmatic goals.

BACKGROUND

The patient (LC) was a 47-year-old English-speaking man who had been a training manager for a large company prior to his stroke. He was premorbidly right-handed and suffered a severe left hemisphere cerebral artery infarction in November 1988. A CT scan revealed the lesion to be in the perisylvian area. His inital symptom of severe expressive aphasia resolved into a mild anomic aphasia within a period of 3 months. Speech therapy commenced 1 week post-onset and continued until the time of his death. LC returned to work after 6 months (in a different capacity), but was frustrated by this experience and elected to take early retirement.

ASSESSMENT

At 18 months post-onset, LC was formally reassessed. At this time, he scored above the Aphasia Quotient cutoff of 93.8 on the Western Aphasia Battery. However in certain clinician-constructed tasks he showed difficulties, specifically in narrative and procedural discourse and in writing tasks (in which he revealed a specific phonological dysgraphia).

On a neuropsychological battery, LC showed organizational and memory problems associated with frontal lobe deficits. These problems included a limited ability to plan or to perform complex tracking tasks. On discourse tasks, his pragmatic deficit became more clearly defined. We used a variety of discourse tasks with this patient, including interactive conversation, narrative discourse (retelling an event), procedural discourse (explaining how to do something), and picture description.

An analysis (of the discourse tasks) using the PCA was undertaken and is summarized in Table 2–3.

Table 2–3. Pragmatic abilities of patient LC on the Profile of Communicative Appropriateness

Scale	Overall Judgment	Specific Behaviors
A: Response to Interlocutor	Appropriate	No difficulties in this area
B: Control of Semantic Content	Some appropriate	Difficulties in sustaining topic due to poor lexical choice
C: Cohesion	Some appropriate	Paucity of cohesive devices — including pronominal references and inappropriate ellipsis
D: Fluency	Mostly inappropriate	Silent pauses, repetitions, incomplete phrases
E: Sociolinguistic Sensitivity	Mostly appropriate	Adequate self-correction Good sense of humor
F: Nonverbal Communication	Some inappropriate	Poor eye contact

Although LC showed excellent interactive skills and followed appropriate rules of turn-taking, as reflected on Scale A, on Scale B some problems were evident in his control of semantic content. This seemed to be linked largely to his word-finding difficulties, which resulted in a great many incomplete ideas. On a procedural discourse task (changing a car tire), all of the essential steps as well as some optional steps were present. However, the order of some of the steps was confused, highlighting not only the linguistic deficit, but a planning and programming deficit probably linked to his frontal lobe signs. On Scale C, LC demonstrated a paucity of cohesive devices, including inappropriate use of ellipsis and inaccurate use of pronouns, for example:

T: What do you think will happen in the country?

LC: Third World

Such features of paragrammatism or fluent aphasia have a major pragmatic impact. Similarly, on Scale D, many areas were felt to be inappropriate. The patient frequently used interjections and repetitions, and there were long unfilled pauses and unsuccessful word-finding attempts. Although some of these symptoms possibly were strategies that LC adopted to compensate for his word-finding deficit, they are not always positive symptoms and were perhaps the largest reason for his pragmatic inappropriateness. This carried over onto Scale F where a lack of eye contact (related to struggle and search behaviors) seemed to account for many judgments of inappropriateness. On Scale E, however, LC's awareness of the listener's needs was reflected as well as a sensitivity to his own conversational failures. He had a well-retained sense of humor and self-corrected where necessary. However, it should be noted that his self-correction was not consistent and was more often linked to his semantic than to his phonologic paraphasias. This is a strong indicator, in my opinion, of the relative pragmatic weighting of these symptoms.

To summarize, although linguistic factors seemed to account for most of the pragmatic deficits observed, there was some evidence in our testing that LC's planning and organization were impaired. Intervention thus took place on both linguistic and cognitive levels.

THERAPY

To achieve the linguistic aims, the following activities were employed:

1. Completing activities to improve lexical search and specificity such as the lexical focus or visualization approach advocated by Linebaugh (1984)

2. Working on synonyms and antonyms
3. Interpreting proverbs and idioms
4. Providing suitable succinct captions to cartoons
5. Practicing summarizing skills (e.g., preparing a book review or providing a précis of a film or TV program each week). (Fortunately therapy sessions happened after "Dallas," which provided ready material).
6. Working on a number of compensatory strategies to improve effectiveness of communication. This included shortening his message, increased fluency monitoring and using circumlocution, or appropriate interjections in lieu of lengthy silent pauses.
7. Increasing active use of the nonverbal channel. Interestingly, his poor eye contact (which he had identified on videotape as interfering with communicative efficiency) was a behavior that was worked on specifically. However, LC found it difficult to control, and through discussion, it appeared that this symptom was actually a strategy which facilitated verbal ability. Guy Wint's (1965) self-report on aphasia is of relevance here:

> I found my speech was much more ready if I did not also have to look at the person spoken to. It was as if the effort of doing the two things at once, talking and seeing, was too much. And so I got in the habit of systematically averting my gaze in conversation. (p. 87)

Such a finding cautions us that we should not view every inappropriate behavior as requiring modification, particularly if it has a pragmatic purpose.
8. Encouraging LC's use of his world knowledge to get a message across. For example, in giving directions to get to his house, he was encouraged to describe the garage on the corner if he could not retrieve the name of his street.
9. Working on cohesion via work on reference and identification of successive verbs. Here, we found the "conversational coaching" approach advocated by Holland (1990) particularly useful, as we called in a third person whose role was to be deliberately quizzical when language was ambiguous.

On the cognitive side, the following activities were encouraged:

1. Stimulating the logical recall of events by using a diary and by recounting particular incidents in a logical and sequential way with insistence on the main steps of narrative (i.e., orientation, the characters involved, and the resolution).

2. Completing multiple-step verbal tasks, such as interpreting maps and giving directions, and monitoring such tasks in terms of explicitness.
3. Planning responses in therapy tasks and life events. This included working out the different options through role play that could be followed in an activity outside the clinic (e.g., in seeking funding for the stroke group), as well as an analysis of others' responses to him.
4. Completing self-correction activities using video recordings. It should be noted that his long silences were the behaviors that he himself found least acceptable and which he was motivated to correct in therapy.

A framework that proved useful for our therapy endeavors is one developed by Biggs and Collis (1982) to characterize the language and learning style of students. Based on Piagetian principles, Biggs and Collis provided a hierarchy of task complexity which allows for graded discourse therapy incorporating both cognitive and linguistic elements. This framework, which we have called "Hierarchical Discourse Therapy" (Penn & Joffe, in preparation), utilizes the presentation of a text (either verbal or written) followed by a series of questions graded for complexity. For example, in response to the following question, based on the reading of a letter written home by a convict in Australia in 1835 (one of Biggs and Collis's tasks), "How difficult was a convict's lot?", LC wrote:

> The convict's lot was fairly easy. Thank God. He had enough to eat. 12 pounds of meat, tea, flour, sugar. Gave them enough to eat for a year. The clothes — three pairs of shoes, shorts and trousers enough for a year. If you misbehaved you got a hundred strokes and you were sent to Port Arthur.

Analyzed according to the framework, this response is multistructural in nature and contains relevant and correct features. However, it lacks integration, cohesion, and orientation, aspects that could be separately identified and addressed in therapy (using similar texts). Extracting a response at a different level of the model can be achieved by asking a different question. For example, "Why do you think a convict's lot was so difficult?" (where the answer is not in the passage) or at an even higher level: "Do you think convicts today are treated well?"

In summary, using such a framework, therapy aimed at elaborating LC's responses and teaching him strategies for both comprehension and organization of text. This type of activity allows management of both the linguistic and extralinguistic sides of the pragmatic coin. Through such tasks, we are able to work on a broad level (e.g., planning the steps for a narrative or a procedure) as well as on a more microcosmic level (e.g., monitoring the dysfluencies in speech or identifying and correcting instances of inappropriate reference).

RESULTS

LC's response to therapy was very positive, as reflected on the PCA. He showed increased awareness and sensitivity to the effects of his impairment on the listener (as reflected on Scale E), and various aspects of his nonverbal behavior (such as eye contact) and fluency behavior were judged to be modified. He was observed to fill pauses (during word search) more frequently to indicate that a search was in progress. He had also developed a variety of conversational starters and comment clauses which ensured his ability to initiate and maintain a conversation when necessary. LC reported an increased ability to cope in a number of domestic and work contexts, an observation confirmed by his family.

His own words (recorded in a speech given to a group of students) perhaps best illustrate this improvement:

> It is not only the speech and writing that affect me but also the problems that go with it. Like not being able to find the right words when speaking or taking a long time to write a letter. Many of the people at work did not understand my problem because I did not look disabled. This year my therapist is L. She has helped me a lot to adjust to my retirement. She asked me to do this speech. It is the first time I have spoken to a group of strangers. It has been difficult adjusting to retirement. B is pleased because I do the housework. When I look back two years I see how much I have improved and am grateful that I have had the chance to learn to speak and also that I am not hemiplegic any more. My family have also learnt to adjust to the problem. There are still times when I feel upset at what has happened but I hope this will get better as time goes on.

Sadly, some two months after this, the patient, unexpectedly to all concerned, took his own life. It was evident that this was carefully planned, but it came as a devastating surprise to everyone, especially to his speech therapists. In an attempt to explain this and to confront the ethical questions that it posed, I have been forced to re-address some of the very basic issues we are taught and expected to imbue as therapists. Among these are: What exactly is one doing by developing, as we did, the judgment and reasoning skills of a patient? Did these cognitive skills actually enable him to recognize his reality and his prognosis, and ultimately choose to opt out of life? What could have been done to prevent this, and is it indeed our role to prevent it?

Given his amazing recovery and his minimal level of impairment, this very sad event illustrates more than anything that a mild deficit, manifested primarily pragmatically, can have severe consequences and that the term "mild" in fact is a misnomer. It is possible that being close to the goal of recovery but never quite making it exacts a far greater toll than we expect (cf. Marshall, 1987).

It also became clear that nothing in my training or textbooks prepared me for this. His mood was in fact quite good before his death — a factor commonly noted in suicide victims (Choron, 1972). I travelled a long and interesting road with this man and feel anger and frustration and a sense of failure that in spite of, and perhaps because of, therapy, he chose the route he did. And yet surely our central role is empowerment of aphasic patients. We work toward the time when it is possible for patients to make and implement independent decisions. Some might argue that there was clinical depression and that the frontal lobe damage was an explanatory factor, but the therapists involved feel convinced that the suicide was a rational decision which we could do little to influence. Very little has been written about grief and death in aphasia patients (Jackson, 1988; Swindell & Hammond, 1991). However, I believe that thoughts of death and suicide are never very far away, yet often remain unspoken by the patients, their families, and the therapists and professionals dealing with such patients. It is my ardent hope that this topic will receive more attention in future teaching and writing, and that this special man whom I was privileged to meet and know will help me to ensure just that.

I digress from the topic but perhaps have shown that a pragmatic approach to therapy does span other aspects, and that the good pragmatic therapist has to leave the safety of structured language tasks and reach out with the patient into real life and death issues.

I hope that the therapy process discussed in these patients serves to highlight some of the principles that I believe guide a pragmatic approach to rehabilitation. Although neither of these cases is particularly typical, each is characteristic of the kind of individual for whom traditional therapy and assessment techniques have limited value. Both patients had mild deficits and were highly motivated and cooperative. They had a specific need: Improvement in conversational competence within a specific communicative setting. Their level of impairment, level of education, and reasoning skills enabled a direct and metalinguistic level of therapy that is not applicable to a wide section of the population. Results from both of these patients, however, demonstrate that carefully and specifically targeted therapy strategies seem to have some significant conversational overflow.

CONCLUSIONS

I would like to conclude by expressing a few personal perspectives on rehabilitation which I have found useful not only with mild aphasic patients such as those discussed here, but in all of the adult neurogenic patients I have seen.

1. Pragmatic assessment by definition is a multilevel assessment. It incorporates linguistic, cognitive, and social factors. The profile of pragmatic abilities found in a patient provides us with insights about the connections among these levels of functioning, particularly if the neurological and cognitive substrates are borne in mind.

2. Assessment should take place at the level of discourse, using a variety of tasks, because task differences, more than anything, can shed light on the nature of the breakdown. Classic picture description does very little to enhance interactive skills. Discourse, if effectively elicited and analyzed, provides considerable insight into the phenomenology of the disorder.

3. Pragmatic assessment, if embedded firmly in the cultural context, using culturally and linguistically matched testers and judges, becomes a tool that seems potentially endlessly versatile and productive for therapy.

4. If language is the primary problem (as in aphasia), pragmatic therapy does not mean that one should ignore structural aspects. However, one should consistently examine how the structural deficit interferes with communication. Some structural deficits (e.g., omission of auxiliaries or phonemic paraphasias) just don't really matter, others make all the difference. Use the patient's cognitive strengths to compensate for the linguistic deficit — enhance compensation and functional strengths, incorporate other channels, enhance turn-taking skills, and develop strategies that are socially appropriate. For example, a filled pause is far more user-friendly than an unfilled pause when a word search is under way. Similarly, if a slower rate is the price to pay for increased fluency (as in both cases described), so be it.

5. If planning and organization are a problem (as in closed head injury), show how linguistic features can compensate for these difficul-

ties. Keeping it short and simple encourages more appropriate turn-taking. Quality, not quantity, of language is important. Identify the main components of a text and help the patient to scaffold the story. Help significant others to develop appropriate interactive conversational strategies (Green, 1984). Teach the power of successive verbs, of self-correction strategies, and of comment clauses. A lovely example comes from one of my patients who suggested to his audience: "If I'm talking too much hogwash, please tell me to shut up."

6. "There is a time for every season under the heaven," especially in aphasia therapy. What should direct our choices of priorities, goals, and activities, however, is not the test score, but the contexts in which the patient operates and what really matters to the individual.

I believe that all too often patients have formed the basis of model-building and theory confirmation at the expense of a focus on rehabilitation, and I believe that a text such as this highlights the central reason for our endeavors as therapists.

I do not think that we need to see a pragmatic approach to therapy as an all or none approach. It is on this point that I take issue with those who have chosen to go back to a more exclusively grammatical and structural approach. I do not believe a pragmatic approach is a threat, a substitute, or even a poor relation to the more structured or traditional approaches to rehabilitation or to the current model-building approaches. It is, instead, an identification at several levels of the patient's strengths and deficits in contexts where it really matters. It is the building up of such strengths and the masking or elimination of such deficits through multifaceted individualized contextual therapy.

Some are disappointed that the pragmatic approach has not simplified the picture but has "attacked our knowledge base, complicated our methods, challenged our conclusions" (Brinton, Craig, & Skarakis-Doyle, 1990), but as these authors point out, the pragmatics revolution can perhaps be compared to a political revolution in that change takes place in phases and reform takes a long time. Coming as I do from a country beset with a history of political upheaval and a university that has taken a very strong anti-government stand for many decades, I would like to take this analogy a little further. Change is slow and painful; it interferes with one's everyday activities. It is uncomfortable but ultimately it is worthwhile. The new era of political reform in my own country, I hope, will, like the field of pragmatics, move from strength to strength, providing answers to old questions, and new questions about old answers. The essence of success in both endeavors should and must remain, in my opinion, humanity oriented.

ACKNOWLEDGMENTS

I am deeply indebted to Victoria Joffe, Liora Tucker, and Ruth Beecham for their therapeutic insights.

Deep gratitude is also due to Shirley Heenen, Director of Hospice Association Johannesburg, for providing me with many new insights.

LC for helping me discover a new and very real side of aphasia.

To Audrey Holland, my friend and mentor who has constantly legitimized therapeutic endeavors and whose support has always been felt across the years and across the miles.

Part of this chapter is reprinted with the permission of Professor Anna Mazzucchi, editor of *New Frontiers in Neurorehabilitation*. Proceedings of a Conference held in Parma, April 1991, 10–13, from a paper entitled "Pragmatic Correlates of Neurogenic Language Disorders."

REFERENCES

Ahlsén, E. (1991). Bodily communication as compensation for speech in Wernicke's aphasia — A longitudinal study. *Journal of Communication Disorders, 24,* 1–12.

Armstrong, E. M. (1991). The potential of cohesion analysis in the analysis and treatment of aphasic discourse. *Clinical Linguistics and Phonetics, 5*(1), 39–52

Armus, S. R., Brookshire, R. H., & Nicholas, L. E. (1989). Aphasic and non-brain-damaged adults' knowledge of scripts for common situations. *Brain and Language, 36,* 518–528.

Behrmann, M., & Penn, C. (1984). Non-verbal communication of aphasic patients. *British Journal of Disordered Communication, 19,* 155–168.

Berko-Gleason, J., Goodglass, H., Obler, L., & Green, E. (1980). Narrative strategies of aphasic and normal speaking subjects. *Journal of Speech and Hearing Research, 30,* 44–49.

Biggs, J. B., & Collis, K. F. (1982). *Evaluating the quality of learning. The SOLO Taxonomy.* New York: Academic Press.

Blomert, L. (1990). What functional assessment can contribute to setting goals for aphasia therapy [Special Issue]. *Aphasiology, The future of aphasia therapy, 4,* 307–320.

Brinton, B., Craig, H. K., & Skarakis-Doyle, E. (1990). Peer commentary on "Clinical Pragmatics: Expectations and Realizations" by Tanya Gallagher. *Journal of Speech-Language Pathology and Audiology, 14*(1), 7–13.

Brookshire, R. H., & Nicholas, L. E. (1984). Comprehension of directly and indirectly stated main ideas and details in discourse by brain-damaged and non-brain-damaged listeners. *Brain and Language, 21,* 21–36.

Brown, C., & Cullinan, W. (1981). Word retrieval difficulty and disfluent speech in adult anomic speakers. *Journal of Speech and Hearing Research, 24,* 358–365.

Busch, C. R., Brookshire, R. H., & Nicholas, L. E. (1988). Referential communication by aphasic and nonaphasic adults. *Journal of Speech and Hearing Disorders, 53,* 475–482.

Chapman, S. B., & Ulatowska, H. K. (1989). Discourse in aphasia. Integration deficits in processing reference. *Brain and Language, 36,* 651–668.

Choron, J. (1972). *Suicide.* New York: Charles Scribner.

Connell, P. (1987). Teaching language form, meaning, and function to specific-language-impaired children. In S. Rosenberg (Ed.), *Advances in applied psycholinguistics. Vol. 1: First-language development* (pp. 60–75). New York: Cambridge University Press.

Davis, G. A., & Wilcox, M. J. (1985). *Adult aphasia rehabilitation: Applied pragmatics.* San Diego, CA: College-Hill Press.

Doke, C. M. (1954). *The Southern Bantu languages.* Cape Town, South Africa: Oxford University Press.

Epstein, N. (1976). *The comprehension ability of a bilingual adult with language impairment: A case study.* Unpublished research report, Department of Speech Pathology and Audiology, University of the Witwatersrand, Johannesburg.

Ernest-Baron, C., Brookshire, R. H., & Nicholas, L. E. (1987). Story structure and retelling of narratives by aphasic and non-brain-damaged adults. *Journal of Speech and Hearing Research, 30,* 44–49.

Fredman, M. (1975). The effect of therapy given in Hebrew on the home language of the bilingual or polyglot adult aphasic in Israel. *British Journal of Disordered Communication, 10,* 61–69.

Fritz, V., & Penn, C. (1992). *Stroke: Caring and coping.* Johannesburg, South Africa: Witwatersrand University Press.

Gallagher, T. M. (1990). Clinical pragmatics: Expectations and realizations. *Journal of Speech-Language Pathology and Audiology, 14*(1), 36.

Glosser, G., Wiener, M., & Kaplan, E. (1986). Communicative gestures in aphasia. *Brain and Language, 27,* 345–359.

Glosser, G., Wiener, M., & Kaplan, E. (1990). Disorders in executive control functions among aphasic and other brain-damaged patients. *Journal of Clinical Experimental Neuropsychology, 12*(4), 485–501.

Green, G. (1984). Communication in aphasia therapy: Some of the procedures and issues involved. *British Journal of Disordered Communication, 19,* 35–46.

Gregorson, E. A. (1977). *Language in Africa: An introductory survey.* New York: Gordon & Breach.

Halliday, M. A. K., & Hasan, R. (1976). *Cohesion in English.* London: Edward Arnold.

Herbert, R. K. (1992). *Sociolinguistics in Africa: Proceedings of International Colloquium.* Johannesburg, South Africa: Witwatersrand University Press.

Hermann, M., Reiche, T., Lucius-Hoene, G., Wallesch, C., & Johannsen-Horbach, H. (1988). Nonverbal communication as a compensative strategy for severely nonfluent aphasics? — A quantitative approach. *Brain and Language, 33,* 41–54.

Hermann, M., Koch, U., Johannsen-Horbach, H., & Wallesch, C. (1989). Communicative skills in chronic and severe nonfluent aphasia. *Brain and Language, 37,* 339–352.

Holland, A. L. (1980). *Communicative abilities in daily living.* Baltimore: University Park Press.

Holland, A. L. (1990). Conversational coaching. Workshop presented at Conference: *Pragmatic Skills in Aphasia,* Stichting Afasie, Rotterdam, Netherlands.

Hough, M. S., & Pierce, R. S. (1989). Contextual influences in aphasia: Effects of predictive versus nonpredictive narratives. *Brain and Language, 36,* 325–334.

Jackson, H. F. (1988). Brain, cognition and grief. *Aphasiology 2*(1), 91–92.

Kacsmarek, B. L. J. (1984). Neurolinguistic analysis of verbal utterances in patients with focal lesions of frontal lobes. *Brain and Language, 21,* 52–58.

Katz, R. C., LaPointe, L. L., & Markel, N. N. (1988). Coverbal behavior and aphasic speakers. Paper presented at the Annual Clinical Aphasiology Conference, South Carolina.

Kertesz, A. (1980). *Western aphasia battery.* New York: Grune & Stratton.

Klippi, A. (1990). Conversational dynamics between aphasics. Poster presented at the Fourth International Aphasia Rehabilitation Congress, Edinburgh, Scotland.

Lanham, L. W. (1978). An outline history of the languages of Southern Africa. In L. W. Lanham & K. P. Prinsloo (Eds.), *Language and communication studies in South Africa.* Cape Town, South Africa: Oxford University Press.

Leonard, L. B., & Loeb, D. F. (1988). Government-binding theory and some of its applications: A tutorial. *Journal of Speech and Hearing Research, 31,* 515–524.

Linebaugh, C. (1984). Mild aphasia. In A. L. Holland (Ed.), *Language disorders in adults.* San Diego, CA: College-Hill Press.

Lomas, J., Pickard, L., Bester, S., Elebard, H., Finlayson, A., & Zoghaib, C. (1989). The communicative effectiveness index: The development and psychometric evaluation of a functional communication measure for adult aphasia. *Journal of Speech and Hearing Disorders, 54,* 113–124.

Mandler, J. M., & Johnson, N. S. (1977). Remembrance of things parsed: Story structure and recall. *Cognitive Psychology, 9,* 111–151.

Marshall, R. C. (1987). Reapportioning time for aphasia rehabilitation — A point of view. *Aphasiology, 1,* 59–73.

McTear, M. F. (1985). Pragmatic disorders: A question of direction. *British Journal of Disordered Communication, 20,* 119–127.

Panzeri, M., Semenza, C., & Butterworth, B. (1987). Compensatory processes in the evolution of severe jargon aphasia. *Neuropsychologia, 25*(6), 919–933.

Penn, C. (1983a). *Syntactic and pragmatic aspects of aphasic language.* Unpublished Ph.D. Thesis, University of the Witwatersrand, Johannesburg, South Africa.

Penn, C. (1983b). Fluency and aphasia: A pragmatic reconsideration. *South African Journal of Communication Disorders, 30,* 3–8.

Penn, C. (1987). Pragmatic profiling of adult language pathology: An exercise in clinical linguistics. *African Studies, 46*(2), 307–327.

Penn, C. (1988). The profiling of syntax and pragmatics in aphasia. *Clinical Linguistics and Phonetics, 2*(3), 179–207.

Penn C. (1991, April). Pragmatic correlates of aphasia. In A. Mazzucchi (Ed.), *New frontiers in rehabilitation: Proceedings of a conference held in Parma,* (pp. 37–54).

Penn, C., & Beecham, R. (1992). Discourse therapy in multilingual aphasia: A case study. *Clinical Linguistics and Phonetics, 6*(1, 2), 11–25.

Penn, C., & Joffe, V. (1992, September). *Discourse therapy in mild aphasia: A framework for interpretation.* Paper presented at 5th International Aphasia Rehabilitation Conference, Zurich, Switzerland.

Prutting, C. A. (1982). Pragmatics as social competence. *Journal of Speech and Hearing Disorders, 47,* 123–134.

Schienberg, S., & Holland, A. L. (1980). Conversational turn-taking in Wernicke aphasia. In R. Brookshire (Ed.), *Clinical Aphasiology Conference Proceedings.* Minneapolis: BRIC Publishers.

Schuell, H. Jenkins, J. J., & Jimenez Pabon, E. (1964). *Aphasia in adults.* New York: Harper & Row.

Semela, J. (1978). *An investigation into the breakdown of the concordial system of Zulu-speaking aphasics.* Unpublished research report, Department of Speech Pathology and Audiology, University of the Witwatersrand, Johannesburg.

Silvast, M. (1990). *Aphasia therapy dialogues.* Paper presented at IVth International Aphasia Rehabilitation Congress, Edinburgh, Scotland.

Sinoff, A. (1992). Verb cohesion in the narratives of deaf children. Manuscript in preparation.

Swindell, C. S., & Hammond, J. (1991). Post-stroke depression: Neurologic, physiologic, diagnostic, and treatment implications. *Journal of Speech and Hearing Research, 34,* 325–333.

Tughendaft, K. (1972). *Luria's test on traumatic bilingual or polyglot aphasics.* Unpublished research report, Department of Speech Pathology and Audiology, University of the Witwatersrand, Johannesburg.

Ulatowska, J. K., North, A. J., & Macaluso-Haynes, S. (1981). Production of narrative and procedural discourse in aphasia. *Brain and Language, 13,* 345–371.

Weisenberg, Y., & McBride, K. E. (1935). *Aphasia: A clinical and psychological study.* New York: The Commonwealth Fund.

Whitney, J. L., & Goldstein, H. (1989). Using self-monitoring to reduce disfluencies in speakers with mild aphasia. *Journal of Speech and Hearing Disorders, 54,* 576–586.

Wilkes, A. (1978). Bantu language studies. In L. W. Lanham & K. P. Prinsloo (Eds.), *Language and communication studies in South Africa.* Cape Town, South Africa: Oxford University Press.

Wint, G. (1965). *The third killer: Meditations on a stroke.* London: Chatto and Windus.

Yorkston, K. M., & Beukelman, D. R. (1980). An analysis of connected speech samples of aphasic and normal speakers. *Journal of Speech and Hearing Disorders, 45*(1), 27–36.

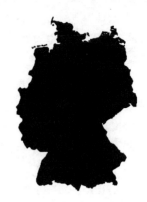

CHAPTER 3

Approaches to Aphasia Therapy in Aachen

WALTER HUBER
LUISE SPRINGER
KLAUS WILLMES
Department of Neurology and School of Logopedics
Rheinisch-Westäflische Technische Hochschule
Aachen, Germany

Our experience with aphasia therapy has developed in the Neurology Department of the Technical University in Aachen under the direction of Klaus Poeck. Aphasia therapy is provided for both in- and outpatients. Inpatients stay either on acute wards, including intensive care, or on a special aphasia ward. Outpatients are seen either for extensive neurolinguistic and neuropsychological diagnosis at the neurological clinic or for aphasia therapy administered at the school of logopedics. The aphasia therapists cooperate with an interdisciplinary group of researchers including linguists, psychologists, and neurologists. Research on therapy has developed from clinical, diagnostic, and theoretical interests. In the past, we have made several attempts to combine different approaches to a comprehensive treatment regimen (cf. Huber, 1988; Huber, 1991, 1992; Huber, Poeck, & Springer, 1991; Huber & Springer, 1989; Poeck,

1982; Poeck, Huber, Stachowiak, & Weniger, 1977; Springer, 1986; Springer & Weniger, 1980; Weniger,Huber, Stachowiak, & Poeck, 1980; Weniger & Springer, 1989). Furthermore, we have been concerned with methodological issues of therapy research using either single case or group designs (Willmes, 1985, 1990).

In this chapter, we first outline our treatment regimen, which is oriented toward the natural course of aphasia. We then report on a group study in which we assessed the efficacy of therapy on the aphasia ward, and finally, we review experimental therapy studies conducted in Aachen. Each of these studies focused on intervention techniques specifically designed for the treatment of impairments at a particular level of linguistic processing. Our approaches range from modality-specific stimulation to relearning of linguistic structures and communicative activation.

CONTENTS AND METHODS OF TREATMENT

From a neurophysiological point of view there are three basic mechanisms of functional recovery in the brain: Restitution, substitution, and compensation (Singer, 1982). Each mechanism appears to correlate in different ways with changes in linguistic behavior at different times post-onset (cf. Rothi & Horner, 1983). Consequently, principles and methods of aphasia therapy vary according to the patient's phase of recovery. In our clinical regimen, we distinguish three phases of aphasia therapy (see Figure 3–1): Activation, symptom-specific training, and consolidation (Huber et al., 1991; Springer & Weniger, 1980).

Of course, all phases of aphasia therapy must be accompanied by family counseling and psychosocial support for the patient. The clinical regimen should always comprise both therapy for aphasia and therapy for the aphasic patient.

ACTIVATION

Restitution of impaired language functions typically occurs during the first 4 weeks and leads to complete recovery in about one third of patients (Biniek, in press). The goal of aphasia therapy during this period is to enhance the evolution of temporarily impaired language functions.

We distinguish the following methods for this phase of treatment:

- direct stimulation;
- indirect stimulation: cuing and deblocking;
- blocking.

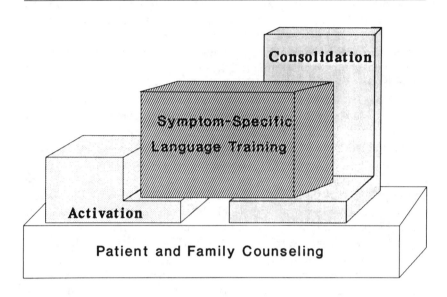

Figure 3–1. Stages of aphasia treatment.

For direct stimulation the patient is asked to imitate nonverbal or verbal acts by mimicking gestures, speaking in unison, or oral repetition. These imitation tasks require the patient simply to give direct and immediate responses without the necessity for internal activation of broader linguistic knowledge and selection among alternatives. In contrast, indirect stimulation makes use of priming effects based on similarity relations between the target and a preceding item (i.e., the "prime"). Cuing techniques in aphasia therapy typically make use of priming effects. For example, confrontation naming stimulates the target name by presenting the initial phoneme or syllable, a semantically related word, a sentence to be completed (closure sentence), or a description of functions and attributes of the object to be named.

The function of direct or indirect stimulation by phonemic cues depends on the nature of the underlying disorder. For postlexical difficulties (e.g., speech apraxia), phonemic cues function as direct stimulation. For lexical difficulties, however, they are a means of indirect stimulation, as they activate not only the target name, but also a set of lexical alternatives, that is, words with phonemic similarity, in which the target name is included.

Each stimulation approach presupposes a detailed analysis of task demands in terms of input, output, and central processing components.

Depending on how many and which components are involved, tasks can be ranked according to their inherent difficulty. The more and the deeper the central processing that is required, the more difficult the task becomes for aphasic patients. Stimulation always starts with modalities that are easy and/or less impaired and proceeds stepwise to the more difficult ones.

Auditory comprehension often appears to be the least impaired modality. This may be due to guessing strategies which enable the patient to use situational information together with some key words for a communicatively adequate reconstruction of what the partner intended to say, rather than to linguistic processing per se. The therapist tries to reinforce these capacities for communication- and situation-based message comprehension at the beginning of each treatment session. This is encouraging for the patient and possibly has a global language activation effect. More specific impairments of the auditory modality may be improved as well. This, in turn, facilitates subsequent stimulation by means of verbal imitation tasks.

It should be clear that, for each aphasic syndrome and possibly even for each individual patient, significant deviations from the general hierarchy of inherent task difficulties must be expected. Some task components can be more impaired than others. Some input or output routes may even appear to be blocked. Weigl (1961) suggested systematic *deblocking* as a therapy method. When a patient performs very poorly on one particular task, the therapist tries to find related tasks in which the patient performs substantially better. The therapist then arranges the tasks into a deblocking chain, with the relatively better preserved tasks preceding the impaired one. This leads to facilitation; the patient now performs well what he or she could not do before. If there is deblocking in the strict sense, improvement occurs immediately and without the patient's awareness.

For example, some aphasic patients are unable to name objects. However, naming becomes possible after the patient has successfully activated the target name in some other task, such as reading the name or indicating comprehension of the spoken name by pointing to the corresponding object. But how does the therapist exclude the possibility that the deblocking effect is brought about by mere retention and verbal imitation? Deblocking effects can also be obtained when the training includes not one, but several words from the same semantic field, in randomized order from task to task. Facilitation is, however, less likely to occur when semantically unrelated words are used (Springer, 1979; Weigl, 1979). Parallel similarity effects have been reported for deblocking syntactic and morphological structures (Weigl & Bierwisch, 1970). From the perspective of cognitive neurolinguistics, it appears that these effects are based on preactivation of units/regularities of central processing components rather than on "deblocking" of impaired output or input routes.

For clinical syndromes that involve a modality-specific disorder such as speech apraxia, agraphia, alexia, conduction aphasia, or pure word deafness, the deblocking method clearly does not work. In these syndromes the modality-specific codes are affected and not merely the dynamics of transmission as presupposed by deblocking theory.

Stimulation is not the only therapy method that is appropriate in the acute phase. In patients with evolving global and Wernicke's aphasia, the therapist attempts to block automatisms, perseverations, jargon, and logorrhea from the very beginning.

With respect to *repetitive verbal behavior* (i.e., automatisms and perseverations) two underlying mechanisms must be distinguished. Repetitive verbal behavior may be brought about as a mode of either disinhibition or failure. When they reflect disinhibition, verbal responses are perseverated across several items with no indication of internal control and self-correction. We found this form to be characteristic in patients with very severe global aphasia, who, as one would expect, showed no practice effects on single word training (Haag, Huber, Hündgen, Stiller, & Willmes, 1985). In contrast, repetitive verbal behavior as a mode of failure was characteristic of patients with less severe global aphasia, who had some residual learning capacities. They used more variable perseverations and automatisms, and quite frequently attempted self-corrections. Most importantly, in these patients, repetitive behavior occurred significantly more often for items on which they had failed on preceding trials. Depending on the characteristics of repetitive behavior, different intervention techniques are used during therapy. With mode of disinhibition, the therapist should always stop and distract the patient. With mode of failure, however, the therapist should try to make the patient aware of the perseveration (e.g., by contrasting the repetitive response with alternatives, including the target).

The overall therapeutic goal during the acute phase is to use all available means to activate the patient to respond as appropriately and as communicatively as possible. Activation techniques should always be applied in a *situational context* that is socially and emotionally relevant to the patient. For example, direct stimulation usually starts with emotional expressions (e.g., in German *au!, mhm, toll, pfui,* etc.) and with overlearned phrases that are used in everyday situations such as greeting and farewell formulas. Words are grouped thematically (e.g., under such topics as breakfast, personal hygiene, weekend, hobby, etc.) rather than according to strict semantic criteria. Since Jackson, aphasiologists have always assumed that emotional and overlearned language is better preserved in aphasia because it is less lateralized to the left hemisphere and therefore easy to reactivate via intact right hemisphere functions. This line of reasoning forms the theoretical assumption underlying Melodic Intonation Therapy (Sparks, Helm, & Albert, 1974). Our experience also suggests that rhythmical tapping, humming, and singing may successfully facilitate temporarily blocked left hemisphere language functions.

SYMPTOM-SPECIFIC TRAINING

The next phase of aphasia therapy begins when the patient is medically stable, and the aphasia can be examined extensively. At that time symptom-specific training is provided, aimed primarily at relearning degraded linguistic knowledge, reactivating impaired linguistic modalities, and learning compensatory linguistic strategies. In other words, language-oriented methods are applied. During the phase of linguistic learning, a gradual functional reorganization of the impaired language system is assumed (cf. Luria, Naydin, Tsvetkova, & Vinatskaya, 1969). This may be achieved by both substitution and compensation for impaired brain functions. It is not clear to what extent functional reorganization presupposes some intact language functions of the left dominant hemisphere and/or carryover to right hemisphere functions (cf. Moore, 1989).

The therapeutic goal is to make the patient indirectly aware (without telling him) of linguistic units and regularities that are specifically lost or, conversely, are available for one item but not for another. By so doing, one hopes to induce learning processes in the patient (cf. Kotten, 1981; Poeck et al., 1977). These techniques are based mainly on careful selection of linguistic problems and material to be practiced. If necessary, the patient is also taught explicit grammatical rules and strategies. To stabilize performance, most patients are required to perform the same or similar items repeatedly. We believe that learning is enhanced when the item context and/or the task demands are varied on these repeated presentations. The target linguistic structure, however, must be the same.

A starting point for therapy planning in this phase is the systematic observation of the patient's verbal behavior across several linguistic modalities. We are also concerned with linguistic units and regularities on different linguistic levels of description. This is reflected by the linguistic design of the Aachen Aphasia Test (AAT) (Huber, Poeck, & Willmes, 1984). We routinely administer the AAT at the beginning of the symptom-specific training. The AAT allows for psychometrically sound analysis of the test profile, standardized ratings of spontaneous language on several levels of description, probabilistic assignment to an aphasia syndrome, and estimation of global, as well as syndrome-specific degrees of severity, by reference to norms.

AAT examinations provide only baseline information. For more detailed assessment, we are developing supplementary tests (Poeck & Göddenhenrich, 1988). In addition to psychometric approaches, clinical exploration of the patient's verbal and nonverbal behavior is necessary. When processing models are available to describe and explain symptoms in terms of underlying mechanisms, as is the case for reading, writing, and naming disorders, these models may guide the planning of therapy (cf. Lesser, 1987). As a rule, further evaluations take place as "process diagnosis" during the course of treatment.

There is no single approach for this phase. But a systematic orientation to linguistic units, structures, and regularities is essential to all therapeutic attempts, irrespective of whether the therapist tries to establish relearning of degraded knowledge, reactivation of impaired modalities, or learning of compensatory strategies. Involving the patient in setting goals for each therapy program is encouraged. For example, personal interests and premorbid language skills must be taken into account. A basic principle for setting up each therapy unit is first to reactivate, second to induce learning and relearning, and third to consolidate. In other words, (re)learning is always embedded within preceding attempts at situational stimulation and/or linguistic activation and succeeding attempts at stabilization and generalization.

In the following sections we outline what we think are the major perspectives of the language-oriented (re)learning approach. The central concepts for therapy planning are:

- linguistic structure;
- linguistic modality;
- linguistic strategy;
- models of linguistic processing;
- processing capacity (working memory).

Linguistic Structure

Beginning in the late 1960s, research on aphasia increasingly used methods taken from descriptive linguistics, and aphasic symptoms were interpreted in terms of grammatical theories. Empirical studies of linguistic behavior in aphasia were conducted to determine which linguistic structures were affected and which were preserved. Based on clinical and experimental findings, hierarchies of inherent linguistic difficulties were proposed. Some of the pioneering work is published in Goodglass and Blumstein (1973).

Aphasia therapy likewise came to be guided by descriptions of language structures taken from general linguistics (Hatfield, 1972; Weniger et al., 1980). Several components of the central language system have been distinguished: Phonology and prosody, lexicon, morphology and syntax, semantics, and discourse grammar. For each component, units and regularities of occurrence and combination are defined.

Two variants of the linguistic structure approach to aphasia therapy can be distinguished. One proceeds mainly in a didactic manner. That is, goals, material, and methods are determined in terms of the grammar of the patient's language. The training material resembles grammatical exercises used in textbooks for second-language learning (e.g., Engl, Kotten, Ohlendorf, & Poser, 1982). The theoretical assumptions underlying this approach are questionable for two reasons. First, brain damage hardly affects linguistic capacities according to the grammar of a language. Neither pathological nor normal brain structures and functions seem to correspond to the logic of the language in a one-to-one fashion (cf. Poeck, 1983). Second, (re)learning in aphasia is not the same as the learning of a second language by a normal adult person, nor is it the same as first language acquisition by a child. The aphasic patient does not lose all linguistic knowledge. Even in global aphasia, residual capacities are preserved. Thus, in aphasia, integration of preserved with lost and relearned linguistic knowledge is required from the very beginning. Interference of intact capacities with knowledge to be learned is not a problem in the same way as it is in second language learning.

In our view, the linguistic structure approach should always be clinically guided. Symptoms and their combination into syndromes must be carefully observed, and their possible underlying mechanisms should be described in terms of linguistic theory. This neurolinguistic description becomes the starting point for planning therapy. The result is that training material is selected with respect to the sound structure, the lexicon, and the grammar of the language itself as well as the patient's specific linguistic impairment. The training material is chosen from the linguistic units and regularities that correspond most closely to a particular aphasic patient's symptoms. For example, if a patient's language output is laden with semantic paraphasias, the corresponding linguistic units and regularities to be worked with are word meanings and their semantic relations. During therapy, items from a few selected semantic fields and their respective classificatory and associative meaning relations are trained through example. This training also involves exercises at the sentence level, in order to treat accompanying disturbances of semantic selection restrictions in sentence planning. The patient must, of course, have sufficient syntactic skills.

Examples of material used in the linguistic structure approach are phonemes and syllables with articulatory contrasts; words with minimal phonemic contrast, with classificatory versus associative meaning relations,
or with grammatical category contrasts such as nouns versus verbs; sentences with constituent structure contrasts, such as intransitive versus
transitive, active versus passive, local versus temporal adverbial complements, coordination versus subordination of clauses; and so forth.

In the linguistic structure approach, it is essential to use metalinguistic
tasks (cf. Springer & Weniger, 1980). These include phonologic and orthographic spelling from memory, sorting words to a given semantic criterion, rearrangement of word or sentence anagrams, sentence completion from multiple-choice sets of content or function words, and so on.
These tasks require the patients to make conscious decisions about phonemic and graphemic, lexical, and grammatical structure, thereby activating their remaining linguistic knowledge. Stimuli should be presented simultaneously in several modalities, mostly as pictures together with
written and/or spoken words or phrases. The target item should be presented with several distractors that resemble it linguistically to varying degrees.

When the patient fails, the therapist gives systematic cues contrasting
increasingly more difficult and incorrect possibilities for resolving the
linguistic problem at hand. The distractor items reflect the linguistic regularities that are most difficult for the patient. In many instances, it is necessary to work specifically on both target and distractor contrasts.

Linguistic Modality

As an alternative to focusing on linguistic structures, therapy may aim
primarily at activating linguistic modalities as described in the stimulation approach for the treatment of acute aphasia. Even if the impairment
in chronic aphasia is multimodal in nature, its severity may differ across
modalities. The therapist tries to capitalize on these differences.

The modality approach requires the therapist to determine when and
why one modality is more affected than others. Each linguistic modality can be divided into input and output components, each of which has
modality-specific codes for processing linguistic information. The
acoustic-phonetic and the articulatory code are primary. The visual-
orthographic and the graphomotor code are secondary. If the analysis
points to a transmission problem (i.e., the level for successful access or
retrieval cannot be attained), then direct and indirect stimulation techniques are appropriate. However, if the modality-specific code is disturbed, then linguistic structure approach is preferable. The therapist

tries to determine which units and regularities in the coding system are impaired and then to select appropriate training material, tasks, and relearning techniques.

Obviously, it is necessary to focus on the coding system of one modality when treating a patient with a modality-specific syndrome. For example, Springer and Luzzatti (1987) proposed a training program for speech apraxia in which the patient learns to mentally anticipate the execution of articulatory gestures. The therapist supports this by making the patient directly aware of the articulators and of movement parameters underlying normal articulation. Visual feedback is given by means of schematic drawings of the vocal tract or by monitoring of tongue movement via ultrasound sonography (Wein, Böckler, Huber, Klajman, & Willmes, 1990).

With severe modality-specific syndromes, only limited progress can be achieved by direct treatment techniques. The patient must develop compensatory strategies. Examples include development of writing in severe speech apraxia, lipreading in pure word-deafness and auditory agnosia (cf. Fechtelpeter, Göddenhenrich, Huber, & Springer, 1990), or finger tracing of letter contours in pure alexia.

In more common, but chronic syndromes of aphasia, disorders are typically multimodal in nature. That is, characteristic symptoms occur in each linguistic modality. Little variation in level of performance is found across modalities, and thus the prerequisites are lacking for a strict modality approach such as Weigl's deblocking method. Nevertheless, the modality approach is useful for the treatment of chronic aphasic syndromes. In contrast to Shewan and Bandur (1986), we do not favor systematic training through one particular modality. Rather, we prefer multimodal stimulation combined with the linguistic structure approach. Central linguistic knowledge is more likely to be activated by input from more than one modality. Likewise, linguistic knowledge can be improved and stabilized when expression is practiced in more than one output modality.

Linguistic Strategy

The linguistic strategy approach offers an alternative to conscious structural relearning in aphasia. Instead of setting the goal in terms of lost or only inconsistently available linguistic units and regularities, the therapist tries to optimize the linguistic processing routines which remain available to patients and which they often use spontaneously (cf. Seron, 1982). In other words, positive rather than negative aspects of the aphasic behaviors become the starting point.

The strategy approach is usually successful for treating word-finding difficulties. The patient is systematically guided to produce circumlocutions that specify the functional and/or situational characteristics of the object or person that cannot be named. In patients with syntactic difficulties, this strategy is, of course, limited. Alternatively, these patients can be encouraged to use semantic search strategies. They are told to enumerate words that come easily to mind because they bear an associative relationship to the target. And they are taught to indicate for each of these associates (by means of interjections like "no," "not quite," etc.) that the intended target is not yet reached. Often, using these compensatory strategies, the intended word is uttered. Linguistic strategies of this kind are built on the positive aspects of word-finding difficulties. Many patients use these strategies spontaneously and the therapist has only to reinforce them in a systematic way.

Disturbances of segmental phonology can be reduced if patients have a relatively preserved orthographic lexicon (sight vocabulary). The therapist suggests that the patient visualize words internally whenever pronunciation difficulties occur. Literature concerning therapy of reading and writing disorders mentions many similar compensatory strategies. They are easily learned by patients as "tricks." Another strategy is use of the so-called link-words applied by Hatfield (1989) to enable English-speaking patients to sound out graphemes and written function words. This trick works just as well for German-speaking patients.

A strategy approach is also useful for the treatment of severe agrammatism. It is assumed that basic thematic relations are still available for sentence planning despite the lack of function words, inflectional endings, and complex phrase structures. The content words used still refer to agents, actions, objects, goals of an action, instruments, location, and so on. Word order still indicates a logical or temporal sequence or a gradation of thematic importance. These positive functions of agrammatism can be systematically enhanced in therapy (cf. Jones, 1986; Kearns, 1990). Patients are told to ignore their grammatical difficulties during sentence planning and to concentrate on the thematically consistent selection of content words. The therapist may introduce a thematic scheme that supports thematic sentence planning. The patient is instructed to consider WHO/IS DOING WHAT/TO WHOM/WHERE/WHEN/WITH WHAT/and so on. This scheme is hierarchically expanded. Only inappropriate selection of content words is corrected by the therapist. Morphological or syntactic errors are ignored. In German we call this method "reduced syntax therapy" (REST) (Springer, Schlenck, & Schlenck, 1991).

In our experience, the strategy approach, despite its initial success and its enhancement of communicative skills, should be applied only with patients who have little remaining linguistic learning capacity or who are not highly motivated to relearn language. For patients without these limitations, the strategy approach should be complemented by treatment methods aimed specifically at remediation of impaired linguistic structures and modalities.

Processing Model

Planning for aphasia therapy often lacks a coherent theoretical framework which allows the therapist to postulate underlying mechanisms for the aphasic symptoms, to predict how impaired linguistic functions interconnect with others, and to judge whether unimpaired functions can possibly compensate for impaired functions. Such a framework, when demonstrated to have observational and explanatory adequacy, can guide the therapist in a step-by-step investigation of the pattern of impairments of an individual patient during the course of therapy (cf. Kotten, 1989; Lesser, 1987; Sasanuma, 1986).

Besides functional localization of the impairment, processing models also support decisions concerning which therapeutic intervention techniques are most appropriate (cf. Huber, 1992). If the impairment primarily involves transmission of information ("routes"), linguistic *modality* or strategy approach methods will be preferred. If, however, the impairment is in knowledge components, which contain linguistic units and complex structures, linguistic *structure* methods are appropriate.

Many unresolved questions remain concerning the application of processing models to aphasia therapy. These include the following:

1. Not all aphasic symptoms can be unequivocally localized within models of *normal* language processing. This is particularly true for symptoms that appear to indicate lack of internal linguistic control such as automatisms, perseverations, jargon, and paragrammatism.
2. Aphasic failure may result from limitations in processing capacity as well as from interrupted transmission routes and degraded knowledge. No processing models that accommodate distinctions among these possibilities are available.
3. Typically, dissociations in performance are directly related to impaired versus unimpaired processing routes and/or components of the model. However, dissociations may simply reflect differences in inherent task difficulties which are not obvious from normal behavior. The task may be so easy for normal control subjects that they always perform at ceiling. To plan therapy, we need models that specify not only routes, units, and regularities involved in processing, but also the quantity of resources required.
4. Most critical, information flow models do not specify how new or lost information is learned or relearned.

Processing Capacity (Working Memory)

Linguistic learning and relearning in the chronic stage of aphasia initially calls for controlled rather than automatic processing. Activated units must be assembled and compared with alternative units, and the units that best fulfill the given goal or purpose of the task must be selected. Processing components of this kind do not function as long-term stores, and, therefore, are not vulnerable to access or knowledge deficits. However, the processing capacity of these control components may be limited either by reduced memory span or by deficits of attention and/or problem solving. Because these deficits frequently co-occur with aphasia (cf. Cramon & von Zihl 1988; Poeck 1989), limited capacity for controlled linguistic processing must be expected. We believe that a general limitation of processing capacity can be managed in three ways, which are discussed below.

First, additional treatment of attention, short-term memory, and general problem solving can be provided. Sturm (1990) argues that patients with left hemisphere lesions are likely to have impairments in selective and divided attention, while right hemisphere patients tend to have disturbances of alertness and vigilance. On the Aachen aphasia ward, patients are provided with comprehensive treatment for their attentional deficits. Preliminary evaluation has suggested that best results are obtained when the training is specific and when it is administered at intervals. At other German rehabilitation centers, specific training programs for deficits in memory span and problem solving (Cramon & von Zihl, 1988) have been developed.

Second, the capacity demands of the tasks used in aphasia therapy must be systematically varied. For example, limitations in auditory memory span can be dealt with by providing additional written stimuli. In patients who pathologically rely on surface routes of repetition, reading, or writing, holistic strategies may be introduced. Patients are taught to attend to lexical units (words and morphemes) rather than sublexical ones (syllables, phonemes, or graphemes). With more complex tasks, trade-off effects must be expected. Treatment of sentence planning usually begins with demands that isolate one of the multiple processing components such as thematic role assignment, lexical selection, phrase structure construction, or morphological marking. When several of these demands require simultaneous attention, trade-off effects are common, (i.e., patients perform more poorly than before). For example, agrammatic patients may be able to handle morphological structures quite well as long as they practice them in isolation (e.g., in an anagram or in a sentence closure task). However, when planning a whole sentence is required (e.g., in picture description or in retelling of narratives) the previous morphological difficulties reemerge.

In addition to demands to process simultaneously in several linguistic components, time constraints are an important factor for trade-off effects. This appears to be specifically true for patients with chronic agrammatism, who need more processing time than is conventionally acceptable in free conversation. Therefore, in "adapting" to the demands of fluent communication, they switch to a processing mode of reduced linguistic complexity. This in turn leads to speaking agrammatic sentences which nevertheless manage to convey the intended message (cf. Heeschen & Kolk, 1988).

A third approach to treating a limitation in processing capacity is to specifically train or develop internal linguistic control (monitoring). As a rule, aphasic patients monitor failure of access better than they monitor overt errors. "Prepairs" are more frequent than repairs (Schlenck, Huber, & Willmes, 1987). An obvious consequence for therapy is that it is beneficial to focus on treatment of comprehension and metalinguistic judgments, using the patient's own output. But success may be limited, even when comprehension improves substantially. This is because limitations in working memory capacity make it difficult for the patient to plan and execute language output while simultaneously monitoring possible errors.

Consolidation

Symptom-specific training is continued as long as comparisons between pre- and post-treatment test results demonstrate substantial improvement. In many patients, treatment can be extended well into the chronic stage of recovery (i.e., beyond 12 months post-onset), until a learning plateau is reached (cf. Hanson, Metter, & Riege, 1989).

The symptom-specific training must be complemented by a phase of consolidation, which has the two therapeutic goals of maintenance and transfer.

Chronic aphasic patients who reach learning plateaus are at risk for deterioration of their linguistic capacities even in the absence of obvious psychosocial problems. Therefore, we have established a maintenance group (cf. Kearns, 1986) of outpatients whose aphasia is 3 to 10 years post ictus. This group has met for several years, with the sole purpose of engaging in verbal communication. At times, conversation must be specifically stimulated by means of prepared topics for discussion, or by games requiring either verbal or social engagement.

A professional aphasia therapist attends the group meetings at regular intervals. The therapist tries to establish conversational rules and strategies (cf. Holland, 1980), such as:

- wait and listen when a partner is about to speak;

- give a clear signal (eye contact, gesture, verbal interjection, or comment) when you want to speak (turn-taking) or when you want to continue;

- take your time when you are speaking, especially when you have trouble with formulation;

- try to convey your message using all available verbal and non-verbal means;

- indicate when you are unable to understand the message of a speaking partner;

- in case of communication misunderstandings try to convey what you have understood so far, but do not act as an overcorrecting teacher.

When several group members spontaneously begin to apply these rules, the therapist reduces his or her participation. In fact, one of our first groups became a local self-help group which is now a member of the German National Aphasia Association.

Another goal of consolidation is to enhance the transfer of practiced linguistic skills to everyday communicative situations (cf. Davis, 1986; Prutting, 1982). Standard techniques are linguistic role playing (De Bleser & Weismann, 1981; Schlanger & Schlanger, 1970) and PACE therapy (Davis & Wilcox, 1985). Current therapy research in Aachen is concerned with specifying contents, scope, and efficacy of these pragmatic approaches to aphasia therapy (cf. e.g., Glindemann & Springer, 1989; Glindemann, Willmes, Huber, & Springer, 1991; Springer, Glindemann, Huber, & Willmes, 1991).

The communicative methods of aphasia therapy are begun during the phase of symptom-specific training to activate stabilization and generalization of practiced linguistic abilities. Training of transfer requires a stepwise procedure. For example, we developed a therapy program for the training of the German modal verbs *can, may, must, want* (Weniger, Springer, & Poeck, 1987). After exercises at the sentence and text level, the patients proceed to role playing (e.g., visit at a doctor's office, negotiation with a salesman). They are instructed specifically to use the practiced modal verbs. Their attempts to do so are videotaped. Later, patients, assisted by their therapists, evaluate the linguistic adequacy of their output and their overall communicative effectiveness.

It may also be helpful to engage patients in actual excursions, where it is often easier to observe the strengths and weaknesses of the patients' communicative coping strategies and to delineate aims and methods for modification of their behavior.

For many patients, the methods of linguistic consolidation must be supplemented by psychosocial support ranging from family counseling to psychotherapy. At the aphasia ward, we regularly offer a two-day seminar for patients and relatives. Doctors, nurses, therapists, and social workers provide detailed information about etiology, general health condition, progress in rehabilitation, prognosis, and social security regulations for each patient. Relatives, alone or with their aphasic partners, have the opportunity to discuss their experiences and everyday difficulties in several group sessions. These group meetings are supervised by a trained psychotherapist as well as an aphasia therapist.

EFFICACY OF APHASIA THERAPY

CLINICAL GROUP STUDY

At the Aachen aphasia ward, the various approaches of the symptom-specific training phase are routinely provided, along with methods of consolidation. An individual patient's treatment lasts 6 to 8 weeks, with nine 60-minute sessions per week (five individual sessions and four group sessions). All patients are beyond the acute stage of neurological illness. Patient selection is based on team decision, guided by reports from neurolinguistic, neuropsychological, and neurological examination. Contents and methods of treatment are tailored to the specific symptom complex observed in a given patient.

In a recent study (Poeck, Huber, & Willmes, 1989), we assessed the efficacy of our treatment regimen in a group of 68 consecutively admitted patients with exclusively vascular etiology. Depending on the time post-onset, the treated patients were divided into early (1–4 months), late (4–12 months), and chronic (>12 months) subgroups. The Aachen Aphasia Test (AAT) was used for pre- and post-therapy assessment. Testing and treatment were always done by different persons.

The control group consisted of 92 patients with vascular etiology from an earlier multicenter study of spontaneous recovery of untreated patients (Willmes & Poeck, 1984). This study was conducted (1979–1980) when aphasia treatment was not generally available in West Germany. Each patient was examined on three occasions at fixed intervals (4–6 weeks, approximately 4 months, approximately 7 months post-stroke). We looked at early (1–4 months post-stroke) and late (4–12 months post-stroke) test scores for the controls. Twenty-three of the initial 92 control patients recovered completely between the first and second examination and were dropped from further study; for this reason the late control group consisted of only 69 patients.

There were no significant differences between the control and treated groups with respect to age or gender. Time post-onset was somewhat shorter in the control group, possibly working against our assumption that treatment is effective beyond the phase of spontaneous recovery. For the early phase (1–4 months post-onset), the control patients were comparable in severity to the treated patients. In the late phase (4–12 months post-onset), aphasia was relatively more severe in the treated group for the following reason: In the spontaneous recovery study, patients evolved to a milder aphasia or recovered completely. In contrast, the treatment study continuously recruited more severely impaired patients.

We evaluated improvement in each individual. A calculation of mean group improvement alone would not have been informative because of large individual variation in improvement. Up to 12 months post-stroke, it was necessary to take into account possible effects of spontaneous recovery. Thus, we quantified the amount of spontaneous recovery observed in the control patients obtained as follows: The difference between a patient's T-score at the beginning of the treatment and the T-score at the end of the treatment was corrected by subtracting the corresponding mean T-score difference obtained in the spontaneous recovery study. The corrections were made only for treatment patients in the early (1–4 months) and late phases (4–12 months) of possible spontaneous recovery. These corrections were done separately for the early and late phases, for each of the five AAT-subtests, and for the overall AAT-profile level. The resulting corrected differences were analyzed by psychometric single case analysis methods (Willmes, 1985).

It should be noted that our procedure for correcting for spontaneous recovery is particularly strict. The expected rate of spontaneous recovery is based on a period of 3 months, whereas the period of intensive therapy was only 6 to 8 weeks. A linear interpolation for the expected rate of spontaneous recovery over 6 to 8 weeks is not feasible because the rates of spontaneous recovery reported in the literature are highly nonlinear (Culton, 1969; Hartmann & Landau, 1987, Kertesz & McCabe, 1977).

The number of treated patients who showed significant improvement beyond the expected amount of spontaneous recovery is summarized in Table 3–1. In the early phase, 78% of the patients benefitted from treatment. In the late phase, the figure was 48%. Both percentages are probably underestimates, given the strict correction that we applied. In the chronic treated group, where no correction was required, the percentage of patients with significant improvement was still quite high (68%).

Table 3-1. Outcome study: Number of individual patients in the treated group with significant Aachen Aphasia Test (AAT) improvement.

	Time Post-onset		
	Early (1-4 months)	Late (4-12 months)	Chronic (>12 months)
n	23	26	19
Significant AAT improvement[a]	22 (96%)	21 (81%)	13 (68%)[b]
After correction for rate of spontaneous recovery	18 (78%)	12 (46%)[b]	no correction

[a] Change in profile level and/or scores in one or more of the five subtests (single case analysis procedures [Willmes, 1985]).

[b] Comparision between improvement rates: $p = .073$ (exact test for 2×3 contingency table).

Although the efficacy of treatment has been demonstrated by several studies (Basso, Capitani, & Vignolo, 1979; Shewan & Kertesz, 1984; Wertz et al., 1981, 1986), the mechanisms or factors that are related to the beneficial efects of treatment remain poorly understood. In this study, age, duration, size and site of lesion on CT, and intelligence as assessed by standard tests were not related to improvement. Intensity and specificity of treatment appear to be of crucial importance.

Many unresolved methodological problems remain. Randomized assignment of patients to treatment versus no treatment with blind assessment of outcome is not acceptable because therapy would be withheld from patients for a rather long period of time. Therefore we felt that a historical control group of untreated patients was preferable to account for the impact of spontaneous recovery. Another alternative would be to study the therapy outcome in outpatients in a day clinic setting with each patient undergoing alternating periods of treatment and no treatment. In the no-treatment condition, physical or occupational therapy should be provided, but it must be unrelated to the specific language impairments of the patient. Such a series of treatment periods should not start before 6 months post-onset (i.e., after the point at which only marginal spontaneous recovery can be expected).

Finally, any attempt to measure global outcome of aphasia therapy in a clinical setting appears to be outdated for three reasons: (1) The possible impact of specific intervention techniques on individual patients is masked by the heterogeneity induced by any group study that is conducted according to a standard clinical regimen; (2) given the many controversial issues regarding contents and methods of aphasia treatment, specifically designed experiments are needed to compare different approaches; (3) any demonstration of differential treatment effects implies, at least for the strongest improvement effect, that it was due to aphasia therapy and not to spontaneous recovery, charm of the therapist, or other reasons.

EXPERIMENTAL STUDIES

Some of our early experimental studies are reviewed in Weniger et al. (1980). In several single case studies, we applied a strictly symptom-specific approach. The results demonstrated not only significant practice effects but also stabilization and generalization. We obtained these effects even for the treatment of severe aphasia. For example, for a 59-year-old stroke patient with phonemic jargon, 6 months post-onset, we developed training material in which minimal phonemic contrasts between words were systematically varied (Huber, Mayer, & Kerscheinsteiner, 1978). Word onset contrasts were found to be more effective for learning than word offset contrasts and no contrasts. The patient was better stimulated to self-correction by auditory error feedback than by writing each phonemic approximation. Thus, materials and modality of intervention both had a specific impact on the patient's learning behavior. Stabilization and generalization of the improvement were achieved only after an interval of no therapy and a second period of intensive training.

In several other controlled observations of therapy, we found material-specific training effects. The linguistic units/regularities investigated were: Lexical structures (semantic similarity and phonemic similarity); syntactic structures (active/passive, lexicalized/pronominalized, and coordination/subordination of clauses); and semantic structures (performative verbs with local/directional event perspective). These structures were chosen to exemplify therapy for impairment on the three levels of linguistic processing.

The therapy design of this early approach was simple. There was one period of treatment, with a pre- and post-test. Half of the control test items were identical to the items practiced, and the other half were structurally similar. Patient selection was based on clinical examination and on level of pre-treatment test performance. Only patients whose pre-treatment performance was low enough to leave room for significant improvement were considered for treatment. Applying the binomial model, our criterion for mastery was that patients perform with 90% accuracy (Klauer, 1987; Willmes, 1990). Mastery was most commonly found in patients with moderate severity of impairment according to pretest performance.

In patients with severe impairment, the frequency and degree of improvement varied widely, with some showing no improvement, some achieving substantial improvement, and only a very few attaining the level of performance we termed mastery. The latter finding, of course, was expected, because the initial floor performance of these patients did not reveal the true degree of impairment. Very poor test performance should not, therefore, necessarily preclude therapy. We believe that a period of "probe therapy" helps to assess the residual learning capacities in these patients.

Another finding was that improvement extended to unpracticed items. Whether this reflects a trivial or a nontrivial learning effect depends on the design of the control test. Theoretically, there are four possibilities for item selection. In comparison to the practiced items, the items of the control test can be: Identical in linguistic units and regularities; partially identical (i.e., the linguistic parameters of the practiced items are held fixed, but the context or the task demands are changed); similar (i.e., one parameter is systematically related to the treatment parameters); or unrelated. Correspondingly, any post-therapy improvement can be labeled as: (simple) practice effect, trivial learning effect, nontrivial learning effect (also called transfer effect), or unspecific treatment effect.

Our experience suggests that simple practice effects are easily obtained by using linguistically structured material. This is generally true except in those patients with severe global or Wernicke aphasia who exclusively use uncontrolled repetitive verbal utterances and who commonly also have severe apraxia and memory and problem solving disorders. In these patients, the therapist may try to improve nonverbal skills and situationally based comprehension. This is best achieved through collaboration with occupational therapy.

Many clinicians argue that transfer of improved linguistic performance should be demonstrated in everyday communication. We certainly agree, but such demonstration raises significant methodological problems. What are the relevant communicative situations to be tested? How can we evaluate communicative behavior with respect to the linguistic units and regularities on which therapy focused? An optimal database would be videotaped samples of communicative behavior in everyday life. But evaluating them is extremely time-consuming and the appropriate methodology for analyzing verbal and nonverbal interactions is not readily available. A practical but overly simple solution is to use protocols containing several rating scales. However, the validity and reliability of such scales are frequently low, especially if they are administered by raters who were not involved in developing them.

Our research concentrates instead on a detailed linguistic analysis of spontaneous language, which we sample during role-playing or in conversations with a familiar or unfamiliar nonaphasic partner on given topics.

Depending on the linguistic content of treatment, we assess parameters such as distribution of word class; number of verb complements and specifications of noun phrases, proportions of inflections, subordinate clauses, and cohesive ties; number of propositions; and so on. Changes in these parameters from pre- to post-treatment samples are viewed as indicative of improvement. Performance at this point can be compared to the ranges achieved by normal speakers. This approach, however, does not answer the question of whether improved linguistic abilities lead to more active communicative behavior, such as more appropriate turn taking, verbal rather than gestural requests, and so forth.

It is important to stress that only the demonstration of non-trivial learning effects (and of subsequent transfer into conversational language) can be safely interpreted as resulting from the treatment as opposed to spontaneous recovery, general communicative stimulation, arousal of motivation, or increased self-confidence in the patient. What cannot be concluded is that the method of treatment applied is better than some alternative one. Comparing alternative methods is methodologically difficult. To compare the results of administering one type of treatment to one patient and another type to another patient requires precisely matched pairs of patients. This is almost impossible given the complexity of aphasic symptoms and the large number of intervening variables that need to be controlled.

A more satisfying approach is the repeated intra-subject crossover design (Coltheart, 1983) with the order of treatment methods systematically varied across patients. Figure 3–2 provides an illustration of this kind

Patient No	Time course				
	T_1	T_2	T_3	T_4	T_5
1	A	B	A	B	
2	B	A	B	A	
3	A	B	A	B	
4	B	A	B	A	
etc					

A,B: different treatment methods
$T_1 ... T_5$: control tests

Figure 3–2. Crossover design for therapy studies.

of design. The differential impact of treatment methods can be tested both within and between subjects. In two recent studies, we used the intra-subject crossover design. We compared the linguistic structure approach both with the stimulation and the communicative activation approach.

LINGUISTIC STRUCTURE VERSUS STIMULATION

In the first study (Springer, Willmes, & Haag, in press), we used a simple crossover design (AB vs. BA). The patients were asked to practice dialogue discourse. The crucial linguistic units were temporal expressions, which were embedded in the dialogues either as Wh-questions (*when, for how long*) or as prepositions (*before, after, since, until,* etc.). Training proceeded in the five steps illustrated in Figure 3–3. Only step 3 was crucial for the comparison of methods. The therapist either demonstrated the linguistic characteristics of target and distractor items (method A) or provided stepwise auditory-verbal stimulation (method B) ranging from tapping, to humming, to singing, and to speaking in a manner similar to Melodic Intonation Therapy.

The control tests included the same units and regularities as the practiced material, but were embedded in different linguistic contexts (i.e., we controlled for trivial learning effects). Furthermore, spatial expressions were introduced (*where, on, under, to,* etc.) to assess nontrivial learning effects. The patient was asked to use these expressions in sentence completion tasks. Twenty items each were included for Wh-questions and prepositions. The whole set was administered in two ways, one requiring oral completion and the other requiring selection from multiple-choice sets of written words.

Each course of training for either method A or B was provided in six sessions distributed over 2 weeks. Twelve patients with either moderate Broca's or Wernicke's aphasia were included in the study, six for each of the two sequences AB and BA. The minimum duration of aphasia was 3 months, the median was 11 months. The results are shown in Figure 3–4.

Irrespective of the sequence, the results of the linguistic structure approach were the more favorable. In the statistical analysis for such a crossover design, aftereffects must first be evaluated (nonparametric tests for the two period crossover design). The differences between pre- and post-treatment performance were calculated for each method of treatment and each of the four linguistic parameters (temporal/spatial Wh-particles/prepositions).

Overall, there were significant differences in aftereffects for practiced but not for unpracticed items. The largest aftereffect was obtained for the sequence stimulation prior to the training of linguistic structures.

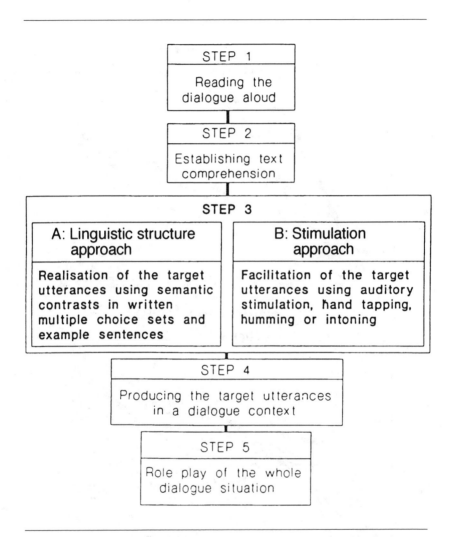

Figure 3–3. Steps for the two treatment approaches in the dialogue study.

Next, we compared the direct effects, that is, we questioned whether the linguistic structure approach was more effective than the stimulation approach at each post-test. For the practiced temporal expressions the linguistic structure approach achieved better results for written performance on Wh-questions and for oral performance on prepositions. For the unpracticed spatial expressions the results of the linguistic structure approach were significantly superior only in oral performance on Wh-par-

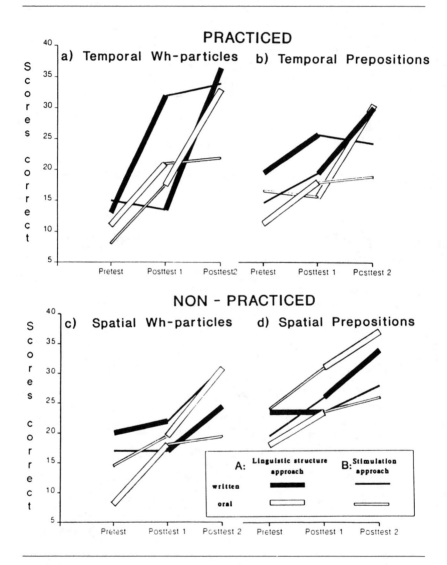

Figure 3-4. Mean performance in control tests (*n* = 6 each) in the dialogue study.

ticles. In addition, there was significant overall improvement in each condition when performance of the second post-test was compared to that of the pretest. This was also true for the unpracticed spatial expressions, even though the amount of overall improvement was again significantly larger for the practiced temporal expressions.

Three conclusions can be drawn from this study. First, specific training irrespective of the method applied led to overall improvement of linguistic performance. Second, trivial learning effects were larger and more widespread than nontrivial ones. Third, the linguistic structure approach was more effective than the stimulation approach. It was most effective when preceded by a period of stimulation. It appears that even beyond the phase of early spontaneous recovery, techniques of verbal activation prepare patients optimally for structured linguistic learning.

LINGUISTIC STRUCTURE VERSUS COMMUNICATIVE ACTIVATION

In a second study (Springer, Glindemann et al., 1991), we used a double crossover design and compared the linguistic structure approach with a communicative activation approach. A well-established paradigm for communicative activation is PACE therapy (Davis & Wilcox, 1981). The patient is encouraged to convey messages by using any verbal or nonverbal means available. This approach does not focus on language system demands such as specific lexical selection, sentence construction, or precise phonological realization. The traditional PACE approach does not try to engage the patient in relearning the structures of language. Rather, it is a purely stimulative approach, in the sense of optimizing the patient's communicative capacities that are unaffected or only mildly affected. Therefore, we wondered whether a modified approach that integrates the demands of the linguistic structure approach into PACE therapy (method B) would be more efficacious than the traditional one (method A).

Method A required patients to identify individual line drawings of objects which were presented in random order. The target name was unknown to the therapist. Patients had free choice of the naming modality. For example, they could say the name, try to write the name, describe the object, use gestures, or even try to draw the object. The therapist never corrected the patient directly, but would tell the patient whether the message was understood or not.

Method B introduced a metalinguistic task and used the training material in a more structured way. Instead of only one picture, the patient was confronted with an array of 22 pictures, a subset of which the patient was asked to sort into a semantic class such as tools, toys, or fruits. The superordinate category was written on a card. This card together with the random array of 22 pictures was given to both the patient and the therapist, who were separated by a screen, as suggested by Clerebaut, Coyette, Feyereisen, and Seron (1984). The screen ensures that subjects are required to convey new information to their partners, which is the essential feature of PACE therapy. Each decision on class membership had to be conveyed to the partner. The therapist gave feedback about the accuracy of classification in addition to the "natural" feedback of the traditional approach.

During control tests, patients' attempts to identify the objects were scored on two scales. In addition to the communication scale of the traditional PACE therapy (Davis, 1980), we introduced a "Language System Scale" taken with a minor modification from the Aachen Aphasia Test (AAT) (Huber et al., 1984). This scale reflected the semantic accuracy of the patient's naming response.

The two methods were compared intra-individually in three patients, two with moderate to mild chronic global aphasia (WB and DZ), and one with moderate Wernicke's aphasia (UZ). All three patients showed marked lexical-semantic difficulties, as reflected by semantic paraphasias on confrontation naming and meaning confusions in word-picture matching. Each training period lasted for 5 days with five full-hour sessions. The results are shown in Figure 3–5.

The modified PACE approach led throughout to significant improvement in both linguistic adequacy and communicative effectiveness. In contrast, the traditional PACE approach was effective only in one patient (DZ) and only in the initial treatment period.

CONCLUSIONS

The results of the two studies led us to the following conclusion: When the linguistic structure approach is aimed at specific impairment of linguistic knowledge in chronic aphasic patients, it is more effective than a purely stimulating or communicatively activating approach. However, several qualifications must be made.

First, the setting for practicing linguistic structure and for pre- and post-training control was always "pragmatic" in the sense that either a discourse pattern (first study) or communicative interactions (second study) were chosen. It is conceivable that this is a prerequisite for the linguistic structure approach to be effective. Learning grammatical structure alone would not do the job. More importantly, pragmatic settings are more likely to induce transfer to everyday communication.

Second, the linguistic structure approach should always be symptom specific. The most promising effects can be expected for patients whose linguistic knowledge is affected as opposed to those who have difficulties of access/retrieval or lower level processing disorders such as speech apraxia, peripheral alexia, or word deafness. It should be understood that some residual linguistic knowledge must be preserved, which precludes use of the linguistic structure approach in severe chronic global aphasia.

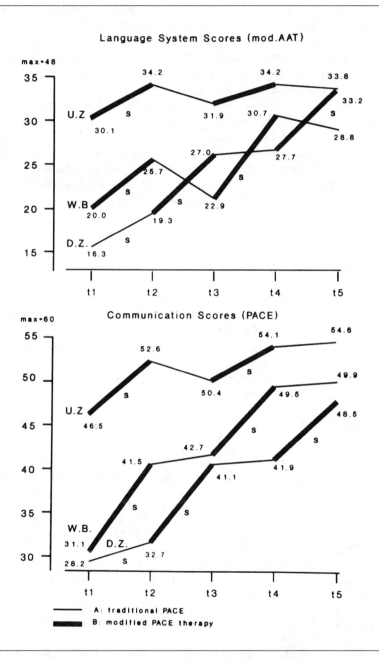

Figure 3–5. PACE study: Performance in control tests of the three patients (UZ, WB, and DZ) (s = significant difference in tests-scores, Randomization Test; Edgington, 1987).

Third, for more complex linguistic demands such as sentence and text production, which require integration of information from several levels of processing, the structure approach may fail completely if the processing capacities of the patients are too limited. In such a situation, the training of strategies is preferable when combined with attempts at improving disorders of working memory.

Fourth, we have not, nor have most others, successfully demonstrated transfer of improved linguistic performance from the therapy setting into everyday spontaneous language and communicative interactions. To achieve this, one must tread a methodologically thorny way. Ultimately, the success or failure of patients and therapists to achieve transfer to everyday language demands will decide whether the symptom-specific and language oriented approaches will remain as central paradigms of aphasia therapy.

ACKNOWLEDGMENT

The work reviewed in this chapter was supported by the Deutsche Forschungsgemeinschaft. We thank Dr. Holland for her thorough reading and improvement of the English. This chapter is gratefully dedicated to Professor Klaus Poeck, former director of the Neurology Department of the Technical University Aachen. Without his expertise, encouragement, and support, there would be no "Aachen approaches" to aphasia therapy.

REFERENCES

Basso, A., Capitani, E., & Vignolo, L. A. (1979). Influence of rehabilitation on language skills in aphasic patients: A controlled study. *Archives of Neurology, 36,* 190–196.

Biniek, R. (in press). *Akute aphasien.* Berlin: Springer.

Clerebaut, N., Coyette, F., Feyereisen, P., & Seron, X. (1984). Une methode de rééducation fonctionelle des aphasiques: la P.A.C.E. *Rééducation Orthophonique, 22,* 329–345.

Coltheart, M. (1983). Aphasia therapy research: A single-case study approach. In C. Code & D. J. Müller (Eds.), *Aphasia therapy.* London: Arnold.

Cramon, D., & von Zihl, J. (Eds.). (1988). *Neuropsychologische Rehabilitation: Grundlagen — Diagnostik — Behandlungsverfahren.* Berlin: Springer.

Culton, G. L. (1969). Spontaneous recovery from aphasia. *Journal of Speech and Hearing Research, 12,* 825–832.

Davis, G. A. (1980). A critical look at PACE therapy. In R. H. Brookshire (Ed.), *Clinical aphasiology conference proceedings.* Minneapolis, MN: BRK Publishers.

Davis, G. A. (1986). Pragmatics and treatment. In R. Chapey (Ed.), *Language intervention strategies in adult aphasia* (2nd ed.). Baltimore, MD: Williams & Wilkins.

Davis, G. A., & Wilcox, M. J. (1981). Incorporating parameters of natural conversation into aphasia treatment. In R. Chapey (Ed.), *Language intervention strategies in adult aphasia*. Baltimore, MD: Williams & Wilkins.

Davis, G. A., & Wilcox, M. J. (1985). *Adult aphasia rehabilitation: Applied pragmatics*. San Diego, CA: College-Hill Press.

De Bleser, R., & Weismann, H. (1981). Übergang von Strukturübungen zum spontanen Dialog in der therapie von aphasikern mit nicht-flüssiger sprachproduktion. *Sprache-Stimme-Gehör, 5*, 74–79.

Edgington, E. S. (1987). *Randomization tests* (2nd ed.). New York: Dekker.

Engl, E., Kotten, A., Ohlendorf, I., & Poser, E. (1982). *Sprachübungen zur aphasiebehandlung: Ein linguistisches Übungsprogramm mit bildern*. Berlin: Marhold.

Fechtelpeter A., Göddenhenrich, S., Huber, W., & Springer, L. (1990). Ansätze zur therapie von auditiver agnosie. *Folia Phoniatrica, 42*, 83–97.

Glindemann, R., & Springer L. (1989). PACE-therapie und sprachsystematische Übungen — Ein integrativer vorschlag zur aphasietherapie. *Sprache-Stimme-Gehör, 13*, 188–192.

Glindemann, R., Willmes, K., Huber, W., & Springer, L. (1991). The efficacy of modelling in PACE-therapy. *Aphasiology, 5*, 425–429.

Goodglass, H., & Blumstein, S. (Eds.). (1973). Psycholinguistics and aphasia. Baltimore, MD: Johns Hopkins University Press.

Haag, E., Huber, W., Hündgen, R., Stiller U., & Willmes, K. (1985). Repetitives sprachliches verhalten bei schwerer aphasie. *Nervenarzt, 56*, 543–552.

Hanson, W. R., Metter, E. J., & Riege, W. H. (1989). The course of chronic aphasia. *Aphasiology, 3*, 19–29.

Hartmann, J., & Landau, W. (1987). Comparison of formal language therapy with supportive counseling for aphasia due to acute vascular accident. *Archives of Neurology, 44*, 646–649.

Hatfield, F. M. (1972). Looking for help from linguistics. *British Journal of Disorders of Communication, 7*, 64–81.

Hatfield, F. M. (1989). Aspects of acquired dysgraphia and implications for reeducation. In C. Code & D. J. Müller (Eds.), *Aphasia therapy: Studies in disorders of communication* (2nd ed.). London: Whurr.

Heeschen, C., & Kolk, H. (1988). Agrammatism and paragrammatism. *Aphasiology, 2*, 299–302.

Holland, A. L. (1980). *Communicative ability in daily living*. Baltimore, MD: University Park Press.

Huber, W. (1988). Methodik und erfolg der aphasietherapie. *Therapiewoche, 38*, 2294–2300.

Huber, W. (1991). Ansätze der aphasietherapie. *Neurolinguistik, 5*, 71–92.

Huber, W. (1992). Therapy of aphasia: Comparison of various approaches. In N. V. Steinbüchel, D. Y. von Cramon, & E. Pöppel (Eds.), *Neuropsychological rehabilitation*. Heidelberg: Springer.

Huber, W., Mayer, I., & Kerscheinsteiner, M. (1978). Phonematischer jargon bei Wernicke-aphasie: Untersuchung zur methode und zum verlauf der therapie. *Folia Phoniatrica, 30*, 199–135.

Huber, W., Poeck, K., & Springer, L. (1991). *Sprachstörungen*. Stuttgart: TRIAS.

Huber, W., Poeck, K., & Willmes, K. (1984). The Aachen Aphasia Test. In F. C. Rose (Ed.), *Progress in aphasiology*. New York: Raven Press.

Huber, W., & Springer, L. (1988). Sprachstörungen und sprachtherapie. In U. Ammon, N. Dittmar, & K. J. Mattheier (Eds.), *Sociolinguistics* (Vol. 2). Berlin: De Gruyter.

Jones, E. V. (1986). Building the foundations for sentence production in a nonfluent aphasic. *British Journal of Disorders of Communication, 21,* 63–82.

Kearns, K. P. (1986). Group therapy for aphasia: Theoretical and practical considerations. In R. Chapey (Ed.), *Language intervention strategies in adult aphasia* (2nd ed.). Baltimore, MD: Williams & Wilkins.

Kearns, K. P. (1990). Broca's aphasia. In L. L. LaPointe (Ed.), *Aphasia and related neurogenic language disorders.* New York: Thieme.

Kertesz, A., & McCabe, P. (1977). Recovery patterns and prognosis in aphasia. *Brain, 100,* 1–18.

Klauer, K. J. (1987). *Kriteriumsorientierte tests.* Göttingen: Hogrefe.

Kotten, A. (1981). Aphasietherapie: Linguistisch gesteuerter Wedererwerb der muttersprache. In G. Peuser (Ed.), *Methoden der angewandten sprachwissenschaft.* Bonn: Bouvier.

Kotten, A. (1989). Evaluation von aphasietherapie. *Neurolinguistik, 3,* 83–106.

Lesser, R. (1987). Cognitive neuropsychological influences on aphasia therapy. *Aphasiology, 1,* 189–200.

Luria, A. R., Naydin, V. L., Tsvetkova, L. S., & Vinatskaya, E. N. (1969). Restoration of higher cortical function following local brain damage. In P. J. Vinken & G. W. Bruyn (Eds.), *Handbook of clinical neurology* (Vol. 3). Amsterdam: North Holland.

Moore, W. H. (1989). Language recovery in aphasia: A right hemisphere perspective. *Aphasiology, 3,* 101–110.

Poeck, K. (1982). *Modern methods of aphasia therapy.* Invited paper read at the 7th Annual Meeting of the Japanese GVD-Society, Hirosaki.

Poeck, K. (1983). What do we mean by "aphasic syndromes"? A neurologist's view. *Brain and Language, 20,* 79–89.

Poeck, K. (Ed.). (1989). *Klinische neuropsychologie* (2nd ed.). Stuttgart: Thieme.

Poeck, K., & Gökddenhenrich, S. (1988). Standardized tests for the detection of dissociations in aphasic language performance. *Aphasiology, 2,* 375–380.

Poeck, K., Huber, W., Stachowiak, F.-J., & Weniger, D. (1977). Therapie der aphasien. *Nervenarzt, 48,* 199–126.

Poeck, K., Huber, W., & Willmes K. (1989). Outcome of intensive therapy in aphasia. *Journal of Speech and Hearing Disorders, 54,* 471–479.

Prutting, C. A. (1982). Pragmatics as social competence. *Journal of Speech and Hearing Disorders, 47,* 123–134.

Rothi, L. J., & Horner, J. (1983). Restitution and substitution: Two theories of recovery with application to neurobehavioral treatment. *Journal of Clinical Neuropsychology, 5,* 73–81.

Sasanuma, S. (1986). Universal and language specific symptomatology and treatment of aphasia. *Folia Phoniatrica, 38,* 121–175.

Schlanger, P. H., & Schlanger, B. B. (1970). Adapting role-playing activities with aphasic patients. *Journal of Speech and Hearing Disorders, 35,* 299–235.

Schlenck, K. J., Huber, W., & Willmes, K. (1987). "Prepairs" and repairs: Different monitoring functions in aphasic language production. *Brain and Language, 30,* 266–244.

Seron, X. (1982). Les choix de stratégies: Rétablir, réorganiser ou aménager l'en-vironment? In X. Seron & C. Laterre (Eds.), *Rééduquer le cerveau. Logopédie, psy-chologie, neurologie*. Bruxelles: Mardaga.

Shewan, C. M., & Bandur, D. C. (1986). *Treatment of aphasia*. San Diego, CA: Col-lege-Hill Press.

Shewan, C. M., & Kertesz, A. (1984). Effects of speech and language treatment on recovery of aphasia. *Brain and Language, 23,* 272–299.

Singer, W. (1982). Recovery mechanisms in the mammalian brain. In J. G. Nich-olls (Ed.), *Repair and regeneration of the nervous system*. Berlin: Springer.

Sparks, R., Helm, N., & Albert, M. (1974). Aphasia rehabilitation resulting from melodic intonation therapy. *Cortex, 10,* 303–316.

Springer, L. (1979). Zur anwendung der deblockierungsmethode in der sprach-therapie. In G. Peuser (Ed.), *Studien zur sprachtherapie*. München: Fink.

Springer, L. (1986). Behandlungsphasen einer syndromspezifischen aphasie-therapie. *Sprache-Stimme-Gehör, 10,* 22–29.

Springer, L., Glindemann, R., Huber, W., & Willmes, K. (1991). How efficacious is PACE-therapy when language systematic training is incorporated? *Aphasi-ology, 5,* 391–399.

Springer, L., & Lazzatti, C. (1987). *Behandlung der sprechapraxie. Eine fallctudie*. Pa-per presented at the Innsbruckner Arbeitsgemeinschaft für Neuropsychol-ogie, Innsbruck.

Springer, L., Schlenck, C., & Schlenck, K. (1991, November). *Reduzierte syntax therapie (REST) als methode zur therapie von chronischem agrammatismus*. Paper presented at the 18th Annual Meeting of the Arbeitsgemeinschaft für Apha-sieforschung und-behandlung, Amsterdam.

Springer, L., & Weniger D. (1980). Aphasietherapie aus logopädisch-linguis-tischer sicht. In G. Böhme (Ed.), *Therapie der sprach-, sprech- und stimmstö-rungen*. Stuttgart: Fischer.

Springer, L., Willmes, K., & Haag, E. (1993). Training the use of wh-questions and prepositons in dialogues: A comparison of two different approaches in apha-sia therapy. *Aphasiology 7,* 251–270.

Sturm, W. (1990). Neuropsychologische therapie von hirnschädigungsbeding-ten aufmerksamkeitsstörungen. *Zeitschrift für Neuropsychologie, 1,* 23–31.

Weigl, E. (1961). The phenomenon of temporary deblocking in aphasia. *Zeitschrift für Phonetik, Sprachwissenschaft und Kommunikationsforschung, 14,* 337–364.

Weigl, E., & Bierwisch, M. (1970). Neuropsychology and linguistics: Topics of com-mon research. *Foundations of Language, 6,* 1–18.

Weigl, I. (1979). Neuropsychologische und neurolinguistische grundlagen eines programms zur rehabilitation aphasischer störungen. In G. Peuser (Ed.), *Stu-dien zur sprachtherapie*. München: Fink.

Wein, B., Böckler, R., Huber, W., Klajman, S., & Willmes, K. (1990). Computer-sonographishe darstellung von zungenformen bei der bildung der langen vokale des deutschen. *Ultraschall in der Medizin, 11,* 55–110.

Weniger, D., Huber, W., Stachowiak, F.-J., & Poeck, K. (1980). Treatment of apha-sia on a linguistic basis. In M. T. Sarno & O. Höök (Eds.), *Aphasia: Assessment treatment*. Stockholm: Almqvist & Wiksell.

Weniger, D., Springer, L., & Poeck, K. (1987). The efficacy of deficit-specific ther-apy materials. *Aphasiology, 3,* 215–223.

Weniger, D., & Springer, L. (1989). Therapie der aphasien. In K. Poeck (Ed.), *Klinische neuropsychologie* (2nd ed.). Stuttgart: Thieme.

Wertz, R. T., Collins, M. J., Weiss, D. G., Kurtze, J. F., Friden, T., Brookshire, R. H., Pierce, J., Holtzapple, P., Hubbard, D. J., Porch, B. E., West, J. A., Davis, L., Matovitch, V., Morley, G. K., & Resurreccion, E. (1981). Veterans Administration cooperative study of aphasia: A comparison of individual and group treatment. *Journal of Speech and Hearing Research, 24,* 580–594.

Wertz, R. T., Weiss, D. G., Aten, J. L., Brookshire, R. H., Garica-Bunnel, L., Holland, A. L., Kurtzke, J. F., LaPointe, L. L., Milanti, F. J., Brannegan, R., Greenbaum, H., Marshall, R. C., Vogel, D., Carter, J., Barnes, N. S., & Goodman, R. (1986). Veterans Administration cooperative study: Comparison of clinic, home, and deferred language treatment for aphasia. *Archives of Neurology, 43,* 653–658.

Willmes, K. (1985). An approach to analyzing a single subject's scores obtained in a standardized test with application to the Aachen Aphasia Test (AAT). *Journal of Clinical and Experimental Neuropsychology, 7,* 331–352.

Willmes, K. (1990). Statistical methods for a single case study approach to aphasia therapy research. *Aphasiology, 4,* 415–436.

Willmes, K., & Poeck, K. (1984). Ergebnisse einer multizentrischen untersuchung über die spontanprognose von aphasien vaskulärer Ätiologie. *Nervenarzt, 55,* 62–71.

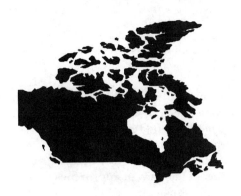

CHAPTER 4

Perspectives on Aphasia Intervention in French-Speaking Canada

GUYLAINE LE DORZE
CLAIRE CROTEAU
École d'orthophonie et d'audiologie, Faculté de Médecine, Université de Montréal

YVES JOANETTE
École d'orthophonie et d'audiologie, Faculté de Médecine, Université de Montréal
Centre de recherche du Centre Hospitalier Côte-des-Neiges

The current status of intervention for aphasic persons in French-speaking Canada shares characteristics with the culture of Québec, the Canadian province where most persons speak French. Although Québec is North American both geographically and in terms of its institutions, historically and linguistically it is French. American and French cultural influences have intermingled to create a unique combination. Thus, just as the legal institutions in Québec proceed both from English and

French influences (the institutions themselves are British but the civil code is Napoleonic), intervention for aphasia proceeds from both the American and the French schools. The result is a unique combination of these two influences.

It is not the purpose of this chapter to provide an exhaustive description of the current approaches used by speech-language pathologists in French-speaking Canada. Rather, the goals are, first, to provide historical background about the origins of current philosophies and orientations in intervention for aphasia and, second, to discuss briefly some contemporary issues raised by clinicians and researchers. Finally, a recent case study conducted by two of the authors will be presented, which serves to illustrate concretely how our concerns about efficacy are related to the issues of aphasia as an impairment in language processing, a disability in communication, and a handicap in daily living.

HISTORICAL BACKGROUND

To discuss recent historical events is a difficult exercise. This is because such a discussion may emphasize certain events which turn out to be of little importance or omit details which may gain importance in a larger perspective. Keeping this reservation in mind, we have elected to begin our brief history of aphasia intervention or aphasia *rééducation*, as it was called in French-speaking Canada in the 1950s. In the mid-1950s, under the guidance of Gustave Gingras, a pioneer of physical rehabilitation medicine in Québec, Germaine Huot, who had received her master's degree in speech pathology from Northwestern University in the United States, established a speech pathology department at the Montréal Rehabilitation Institute, the first to specialize in the rehabilitation of aphasic patients. Concurrently, Gingras established the first program in Canada for the training of speech-language pathologists and audiologists. This program, in the School of Rehabilitation of the Faculty of Medicine of the University of Montréal, was directed by Huot until the early 1960s.

Some years later, Louise Coderre,[1] one of Huot's students, became an influential figure. She devoted her efforts to the rehabilitation of aphasic patients, following the British and American approaches as represented

---

[1] In the mid-1960s, Louise Coderre became the director of the program of studies in speech-language pathology and audiology at the Université de Montréal. The program she developed and directed for 26 years is still the only program on the North American continent that offers training in speech-language pathology and audiology in the French language. Now an autonomous department of the Faculty of Medicine, it offers a program of studies at the undergraduate and graduate levels.

by Weisenburg and McBride (1935), Schuell (Schuell, Carroll, & Street, 1955), and Eisenson (1954). She was also, however, much influenced by the writings of Ombredane (1951). Through meticulous clinical observations and linguistic analysis, together with an interest in the use of language in different contexts, she developed an approach to intervention later recognized as a precursor to the contemporary neurolinguistic and pragmatic approaches. Her clinical work and her teachings have influenced many French-speaking clinicians in Canada. In 1970, Coderre, with an experienced clinician and colleague, Michèle Bergeron, studied in France with Blanche Ducarne de Ribaucourt. Ducarne was responsible for the Rééducation Center for Language Disorders at L'Hôpital de la Salpêtrière in Paris, under the direction of François Lhermitte. Coderre and Bergeron thus were able to compare the approaches to intervention used in Québec and France. The distinctiveness of the approach used in Québec was apparent, as it arose from the contributions of both the American and the European aphasiological literature. The essence of the approach developed in Québec is described in a chapter written by Coderre and colleagues (Lecours, Coderre, Lafond, Bergeron, & Bryans, 1979).

The approach to aphasia intervention put forth by Ducarne (Ducarne, 1967; Ducarne, 1986; Lhermitte & Ducarne, 1965) was quite similar to that suggested by Schuell (Schuell, Jenkins, & Jiménez-Pabon, 1964) (see Lecours et al., 1979a, and Joanette et al., 1987, for further discussion) in that intervention was essentially focused on the symptoms of language disturbance, with the task of the clinician being to create an individualized treatment program. Schuell's approach strongly emphasized auditory stimulation, which Ducarne's approach did not. Rather, Ducarne considered that therapy should proceed from a careful linguistic analysis of aphasics' oral expression. For example, she suggested that oral expression should be examined at the levels of phonetics, phonemics, lexicon, syntax, and as a "whole" in narrative tasks. She also was concerned with the problem of generalization, and included family members in therapy so that they could reproduce elements of therapy at home. The approaches used in Québec also emphasized analysis of these various levels of verbal output as well as the problem of generalization.

Ducarne's approach can also be characterized as oriented toward the needs of the individual. This "humanistic" dimension was so deeply rooted in clinical practice in Québec, that when the pragmatic revolution occurred in aphasiology, speech-language pathologists in Québec were easily able to incorporate the new terminology into their work. In effect, the terminology echoed the objectives of generalization, communication-at-large, and social readjustment that speech-language pathologists already pursued in their clinical practice.

Another significant figure in the history of aphasiology in Québec is André-Roch Lecours. After completing his studies in medicine in Montréal, Lecours studied in Boston with Paul Yvan Yakovlev and in Paris with François Lhermitte. Upon his return, Lecours established the Centre de Rééducation du Langage et de Recherche Neuropsychologique de l'Hôtel-Dieu de Montréal in 1972 and later, in 1982, the Centre de Recherche du Centre Hospitalier Côte-des-Neiges. Both of these centers conducted research aimed at furthering the understanding of aphasia. Lecours played a significant role in teaching and training students interested in aphasiology and speech-language pathology. His textbook on aphasia is a basic reference (Lecours & Lhermitte, 1979).

Although there are clearly French influences in Québec, clinical practice is organized very differently in France and Québec. In fact, the profession of speech-language pathology in Québec is similar to the profession as practiced in other parts of Canada and in the United States. Speech-language pathologists are trained in undergraduate and graduate programs in speech-language pathology and audiology at the Université de Montréal. They become eligible for membership in the Corporation des Orthophonistes et Audiologistes du Québec once they have obtained a Master's degree, which is legally required to practice.

Speech-language pathology as currently practiced in Québec incorporates both French and American influences. Historically, although intervention for aphasia was influenced by a French perspective, American perspectives have always been present, especially since the development of scientific literature in the field of human communication disorders. Such a development has not occurred in France because speech-language pathology is not well established as a scientific discipline within the universities. Other influences are at play in Québec. For example, Luria's work on rehabilitation and the more recent concept of cognitive rehabilitation, as it originates from Belgium, the United Kingdom, and the United States, are taught to students and therefore influence, to some degree, clinical practice in Québec. This original and eclectic philosophy of intervention is implemented in a professional structure that is essentially American.

In general terms, the approach to intervention is still very much centered on patients' individual needs. Most clinicians plan therapy after having identified the linguistic deficit(s) underlying the aphasia. Therapy which will reactivate, reorganize, or compensate for the deficit(s) is then provided (see Joanette et al., 1987). Moreover, intervention is considered effective if there is concurrent improvement in communication in other situations. Therefore, specific goals to foster such generalization are included in the treatment plan. Available and interested family members are included in the intervention process, and group therapy is often provided as a supplement to individual treatment. There has always been great concern for intervention which leads to significant functional and useful changes for daily living. Nevertheless, there is probably much more interest now than ever before in defining and measuring in a scientific manner the therapy procedures that are likely to result in significant changes. The growing body of scientific literature on intervention effects has helped to foster this interest.

CURRENT ISSUES IN LANGUAGE INTERVENTION

Today, the efficacy of aphasia intervention is a concern of many researchers as well as clinicians. The next section briefly outlines some of the current issues related to efficacy. The topics we have selected for discussion are not exhaustive, but serve to illustrate the types of questions we and other colleagues have raised.

THE BASIC QUESTION OF EFFICACY

The question of the effects of intervention has been central in the field from both clinical and scientific perspectives. First has been the crucial matter of what treatment aphasic persons should be receiving. In 1970, Sarno, Silverman, and Sands published a study showing that intervention may not be very beneficial for some global aphasics. In reaction to the overgeneralization that followed this study, many subsequent studies have led to a better understanding of the variables associated with significant effects of therapy (see the reviews of Basso, 1989; Shewan, 1986; and Wertz, 1987). The conclusions of these studies, especially those of the Italian group (Basso, Capitani, & Vignolo, 1979), have been useful in determining the intensity and duration of therapy and the advisability of using volunteers to deliver treatment. The current consensus concerning the minimal conditions necessary for efficacious treatment is well described by Wertz (1987). Aphasia therapy needs to be intensive, from three to five sessions per week, as patients in the studies that offered two sessions or fewer showed no improvement (David, Enderby, & Bainton, 1982; Hartman & Landau, 1987; Lincoln et al., 1984; Prins, Schoonen, & Vermeulen, 1989). Therapy also needs to last a minimum number of months and should be conducted by a speech-language pathologist rather than a nonprofessional volunteer. Most rehabilitation centers in the Montreal area (which is the largest city in French-speaking Canada) offer speech and language therapy according to these guidelines (i.e. intensive [daily] treatment sessions for 3 to 6 months provided by a speech-language pathologist). Some patients also receive therapy for a longer period of time on an outpatient basis, but this is not a general rule.

Outside of the Montréal area, these minimal conditions are not always met and the availability of therapy services varies considerably, even to the extent that no services are available in some places. In acute care hospitals in Montréal and other larger cities, intensive speech-language therapy services are rarely available. In the best situations, speech-language pathologists are able to perform inpatient evaluations and to recommend follow-up services. Speech-language therapy services are hospital-based in a system of socialized medicine and are delivered in a rehabilitation setting. Part of the explanation for inadequate services is understaffing and insufficient financing of many clinics. Moreover, few private practitioners serve the neurologically impaired population.

From the perspective of the science of intervention, group studies on the efficacy of aphasia rehabilitation have essentially shown that language intervention is beneficial for aphasic patients in general (Basso et al., 1979; Broida, 1977; Hagen, 1973; Poeck, Huber, & Willmes, 1989; Shewan & Kertesz, 1984; Wertz et al., 1981; Wertz et al., 1986). Yet, other more specific questions need answers; for example, questions about which approach is likely to produce the maximum effects for an individual presenting with a particular aphasia or a particular symptom (Howard, 1986). This quest for answers to more specifically focused questions has led researchers to adopt single-subject methodology (Hegde, 1987). This approach to intervention is vital to our understanding of how therapy improves the aphasic condition, although it does present some difficulties. For example, generalization to similar subjects is possible only if replications of a particular single-subject study are undertaken (Hegde, 1987). This may be problematic, as aphasic subjects are thought to vary considerably. Nevertheless, the development of the single-subject methodology has made it possible to conduct research in this area because it removes the considerable ethical problem associated with group approaches that require a control (untreated) group of subjects. The establishment of single-subject research is consistent with the overall goal of the development of a scientific discipline of speech-language pathology intervention. Intervention research is vital to the development of the discipline of communication disorders. Our future as a scientific discipline, as well as a clinical science, rests to some extent on our ability to explain under what conditions therapy improves communication disorders.

In determining intervention effects for aphasic patients, efficacy cannot be defined as a return to normally functioning language and communication. If this were the case, the problem of identifying good therapy would be relatively simple; we would need only to count the number of subjects who are "normal" after one type of therapy and compare this group to those treated with other approaches. Because recovery from aphasia is most often partial and incomplete, however, the problem becomes one of measurement of behavior. This problem is compounded by the inherent complexity of language processing and verbal communication and by the fact that recovery, as a neurophysiologically based process, is not well understood.

The model of chronic diseases of the World Health Organization, applied to rehabilitation (Frey, 1984), may serve to crystallize some of the issues involved in aphasia intervention. This model describes the outcomes of rehabilitation at three levels: The impairment, the disability and the handicap.[2] It may help in understanding therapy itself. For example, intervention has been depicted as seeking to improve either language processing, without consideration for communication (direct language approach), or communication (pragmatic approach), without consideration for language processing (see Joanette et al., 1987). These two approaches have been contrasted (Aten, 1986), when in fact they are *both* necessary; the focus of each is at a different level. That is, language processing approaches aim to treat the impairment, whereas pragmatic approaches aim to reduce the disability. On the one hand, it is true that insufficient attention has been paid to the conditions and variables that enhance or modify communication abilities in aphasics. On the other hand, a clear understanding of the nature of the impairments a patient presents is also essential in order to determine ways to reduce language impairments and thus enhance communication abilities.

All clinicians have encountered individuals who, in spite of severe aphasia, appear to be relatively good communicators as well as some clients with mild aphasia who appear to be unable to function as communicators. A better understanding of these paradoxical clients might clarify the relationships among impairment, disability, and handicap. Clinical practice could be adapted even more specifically to needs of individual aphasic patients if appropriate instruments for measuring the disability and the handicap associated with aphasia were developed.

Various avenues of research are open for studying the effects of intervention. Recent advances in psycholinguistics have much to offer and

---

[2] With respect to aphasia, the *impairment* can be defined as the disruption of the various processes and representations necessary for language. The *disability* is related to the communication disorder, defined by the restrictions and limitations in (1) verbal expression of ideas, opinions, needs, (and more); (2) auditory comprehension of diverse types of messages; (3) reading; and (4) written expression. The *handicap* can be defined as the language impairment and communication disorder that prevent the aphasic individual from fulfilling his or her role in society. Yorkston, Beukelman, and Bell (1988) have made an elegant application of these concepts to define dysarthria, another neurological communication disorder.

need to be explored for their capacity to define linguistic processing impairments and to structure therapy. This type of research will determine the potential of therapy for improving deficient language processing. Promising case studies have been published, for example, on agrammatism (Jones, 1986), dyslexia (de Partz, 1986), and auditory comprehension (Cyr-Stafford, 1986). Another avenue is to explore which strategies can reduce the disability associated with aphasia, that is, which strategies can enhance communication. Considerably less has been published along these lines. Still another path researchers may embark on is the identification of approaches whose objectives are to reduce the handicap associated with aphasia. Strategies seeking to modify the environment or to permit aphasic persons self-expression in spite of limited language also can be evaluated in a scientific manner. This notion of aphasia as consisting of three aspects needing treatment — impairment, disability, and handicap — holds the potential for furthering our understanding of possible goals and methods of intervention. This concept has not yet been integrated into our therapy, nor have instruments for measuring the three levels been developed.

NEUROBIOLOGICAL BASES OF RECOVERY FROM APHASIA

Whether the aphasic person recovers spontaneously or benefits from intervention is a classical question that has always haunted those who are interested in aphasia rehabilitation, especially with respect to the neurobiological bases of recovery. As early as 1865, Broca himself was puzzled by this question:

> Comment se fait-il donc que l'individu rendu aphémique par la destruction partielle ou totale de la troisième circonvolution gauche, n'apprenne pas à parler avec l'hémisphère droit?[3] (p. 18)

Some early aphasiologists thought the question was easy to answer. They postulated that a right hemispheric involvement was responsible for linguistic changes observed in recovery. For example, such was the concept of von Mayendorf (1911) and Henschen (1926). But it is now known that this question cannot be answered simply (Joanette, Goulet, & Hannequin, 1990). In fact, the question remains unsolved today as it was in Broca's time. Some research undertaken in Québec centers on this general issue.

---

[3] Translation of the quotation: "Why is it that an individual who has become aphemic following the partial or total destruction of the left third frontal convolution does not learn to speak with the right hemisphere?"

The question of the neurobiological bases of aphasia recovery can be addressed in many ways. In this context, it is vital that the respective roles of each hemisphere for language be better understood. One of the first means by which this question was explored involved the analysis of exceptional cases of aphasia. Patients with extremely large left-hemisphere lesions were studied (e.g., Cambier, Elghozi, Signoret, & Henin, 1983; Landis, Cummings, & Benson, 1980), because in such patients recovery of language could logically be attributed to the right hemisphere. Also studied was a group of patients who suffered a second lesion, affecting the right hemisphere, during the course of recovery (e.g., Cambier et al., 1983; Lee, Nakada, Deal, Lin, & Kwee, 1984). In these cases, if the second lesion changed language function, it could be taken to indicate the contribution of the right hemisphere to language recovery. Some researchers have extended their methodology to the point of inducing "functional" and transitory lesions of the right hemisphere in recovering aphasics, with sodium amytal injections (e.g., Czopf, 1979; Kinsbourne, 1971). Although the ethics of such an approach may be questioned, these studies have provided interesting data about the role of the right hemisphere.

Another method used to examine this question was to obtain functional indicators of brain lateralization using dichotic listening techniques designed to identify ear advantage in aphasics (e.g., Niccum, Selnes, Speaks, Risse, & Rubens, 1986; Niccum, Speaks, Rubens, et al., 1986). However, these studies suffer from associated methodological problems. Finally, another way of approaching the problem is to search for any neurophysiological indications of changes in lateralization as aphasia recovery takes place. Thus, studies have been completed using regional cerebral blood flow techniques (e.g., Demeurisse & Capon, 1985), metabolism studies based on the PET-scan (Heiss, Herholz, Pawlik, Wagner, & Wienhard, 1986), and evoked potential techniques (Brandeis & Lehmann, 1986). All of these methods share the limitations associated with dynamic brain imaging techniques.

In contrast to these approaches, one line of research currently being explored in Montréal seeks to increase the body of knowledge about the exact nature of the contribution of the right hemisphere to language and verbal communication. This line of research, which is being pursued by Joanette and colleagues (see Joanette et al., 1990 for a comprehensive and critical review of this domain of research), may contribute to the understanding of the role of the right hemisphere in aphasia recovery. What is needed is an understanding of those aspects of language and verbal communication to which the right hemisphere normally contributes, and of those aspects to which it normally does *not* contribute. For example, if the question of left and right hemisphere capabilities for processing abstract and concrete nouns could be resolved, an indicator of the contribution of the right hemisphere to aphasia recovery could be gained. If the right hemisphere developed a superior ability to process abstract nouns in recovering aphasic subjects, this could indicate a truly qualitative difference from the usual role of the right hemisphere and, thus, testify to its genuine contribution to recovery. In the future, studies seeking to qualify the role of the right hemisphere in recovery will likely supplement research that merely quantifies differences between left and right hemisphere contributions to language.

PSYCHOLINGUISTIC THEORIES AND APHASIA INTERVENTION

The interest in linguistic aspects of disturbed language prevalent in the 1970s (Lecours & Lhermitte, 1979, chapter on intervention) has shifted to focus more on the psycholinguistic and cognitive aspects of aphasia. Psycholinguistic models such as Garrett's language production model (Garrett, 1982, 1984) and Lesser's cognitive model of naming (Lesser, 1989), among others, have enhanced our understanding of the underlying processes that may be responsible for some of the observed behavior in aphasia. This shift in interest has resulted in a number of changes in clinical practice with respect to both the evaluation of patients and intervention strategies. For example, clinical instruments have been developed to identify the processes affected by aphasia by reference to a model of normal production. One such instrument, *l'Examen des dyslexies acquises* (Lemay, 1990), permits in-depth evaluation of reading disorders. Another, the *Protocole d'évaluation des troubles lexico-sémantiques* (Le Dorze, currently under development), will be used to analyze the processes involved in lexical production.

In addition, intervention strategies based on a hypothesis about which language processing mechanisms are defective (Joanette et al., 1987) are devised individually for each patient to the best of the clinician's ability. Some of the work that has been done along these lines in Montréal relates to agrammatism (Le Dorze, Jacob, & Coderre, 1991) and to lexical production (Le Dorze, in press; Le Dorze & Nespoulous, 1989). A basic influence from the psycholinguistic perspective has been the work of Garrett (1982, 1984) on the processes and levels of representation involved in sentence production. Lexical access, in Garrett's model, is thought to proceed from two separate processes. First, lexical selection involves the identification of (1) a semantic representation or "meaning," and then (2) a phonological representation or "form." This basic duality of processing is compatible with current views on semantic memory (see Klatzky, 1988) which distinguish between conceptual memory, where meanings are represented, and lexical memory, where phonological forms are represented.

Considering lexical processing in this fashion holds the potential for furthering our understanding of anomia. The implication is that there may be different types of anomia of different origins, requiring different modes or strategies for successful intervention.

Recent work we have conducted on this topic suggests that moderate anomia is essentially related to failures in accessing lexical forms with relative sparing of semantic access and representations (Le Dorze & Nespoulous, 1989). A single-case study with a conduction aphasic was undertaken after an in-depth evaluation showed that the major difficulty involved the accessing of information about word form. The patient was encouraged to use the initial letter to facilitate access when naming (Le Dorze, in press). The results essentially supported the idea that treatment was effective in producing changes in lexical access. Replications are needed, and many more studies of different intervention strategies should be contrasted and compared for their relative effects. It will then be possible to develop a theory of intervention for this impairment. Much more research on the various language impairments associated with aphasia will allow the emergence of a science of intervention.

APHASIA AS A HANDICAP

As mentioned in the historical section of this chapter, speech-language pathologists in Québec have long invested efforts in the reintegration of patients into their families and professional worlds (see Lecours & Lhermitte, 1979). The development of the concepts of impairment, disability, and handicap, as they relate to rehabilitation outcomes (see Frey, 1984), places clinical interest in reintegrating aphasic individuals into everyday life in a proper perspective. According to this conceptualization, aphasia is a significant handicap which prevents the aphasic person from functioning normally in society. Moreover, this handicap can also be thought of as society's inability to integrate individuals who function differently from most others. Thus, the role of speech-language pathology involves not only the remediation of linguistic impairments and the reduction of communication disabilities, but also the modification of the handicaps associated with aphasia. This expanded approach to intervention includes relatives, friends, and colleagues of aphasic individuals, in the sense that compensatory mechanisms leading to more effective communication between aphasic and nonaphasic persons could be identified and implemented to decrease aphasia's handicap. This view of aphasia is also compatible with the role of public advocacy for aphasic persons as another mode of intervention. Better public understanding of aphasia could lead to better recognition and fulfillment of aphasic persons' needs.

The concern for reintegration of aphasic persons into society has led to the creation of associations for aphasic persons. These began to emerge in the early 1980s, with the help of speech-language pathologists and family members of aphasic persons. Quite a few of these groups are currently active in some cities in Québec. Many speech-language pathologists share the impression that participation in such associations is a means by which aphasic persons can initiate and develop their social reintegration. These associations represent genuine micro-societies that meet regularly to initiate and carry out common projects. In addition, such associations represent a first step in assisting aphasic persons to gain confidence in participating in society.

We must increase our understanding of the disabilities and the handicap the aphasic person experiences to ensure that intervention is better suited to the needs of aphasic individuals. A recent book edited and written by some speech-language pathologists and researchers from Québec, France, and Belgium represents a first step in that direction. *L'aphasique* (Ponzio, Lafond, Degiovani, & Joanette, 1991), published in English under the title *Living with Aphasia, Psychosocial Issues*, discusses the handicap and disabilities associated with aphasia, with particular emphasis on the psychological effects of aphasia on the individual (Létourneau, 1991). Discussions of the changes in family relationships (Boisclair-Papillon, 1991; Labourel & Martin, 1991; Ponzio & Degiovani, 1991), aphasic persons' ability to function in society in general (Lemay, 1991) and at work (Rolland & Belin, 1991), legal problems associated with aphasia (Cot & Degiovani, 1991), and associations for aphasic persons (Hubert & Degiovani, 1991) are also presented. Although these contributions are limited by a lack of research, it is hoped that they will soon be addressed as scientific enquiries in their own right, so that we will continue to see advancement in our field.

A CASE STUDY

A case study of a recent intervention is presented here as an illustration of how language impairments, communication disabilities, and handicap are related in intervention. An analysis of our subject's linguistic impairments allowed us to devise a specific compensation approach to therapy. The treatment was implemented in a structure that emphasized real communicative exchange. Observations of generalization were made, including a change at the level of the handicap the aphasic subject and her family were experiencing.

BACKGROUND

Anomia is considered a central impairment of aphasia (Goodglass & Kaplan, 1983), and based on clinical observations (Benson, 1988), various sub-types of anomia are thought to exist. Models of lexical access and naming are also available (Lesser, 1989). Because the ability to access and produce meaningful words is essential to any verbal exchange, anomia is one of aphasia's most incapacitating expressive impairments. It follows logically that intervention for anomia needs to be provided to most aphasic patients. Although the literature contains general indications about effective therapy for this problem (Howard, Patterson, Franklin, Orchard-Lisle, & Morton, 1985), more specific information is lacking about which therapy is most effective for a particular type of anomia. There is also a lack of information concerning which therapy will have effects that will generalize best to communication in general.

A general objective of this study was to contribute information to the question of defining what is effective therapy. We recently provided therapy for a person who was one of our relatives. The outcome was quite interesting because of the unique viewpoint that one of us had as a family member and because of the continuous and informal observations we made over time, extending well beyond the end of the experiment. It is our impression that the case we report is interesting both as an attempt to demonstrate the effectiveness of therapy and also because of the generalization effects that were observed. First, anomia appeared to decrease in spontaneous speech and second, the structure of the interaction used during therapy was utilized spontaneously by the patient with the therapist. After therapy ended, the patient became more active in the resolution of breakdowns in communication.

METHODS

The study began with an in-depth evaluation. The intervention was planned in terms of objectives, tasks, facilitators, and stimuli to be used. The specific design was outlined and baseline measures were prepared.

CASE PRESENTATION

Mrs. TR is a right-handed 62-year-old individual who abruptly became aphasic in November 1986. She had a left fronto-parietal CVA confirmed by CT-scan, resulting in a slight right hemiparesis, right-sided neglect, and severe aphasia. In the weeks following the CVA, she was evaluated and shown to have a severe mixed aphasia with mild oral apraxia. Mrs. TR was seen for intensive speech-language therapy for 6 months, then weekly for the next 2 years, and finally, bi-weekly until she was approached for this experiment. Although her therapist agreed that she had attained a plateau, she was still receiving speech-language therapy. During this investigation, regular therapy was discontinued.

We first evaluated Mrs. TR 3½ years after the onset of her aphasia. Diagnostic testing was conducted using the *Protocole Montréal-Toulouse d'examen linguistique de l'aphasie* (MT-86) (Nespoulous et al., 1986). She was found to have a moderate-to-severe Wernicke's aphasia. An evaluation of her spontaneous language revealed that she still had significant limitations in oral expression due to severe anomia. Sporadically, some adequate and relatively long utterances were produced. Most of the time, though, multiple hesitations were associated with episodes of word-finding difficulties. TR often commented on her incapacity to produce words and to communicate. She produced occasional verbal paraphasias and somewhat fewer phonemic paraphasias. Auditory comprehension problems persisted at the sentence level. The Token Test (DeRenzi & Vignolo, 1962) confirmed the relative severity of the comprehension disorder (Part I, 9/10; Part II, 5/10; Part III 4/10; Part IV, 6/10; Part V, 8/22). Written language comprehension, repetition, and oral reading were relatively better preserved.

Further testing for anomia with the *Protocole d'évaluation des troubles lexico-sémantiques* (PETLS) (Le Dorze, 1990) revealed that she had a moderately severe confrontation naming problem (52/120). The most frequent errors were semantic paraphasias, half of which were accompanied by comments or other attempts at naming. She also produced many "I don't know" responses, some circumlocutions, which were not particularly informative, and occasional perseverations. On another testing task of the PETLS, she had mild difficulty identifying semantic properties of words she was unable to name (19/24) and a slightly more significant problem identifying the syllables of words she was unable to name (12/24). In contrast, when she was capable of naming correctly, she was successful at identifying all properties (semantic, 16/16 and syllabic, 16/16) of words. Such a performance suggested a mild access problem to the semantic lexicon (also called the verbal semantic system, in Lesser's [1989] terminology), and a more significant problem in accessing formal-lexical information (also called the output phonological lexicon in Lesser's model [1989]).

Spontaneous speech was assessed with the Cookie Theft picture from the Boston Diagnostic Aphasia Examination (BDAE) (Goodglass & Kaplan, 1983) which confirmed that the anomia was relatively severe in a more spontaneous production task.

TR was described as experiencing few successful moments of communication. When she encountered word-finding problems, she depended on her spouse to verbalize her message. She also depended on all family members to guess what she wanted to say. This was a problem as her spouse had a tendency to speak for her, and her relatives were often unable to guess correctly. She tended to give up quickly when she could not communicate, and neither she nor her family members appeared to have developed strategies to overcome these failures. For example, if she did not get her message across when she was using the telephone, she would end the conversation abruptly by hanging up without saying good-bye. These communication breakdowns were a source of considerable frustration for her and for family members.

Following this evaluation, we reasoned that since TR had significant problems accessing the formal-lexical information for words, therapy should be directed toward using the relatively more intact semantic information for formulating circumlocutions. She was already attempting to access semantic information about words in her circumlocutions, but with limited success. This justified devoting some attention to developing more informative circumlocutions. In that sense, this therapy approach could be called compensatory (Joanette et al., 1987). We also thought that, with respect to communication in general, circumlocutions could be used as a strategy of substitution for missing words (Holland, 1988); normal subjects produce circumlocutions when words are missing. Circumlocutions can be sufficiently informative in the context of a verbal exchange for an interlocutor to identify the speaker's intention and possibly supply the right word in communication. Moreover, we considered it would be useful for TR to learn to use this strategy because: (1) she was not using a systematic strategy to overcome her anomic problems; (2) her previous intervention, like most anomia therapy, had emphasized finding the word rather than defining words; and (3) not all patients spontaneously discover useful strategies for effective communication. It was also our impression that aphasic patients need to experience successful communication using circumlocutions in a variety of situations to encourage them to use such a strategy.

DESIGN

The design that was intended was a single-subject ABAB withdrawal design (Hegde, 1987). Unfortunately, TR was hospitalized for anemia when the second B phase was due to begin. It was therefore cancelled and a ABA design was the result.

THERAPY

The therapy provided was inspired by the work of Davis and Wilcox (1985) and Belliol (1990). It was very similar to PACE treatment in that some of its basic principles were respected, such as (1) the exchange of new information was the basis of the therapy, (2) each person acted as an equal participant in the exchange, and (3) feedback was related to comprehension of the message. It was different from PACE in that (a) there was a specific objective of teaching circumlocutions in the exchange, (b) the patient received instructions about how to perform the tasks, and (c) precise facilitation procedures were provided to help maximize the accomplishment of the task. These are described below. TR had not received PACE therapy before this experiment.

First, therapy objectives were explained to the patient. She was told that giving a "definition" (circumlocution) could help her communicate more effectively because when one cannot produce the intended word, circumlocution gives more information to the other person than saying nothing. She was also given information about how a definition can be constructed. She was taught that a definition can include the category name of the object, the use of the object, and a number of characteristics or attributes. Some examples were provided.

Therapy consisted of two parts: (a) when TR was the sender of information, with the task of producing definitions (circumlocutions) and (b) when TR was the receiver of information, with the task of naming after hearing a definition (circumlocution). TR and the experimenter alternated in these roles. When the experimenter was the sender of information, her definitions were a model of the desired behavior.

Production of Circumlocutions

When she was the sender, TR was given the following instructions: "give a definition of the word which will enable me to guess what the word is, but do not say the word."

After hearing TR's definition, the experimenter tried to guess the word. If she was unsuccessful, the following facilitation procedures were provided to elicit the category name, the use, and one characteristic:

1. The experimenter inquired about category membership, while presenting a color-coded card with the written cue, "It's a kind of . . . ." If TR was unable to respond, a list of possible category names was presented to her. She was required to select the category from that list.
2. The experimenter inquired about the use of the object, while presenting a color-coded cue card with the written cue, "It is used to . . . "
3. The experimenter inquired about the characteristics of the stimulus, presenting a color-coded cue card, saying, "It looks like a . . ."

After attempting to elicit these three basic informative elements, the experimenter guessed at the word. Unsuccessful attempts were followed by very specific questions about the stimulus to elicit information about its use or its characteristics. The experimenter then guessed again.

Naming to Description

When the experimenter was the sender and TR was the receiver, TR's instructions were to try to guess the word after listening to the definition. The experimenter gave a definition comprising three standard elements (category, use, and characteristic), and allowed 30 seconds for TR to respond. If facilitation was required, the following cues were provided in this order:

1. repetition of the definition;
2. addition of another piece of information to the definition;
3. a sentence cue, for example, pass the salt and . . . (pepper);
4. a phonemic cue, first sound of word; and lastly,
5. saying the target word.

Stimuli

A pool of 300 pictures representing words that could be defined by category, use, and characteristics, served as stimuli. Monosyllabic, bisyllabic, and polysyllabic words corresponded to the pictures and were placed in separate envelopes. We decided to use length as a gross estimate of difficulty because length and word frequency are correlated (Zipf, 1984). Each therapy session comprised 20 randomly selected stimuli from these envelopes: 6 were monosyllabic, 8 to 10 were bisyllabic, and 4 to 6 were polysyllabic. This allowed for some uniformity in the difficulty of items across treatment sessions as 20 new stimuli were used for each session. Of these 20 stimuli, 10 were used for eliciting the production of circumlocutions and the other 10 stimuli served to elicit naming responses.

Procedures

Baselines. Three baseline tests were constructed in the same fashion as the therapy stimuli. Twenty different stimuli were used for each baseline session and none of these stimuli was presented in the treatment sessions.

Therapy Procedures and Measures. Each session began with a repetition of the therapy objectives and instructions about the tasks. TR and the experimenter took turns being the sender and receiver of information. The first response TR produced as sender was used to describe her performance before each therapy session and is referred to here as the daily pre-session measure for production of circumlocutions. Her first response as the receiver of information also served as the daily pre-session measure of naming. Therapy and facilitations were then provided as described above. Encouragement and positive reinforcement were given as needed.

Once all of the stimuli had been used in therapy, the effects of therapy were measured. Thus, each session ended with a second presentation of all of the stimuli used in that session, but in a different order, with identical instructions for both producing circumlocutions and naming, except that no feedback was given. Thus we obtained a daily post-session measure for the production of circumlocutions and a daily post-session measure for naming.

All therapy sessions were recorded and transcribed for analysis.

Coding of Responses. Each element of a circumlocution describing the category, the use, or a characteristic of the object was attributed 1 point. Circumlocutions that conveyed personal information were scored ½ point, because, although they were informative, they were only so to family members. An example of a personal circumlocution is, "Jules le prend pour aller voir le monde" ("Jules [her husband and an amateur photographer] takes it to go see people"), produced for the stimulus, "camera." For the naming to description task, the correct responses produced were counted.

Analysis of Results. Each baseline measure consisted of two scores. The first was the information score for the circumlocutions the patient produced in the role of sender, and the second was the number of correct responses she produced in the role of receiver. These scores are represented on separate graphs. Figure 4–1 represents the information scores for the circumlocutions, and Figure 4–2 represents the naming scores. Figure 4–1 charts the information scores of the daily pre- and post-session measures in the production of circumlocutions task. Figure 4–2 charts the naming scores of the daily pre- and post-session measures for naming to description task.

Generalization Measures. After the experiment, the patient was tested again with the Cookie Theft picture, the Protocole Montréal-Toulouse (Nespoulos et al., 1986) and the Protocole d'Évaluation des Troubles Lexico-Sémantiques (LeDorze, under development).

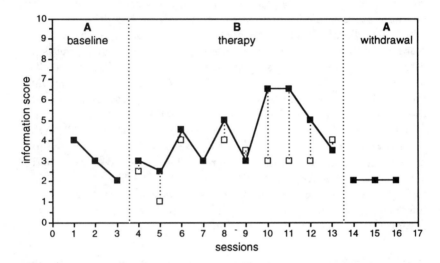

Figure 4–1. Total information score obtained for daily sessions during baseline, therapy, and withdrawal phases, represented by the shaded square. The small dot represents the daily pre-session score obtained before therapy. The dotted line unites the pre- and post-session scores and thus represents the change observed after the therapy session as compared to before the therapy session.

RESULTS AND DISCUSSION

Direct Effects of Therapy

Circumlocutions. The first portion of Figure 4–1 represents baseline measures (A phase), presented without feedback or therapy. The second part represents measures taken during therapy (B phase). The third portion is associated with the withdrawal phase (A phase), which involves a repetition of the baseline measures without feedback or therapy.

In the baseline measures, the information scores produced for the ten stimuli are 4, 3, and 2, with an average of 3. This performance determined the criterion for terminating the treatment phase. We selected an information score of 6 as indicative of improvement, as this was double the average performance at baseline. The criterion was to be achieved for 3 consecutive treatment days. A maximum of 10 sessions was to be conducted before the withdrawal phase was introduced.

Because the criterion was reached but not maintained for 3 days during the treatment phase, the full 10 sessions were conducted. During the treatment phase, the daily post-session measures generally were superior to the average score obtained on the baselines, except for session 2 which was slightly less than the average and sessions 1, 4, and 6 which were equal to the average. It was notable also that, in general, the post-session scores were significantly superior to the pre-session scores (Wilcoxon test, $T+ = 37.5, N = 9, p < .05$) (Siegel & Castellan, 1988). During the withdrawal phase, the scores on the baseline measures reverted to the pre-treatment level. The average information score was 2.5.

A Kruskal-Wallis analysis of variance (Siegel & Castellan, 1988) on the scores obtained before, during (using the best score pre- or post-session to calculate the statistic), and after therapy, demonstrated that the medians were significantly different ($KW = 6.49, p < .05$).

These results suggested that there was significant improvement in the informativity of circumlocutions associated with therapy, although the criterion we had set was not reached.

Naming. Figure 4-2 presents correct scores for naming at baseline during treatment and post-treatment. The difference between the pre- and post-session scores for each day of therapy was significant (Wilcoxon, $T+ = 50, N = 10, p < .01$). When the withdrawal phase was introduced, the naming score decreased, although to a level that was .5 higher than baseline.

A Kruskal-Wallis analysis of variance was performed on the number of correct responses obtained before (A phase), during (using the best performance obtained in the B phase to calculate the statistic), and after therapy (withdrawal A phase). This analysis demonstrated that there was a significant difference between the medians ($KW = 7.96, p < .05$). These results suggest there was also improvement in naming to description associated with therapy.

Generalization

Naming. TR obtained essentially the same score on the naming test of the PETLS after therapy (50/120). Moreover, the same number of circumlocutions were produced after therapy as before on this test. Therefore, she did not appear to generalize the improved naming abilities and

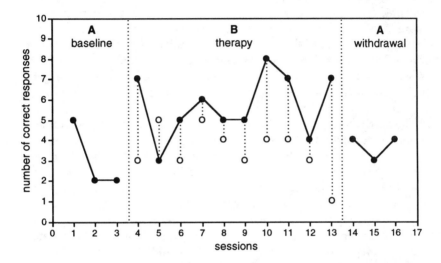

Figure 4–2. Total number of correct responses produced in naming for daily sessions in baseline, therapy, and withdrawal phases represented by the shaded square. The small dot represents the daily pre-session score in naming obtained before therapy. The dotted line unites the pre- and post-session scores and thus represents the change observed after the therapy session as compared to before the therapy session.

the improved circumlocution ability observed in treatment to untreated items presented outside of the therapy context. Her performance did not change on the task of identifying semantic and syllabic properties of words. This suggests no basic change in lexical processing.

Spontaneous Discourse. The Cookie Theft production was transcribed in full and five independent judges were asked to rate the degree of informativeness and the severity of anomia of both samples, before therapy and after therapy. They were unaware of which sample was taken before therapy and which was taken after therapy. All five judged the post-therapy sample more informative and less anomic than the pre-therapy sample. Mean degree of information on a 7-point scale was 2.6 before therapy and 4.2 after therapy. This difference is significant (Wilcoxon $T+ = 15, p < .05$) (Siegel & Castellan, 1988). Mean ability to produce adequate words was rated 2.6 before therapy and 4.0 after therapy. This difference was also significant (Wilcoxon $T+ = 15, p < .05$). No changes in comprehension were noted through another study.

Functional Changes and Longitudinal Observations. When therapy was initiated, TR was severely frustrated by her communication breakdowns. When she was incapable of producing information, she would sometimes throw the stimulus card or appear unhappy with the facilitation procedures we had planned. We persevered, and after a few therapy sessions, TR was much more cooperative and finally enjoyed the treatment. She was quite disappointed when the experiment was terminated because of her health.

Because of our privileged relationship with TR, we continued to have frequent contact with her over the year that followed this experiment. During that time she became less passive as a communicator, and seemed to expect less from other speakers. She became more aware that other persons cannot guess the content of her message. As a result, she is now less likely to become angry when failures to communicate occur. She is generally more responsive in communicative situations. Overall, she is less aggressive when failures occur, and no longer abruptly hangs up the telephone. In her interactions with her former therapist, she indicates that she would like the exchange to follow the pattern developed in therapy. The exchanges usually take the form of first, a general question about the category or about the topic, followed by questions about the specific characteristics or possible use of the word. If a word cannot be found, she will sometimes say, "I cannot find it now, maybe it will come later." Although this generalization is quite remarkable, it has occurred only with the therapist who conducted the experiment.

When asked for her impressions of the intervention, she said that she now spoke better, although she did not always think of producing a definition when she could not find a word. She thought that she was less angry when unable to find words and that she spoke more with other family members. She added that her spouse still had problems in letting her speak but she thought he was "too old to change." Her only regret was that the therapy did not last longer.

Comment

Our original question was whether treatment with the objective of teaching the production of circumlocutions in a pragmatic context could reduce the word-finding difficulties of a moderately severe aphasic. Our results tend to indicate that there was improvement in both therapy tasks: circumlocutions became more informative and naming became more successful. We could state this conclusion with more confidence if we had been successful in implementing the second B phase of the study.

No changes were observed in confrontation naming, untreated in this experiment, but nevertheless dependent on the processes and representations involved in producing words. This suggests that no basic change occurred in lexical processing and production. In that sense, the originally identified impairment remained unchanged.

However, there appears to be some generalization after therapy. TR demonstrates improved ability to produce informative discourse in picture description. Because description involves more spontaneous expression than picture naming, it is possible that improvement occurred in contexts similar to the one developed in therapy, where expression relies more on internal stimulation. Thus, she may have increased her skill at using her residual language processing abilities for communication purposes. In that sense, it is possible to postulate that the communicative disability was reduced.

Our qualitative observations of changes in the patient's behavior as a communicator lead us to think that there was generalization of the structure of the therapy interaction for resolving communication breakdowns. This occurred only with the person who conducted the therapy. Possibly, since Mrs. TR's other relatives and family members did not receive the treatment, they could not be expected to know how to structure an exchange for resolution of breakdowns. After all, the responsibility for successful communication does not rest only on the aphasic individual. This suggests that to attain certain goals, aphasia therapy should involve persons other than the aphasic patient. Under such circumstances, the role of the aphasia therapist would be to act as an observer and teacher of communication strategies to two or more individuals. This represents a shift from the usual role of the speech-language pathologist as the exclusive communication partner of the aphasic person, to a focus on other partners. Therapy conducted in this manner holds the potential for significantly improving a patient's and his significant others' abilities as communicators, as well as for enhancing family members' abilities to create contexts in which the aphasic person becomes a better communicator. This type of approach to treatment could have the effect of reducing the handicap associated with aphasia. Further research along these lines is required to be better able to delineate the most favorable conditions for reducing communicative handicaps.

CONCLUDING REMARKS

This patient highlighted several aspects of the efficacy of therapy that we perceive as central to the field of aphasia intervention. We believe that a better understanding of the conditions, variables, and therapies that allow aphasic patients to function optimally in the communicative world will be obtained only if the broadest perspectives on intervention are developed. Research about intervention effects is necessary, especially as we refine our insights into language impairments. New lines of investigation of intervention are open, including the perspectives of individual communicative disabilities and handicaps associated with aphasia. Also, further research on the role of the right hemisphere in language recovery holds the promise of greater understanding of the mechanisms underlying functional changes.

Finally, the particular geographical and linguistic situation of Québec favors the continuation of input from Europe and the United States in the development of a scientific discipline of aphasia intervention. The perspectives developed in French-speaking Canada are likely to provide fruitful avenues of research and collaboration with researchers in other parts of the world. As our traditions show, our bilingual circumstances put us in a strong collaborative position. Our endeavors, along with the others presented in this book, should further understanding of the best means to treat language impairments, reduce communication disabilities, and improve the quality of life of aphasic patients.

ACKNOWLEDGMENT

This work was supported by a grant from the Fonds de la Recherche en Santé du Québec, awarded to the first author.

REFERENCES

Aten, J. L. (1986). Functional communication treatment. In R. Chapey (Ed.), *Language intervention strategies in adult aphasia* (2nd ed., pp. 266–276). Baltimore, MD: Williams & Wilkins.

Basso, A. (1989). Spontaneous recovery and language rehabilitation. In X. Seron & G. Deloche (Eds.), *Cognitive approaches in neuropsychological rehabilitation* (pp. 17–37). Hillsdale, NJ: Lawrence Erlbaum.

Basso, A., Capitani, E., & Vignolo, L. (1979). Influence of rehabilitation on language skills in aphasic patients: A controlled study. *Archives of Neurology, 36,* 190–196.

Belliol, M. (1990). *Évaluation d'un traitement basé sur une stratégie compensatoire au manque du mot chez l'aphasique.* Mémoire de maîtrise, École d'orthophonie et 'audiologie, Faculté de Médecine, Université de Montréal, Québec.

Benson, D. F. (1988). Anomia in aphasia. *Aphasiology, 2,* 229–236.

Boisclair-Papillon, R. (1991). La famille de l'aphasique. In J. Ponzio, D. Lafond, R. Degiovani, & Y. Joanette (Eds.), *L'aphasique* (pp. 163–176). St-Hyacinthe, Québec: Edisem; Paris: Maloine S.A.

Brandeis, D., & Lehmann, D. (1986). Event-related potentials of the brain and cognitive processes: Approaches and applications. *Neuropsychologia, 24,* 151–168.

Broca, P. (1865). Sur la faculté du langage articulé. *Bulletin de la Société d'Anthropologie, 6,* 337–393.

Broida, H. (1977). Language therapy effects in long term aphasia. *Archives of Physical Medicine and Rehabilitation, 58,* 248–253.

Cambier, J., Elghozi, D., Signoret, J. L., & Henin, D. (1983). Contribution de l'hémisphère droit au langage des aphasiques. Disparition de ce langage aprbès lésion droite. *Revue Neurologique, 139,* 55–63.

Cot, F., & Degiovani, R. (1991). L'aphasique et la loi. In J. Ponzio, D. Lafond, R. Degiovani, & Y. Joanette (Eds.), *L'aphasique* (pp. 213–234). St-Hyacinthe, Québec: Edisem; Paris: Maloine S.A.

Cyr-Stafford, C. (1986). Recovery of auditory comprehension in aphasia: Is language therapy effective? *Journal of Neurolinguistics, 2,* 48–88.

Czopf, D. (1979). The role of the non-dominant hemisphere in speech recovery in aphasia. *Aphasia Apraxia Agnosia, 2,* 27–33.

David, R., Enderby, P., & Bainton, D. (1982). Treatment of acquired aphasia: Speech therapists and volunteers compared. *Journal of Neurology, Neurosurgery, and Psychiatry, 45,* 957–961.

Davis, G. A., & Wilcox, M. J. (1985). *Adult aphasia rehabilitation: Applied pragmatics.* San Diego, CA: College-Hill Press.

Demeurisse, G., & Capon, A. (1985). *Does the right hemisphere contribute to language recovery in Broca's and Wernicke's aphasia?* Paper presented at the 8th European Conference of the International Neuropsychological Society, Copenhagen.

de Partz, M. P. (1986). Re-education of a deep dyslexic patient: Rationale of the method and results. *Cognitive Neuropsychology, 3,* 149–177.

DeRenzi, E., & Vignolo, L. A. (1962). The Token Test: A sensitive test to detect receptive disturbances in aphasia. *Brain, 85,* 665–678.

Ducarne, B. (1967). La rééducation des troubles du langage d'origine cérébrale. *Acta Neurologica Belgica, 67,* 1059–1072.

Ducarne, B. D. R. (1986). *Rééducation sémiologique de l'aphasie.* Paris: Masson.

Eisenson, J. (1954). *Examining for aphasia.* New York: The Psychological Corporation.

Frey, W. D. (1984). Functional assessment in the '80s. In A. S. Halpen & M. J. Fuhrer (Eds.), *Functional assessment in rehabilitation* (pp. 11–43). Baltimore, MD: Paul H. Brookes

Garrett, M. F. (1982). Production of speech: Observations from normal and pathological language use. In A. W. Ellis (Ed.), *Normality and pathology in cognitive functions* (pp. 19–76). London: Academic Press.

Garrett, M. F. (1984). The organization of processing structure for language production: Applications to aphasic speech. In D. Caplan, A. R. Lecours, & A. Smith (Eds.), *Biological perspectives on language* (pp. 172–193). Cambridge: The MIT Press.

Goodglass, H., & Kaplan, E. (1983). *The assessment of aphasia and related disorders* (2nd ed.). Philadelphia: Lea & Febiger.

Hagen, C. (1973). Communication abilities in hemiplegia: Effects of speech therapy. *Archives of Physical Medicine and Rehabilitation, 54,* 454–463.

Hartman, J., & Landau, W. (1987). Comparison of formal language therapy with supportive counseling for aphasia due to acute vascular accident. *Archives of Neurology, 44,* 646–649.

Hegde, M. N. (1987). *Clinical research in communicative disorders.* Boston: College-Hill Press.

Heiss, W. D., Herholz, G., Pawlik, G., Wagner, R., & Wienhard, K. (1986). Positron emission tomography in neuropsychology. *Neuropsychologia, 24,* 141–149.

Henschen, S. E. (1926). On the function of the right hemisphere of the brain in relation to the left in speech music and calculation. *Brain, 49,* 110–123.

Holland, A. (1988). A pragmatic perspective for aphasia therapy. *L'orthophonie, ici, ailleurs, autrement: Approches cognitivistes et pragmatiques* (pp. 199–204). Isbergues, France: L'ortho-Edition.

Howard, D. (1986). Beyond randomised controlled trials: The case for effective case studies of the effects of treatment in aphasia. *British Journal of Disorders of Communication, 21,* 89–102.

Howard, D., Patterson, K., Franklin, S., Orchard-Lisle, V., & Morton, J. (1985). Treatment of word retrieval deficits in aphasia. *Brain, 108,* 817–829.

Hubert, M. D., & Degiovani, R. (1991). Les associations de personnes aphasiques. In J. Ponzio, D. Lafond, R. Degiovani, & Y. Joanette (Eds.), *L'aphasique* (pp. 235–257). St-Hyacinthe, Québec: Edisem; Paris: Maloine S. A.

Joanette, Y., Cot, F., Cyr-Stafford, C., Hubert, M., Lafond, D., Lemay, A., & Lecours, A. R. (1987). Intervention orthophonique auprès des aphasiques. In M. I. Botez (Ed.), *Neuropsychologie clinique et neurologie du comportement* (pp. 383–393). Montréal, Québec: Les Presses de l'Université de Montréal; Paris: Masson.

Joanette, Y., Goulet, P., & Hannequin, D. (1990). *Right hemisphere and verbal communication.* New York: Springer Verlag.

Jones, E. V. (1986). Building the foundations for sentence production in a nonfluent aphasic. *British Journal of Disorders of Communication, 21,* 63–82.

Kinsbourne, M. (1971). The minor hemisphere as a source of aphasic speech. *Archives of Neurology, 25,* 303–306.

Klatzky, R. L. (1988). Theories of information processing and theories of aging. In L. L. Light & D. M. Burke (Eds.), *Language, memory, and aging* (pp. 1–16). New York: Cambridge University Press.

Labourel, D., & Martin, M. M. (1991). L'aphasique et sa famille. In J. Ponzio, D. Lafond, R. Degiovani, & Y. Joanette (Eds.), *L'aphasique* (pp. 141–161). St-Hyacinthe, Québec: Edisem; Paris: Maloine S. A.

Landis, T., Cummings, J. L., & Benson, D. F. (1980). Le passage de la dominance du langage à l'hèmisphére droit: Une interprétation de la récupération tardive lors d'aphasies globales. *Revue Médecine Suisse Romande, 100,* 171–177.

Lecours, A. R., Coderre, L., Lafond, D., Bergeron, M., & Bryans, B. (1979). Rééducation des aphasiques. In A. R. Lecours & F. Lhermitte (Eds.), *L'aphasie* (pp. 535–604). Paris: Flammarion Médecine-Sciences.

Lecours, A. R., & Lhermitte, F. (1979). *L'aphasie*. Paris: Flammation Médecine-Sciences.

Le Dorze, G. (1990). Protocole d'évaluation des troubles lexico-sémantiques. Version expérimentale. Université de Montréal, Québec.

Le Dorze, G. (1991, September). Étude des effets de l'intervention auprés d'un cas d'aphasie de conduction avec trouble d'accés au lexique. *Journal of Speech-Language Pathology and Audiology, 15*(3), 21–29.

Le Dorze, G., Jacob, A., & Coderre, L. (1991). Aphasia rehabilitation with a case of agrammatism: A partial replication. *Aphasiology, 5*, 63–85.

Le Dorze, G., & Nespoulous, J. L. (1989). Anomia in moderate aphasia: Problems in accessing the lexical representation. *Brain and Language, 37*, 381–400.

Lee, H., Nakada, T., Deal, J. L., Lin, S., & Kwee, I. L. (1984). Transfer of language dominance. *Annuals of Neurology, 15*, 304–307.

Lemay, M. A. (1990). *Examen des dyslexies acquises, (EDA)*. Montréal: Les Éditions PointCarré.

Lemay, M. A. (1991). L'aphasique et la société. In J. Ponzio, D. Lafond, R. Degiovani, & Y. Joanette (Eds.), *L'aphasique* (pp. 177–191). St-Hyacinthe, Québec: Edisem; Paris: Maloine S. A.

Lesser, R. (1989). Some issues in the neuropsychological rehabilitation of anomia. In X. Seron & G. Deloche (Eds.), *Cognitive approaches in neuropsychological rehabilitation* (pp. 65–104). Hillsdale NJ: Lawrence Erlbaum.

Létourneau, P. Y. (1991). Conséquences psychologiques de l'aphasie. In J. Ponzio, D. Lafond, R. Degiovani, & Y. Joanette (Eds.), *L'aphasique* (pp. 63–83). St-Hyacinthe, Québec: Edisem; Paris: Maloine S. A.

Lhermitte, F., & Ducarne, B. (1965). La rééducation des aphasiques. *La Revue du Praticien, 15*, 2345–2363.

Lincoln, N. B., McGuirk, E., Mulley, G. P., Lendrem, W., Jones, A. C., & Mitchell, J. R. A. (1984). Effectiveness of speech therapy for aphasic stroke patients: A randomised controlled trial. *The Lancet, 1*, 1197–1220.

von Mayendorff, N. (1911). *Die aphasischen symptome*. Leipzig: Engelman.

Nespoulous, J. L., Lecours, A. R., Lafond, D., Lemay, A., Puel, M., Joanette, Y., Cot, F., & Rascol, A. (1986). *Protocole Montréal*-Toulouse d'examen linguistique de l'aphasie (MT86). Centre de Recherche du Centre Hospitalier Côte-des-Neiges, Montréal.

Niccum, N., Selnes, O. A., Speaks, C., Risse, G. L., & Rubens, A. B. (1986). Longitudinal dichotic listening patterns for aphasic patients (Vol. III). Relationship to language and memory variables. *Brain and Language, 28*, 303–317.

Niccum, N., Speaks, C., Rubens, A. B., Knopman, D. S., Yock, D., & Larson, D. (1986). Longitudinal dichotic listening patterns for aphasic patients (Vol. II). Relationship with lesion variables. *Brain and Language, 28*, 289–302.

Ombredane, A. (1951). *L'aphasie et l'élaboration de la pensée explicite*. Paris: Presses Universitaires de France.

Poeck, W., Huber, W., & Willmes, K. (1989). Outcome of intensive language treatment in aphasia. *Journal of Speech and Hearing Disorders, 54*, 471–479.

Ponzio, J., & Degiovani, R. (1991). De quelques comportements observés chez l'aphasique et sa famille. In J. Ponzio, D. Lafond, R. Degiovani, & Y. Joanette

(Eds.), *L'aphasique* (pp. 129-139). St-Hyacinthe, Québec: Edisem; Paris: Maloine S. A.

Ponzio, J., Lafond, D., Degiovani, R., & Joanette, Y. (Eds.). (1991). *L'aphasique.* St-Hyacinthe, Québec: Edisem; Paris: Maloine S. A.

Prins, R. S., Schoonen, R., & Vermeulen, J. (1989). Efficacy of two different types of speech therapy for aphasic stroke patients. *Applied Psycholinguistics, 10,* 85–123.

Rolland, J., & Belin, C. (1991). L'aphasique et le monde du travail. In J. Ponzio, D. Lafond, R. Degiovani, & Y. Joanette (Eds.), *L'aphasique* (pp. 193–211). St-Hyacinthe, Québec: Edisem; Paris: Maloine S. A.

Sarno, M. T., Silverman, M., & Sands, E. (1970). Speech therapy and language recovery in severe aphasia. *Journal of Speech and Hearing Research, 13,* 607–623.

Schuell, H. M., Carroll, V., & Street, B. S. (1955). Clinical treatment of aphasia. *Journal of Speech and Hearing Disorders, 20,* 43–53.

Schuell, H., Jenkins, J., & Jiménez-Pabon, E. (1964). *Aphasia in adults.* New York: Harper.

Shewan, C. M. (1986). The history and efficacy of aphasia treatment. In R. Chapey (Ed.), *Langugae intervention strategies in adult aphasia* (2nd ed., pp. 28–43). Baltimore, MD: Williams & Wilkins.

Shewan, C. M., & Kertesz, A. (1984). Effects of speech and language treatment on recovery from aphasia. *Brain and Language, 23,* 272–299.

Siegel, S., & Castellan, N. J. (1988). *Non-parametric statistics for the behavioral sciences* (2nd ed.). New York: McGraw-Hill.

Weisenburg, T. H., & McBride, K. E. (1935). *Aphasia.* New York: Commonwealth Fund.

Wertz, R. T. (1987). Language treatment for aphasia is efficacious, but for whom? *Topics in Language Disorders, 8,* 1–10.

Wertz, R. T., Collins, M. J., Weiss, D., Kurtzke, J. F., Friden, T., Brookshire, R. H., Pierce, J., Holtzapple, P., Hubbard, D. J., Porch, B. E., West, J. A., Davis, L., Matovich, V., Morley, G. K., & Resurrection, E. (1981). Veterans administration cooperative study on aphasia: A comparison of individual and group treatment. *Journal of Speech and Hearing Research, 24,* 580–594.

Wertz, R. T., Weiss, D. G., Aten, J. L., Brookshire, R. H., Garcia-Bunuel, L., Holland, A. L., Kurtzke, J. F., LaPointe, L. L., Milianti, F. J., Brannegan, R., Greenbaum, H., Marshall, R. C., Vogel, D., Carter, J., Barnes, N. S., & Goodman, R. (1986). Comparison of clinic, home, and deferred language treatment for aphasia. *Archives of Neurology, 43,* 653–658.

Yorkston, K. M., Beukelman, D. R., & Bell, K. R. (1988). *Clinical management of dysarthric speakers.* Boston: College-Hill Press.

Zipf, G. K. (1984). *La psychobiologie du langage.* Paris: Retz.

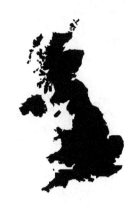

CHAPTER 5

Hypothesis Testing and Aphasia Therapy

SALLY BYNG

Department of Clinical Communication Studies
City University
London, England

To describe my perspective on aphasia therapy, I first consider some aspects of the development of aphasia therapy in Britain to indicate what has motivated my current approach to therapy. Then I describe the basis of this approach and how it has developed. Finally, I underline some of the issues that most currently concern me.

A PERSPECTIVE ON THE DEVELOPMENT OF APHASIA THERAPY IN BRITAIN

As in many other countries, services to people with aphasia developed in Britain subsequent to the World War II, when men who had sustained brain damage from head injuries were surviving with language impairments. In 1946, Butfield and Zangwill published a review of their retraining methods and of the outcome of therapy, which served to focus attention on this population. The services gradually developed, and speech therapists became increasingly concerned with people with aphasia.

In the late 1970s, the use of volunteers in therapy for people with aphasia was becoming increasingly popular. A charity, then called the Chest Heart and Stroke Association (now the Stroke Association) set up a series of stroke clubs, through the "Volunteer Stroke Scheme," which continue today with new clubs still being set up. The majority of these clubs do not attempt to provide "therapy" for aphasia, but some do run language-activity based groups. The *British Medical Journal*, not well known for its interest in aphasia or therapy, has published two papers (Eaton Griffiths, 1975, 1980) describing the work of the stroke clubs. Volunteers are now widely used in speech and language therapy services to people with aphasia, in a supplementary as well as complementary role (Rossiter & McInally, 1989). In a survey of aphasia therapy services, many therapists commented that the service could not run without the help of volunteers (Rossiter & McInally, 1989).

Partly as a result of this initiative, aphasia therapy focused on evaluating the outcome of services provided to people with aphasia. A number of large clinical trials of the efficacy of aphasia therapy were implemented, with results that have become well known (e.g., David, Enderby, & Bainton, 1982; Lincoln et al., 1984; Meikle et al., 1979). The results of such studies have often been taken to reinforce the "belief-system," identified by Holland and Wertz (1988), that aphasia therapy is largely ineffective at remediating the language deficit in aphasia. This belief system has been resistant to change despite criticisms about both the nature of the research questions and the design of the studies (see Howard, 1986; Pring, 1986). The negative results of these early trials remain paramount in the minds of many people responsible for services to aphasic people. Although these issues now represent well-trodden ground, I want to clarify some of them here because they have been important in the development of services to people with aphasia in Britain.

The clinical trials of the efficacy of aphasia therapy focused on a range of questions, such as the following:

"Whether any improvement relating to speech therapy was associated with the specific skills and experience of the speech therapist or was a consequence of the general stimulation and support which most therapeutic relationships provide" (David et al., 1982, p. 957);

"Are there differences in the progress made by people with aphasia who received 'formal, conventional treatment' compared with people receiving treatment from nonprofessional volunteers working under guidance from an experienced speech therapist" (Meikle et al., 1979, p. 87);

and "Whether speech therapy produces a better language outcome than does natural recovery alone [in people with aphasia]" (Lincoln et al., 1984, p. 1197).

The answers to all of these questions provided by the large clinical trials have been largely negative.

Interpretation of the results of the studies, however, has not been confined to answering the questions asked. For example, a popular quotation from the paper by Lincoln and her colleagues (1983) is as follows:

> Our study indicates that speech therapy did not improve language abilities more than was achieved by spontaneous recovery. . . . (Our results) suggest that one aspect of the speech therapy service for aphasic patients—namely, individual treatment—is ineffective (p. 1199).

If we accept the findings of the Lincoln study, speech therapy, as provided in their study, was found not to be useful or effective. People have been quick to interpret this as demonstrating that individual speech therapy cannot affect the language deficit in aphasia. However, Lincoln et al.'s results do not imply that all individual speech therapy in aphasia is necessarily ineffective, but rather that the therapy, as carried out in their study, was ineffective, so that a new set of questions is raised. Is *any* amount or type of individual aphasia therapy ineffective, or would different treatment regimens or different treatments be more successful? Was the poor outcome in the study due to content of therapy, service delivery, or genuinely because any type or amount of individual therapy is ineffective? These alternatives were not addressed by the Lincoln study, but it has been widely accepted as a demonstration of the ineffectiveness of aphasia therapy (and even speech therapy per se).

Another question that these studies have asked, either implicitly or explicitly, is: "Does therapy in general improve aphasia in general?" (Howard & Hatfield, 1987, p. 110). It might be considered unlikely that a study designed to ask such a question would show positive results; why should therapy in general benefit aphasia in general? I would assume that no doctor would expect much of a study that aimed to investigate the effect of medication on headache when a number of different, but unspecified medications were used, and when many of those different medications were untested. I imagine that ethical approval for such a study would not be given. This is, however, a reasonable analogy with the large group efficacy studies for aphasia therapy that have been carried out; we know little of the content, range, variety, or effectiveness of the types of therapies provided. It is, of course, of paramount importance that we evaluate the effectiveness of both the therapy and the service we provide. To do this, very specific research questions should be asked in order to provide the purchaser, the provider, and the user of a service with relevant information about both the content and the delivery of the service.

It is not surprising then that the way the findings of these studies were reported had a considerable impact on the view of aphasia therapy taken both within and outside the speech and language therapy profession.[1] In the mid-1980s there was a detectable decline in interest and enthusiasm for the treatment of aphasia among many speech and language therapists. Many therapists began to doubt the effectiveness of intervention in aphasia and to lose confidence in bringing about some modification of the language deficit itself. The prevailing attitude seemed to be that the language impairment was largely irremediable, and this seemed to have a direct impact on the provision of services for people with aphasia. The type of therapy provided changed too. There was a discernible shift away from treating the language disorder per se and toward providing strategies to circumvent the language problems. During the same period there was considerable growth in the provision of speech and language therapy, but this was predominantly in the provision of pediatric services.

These large scale efficacy studies in aphasia therapy provoked a lot of debate and discussion within the speech therapy profession in Britain. What especially concerned me then about the studies, apart from the fact that I thought there was a discernible impact on the availability of therapy, was that I felt they were premature. Were we confident enough in our knowledge about the nature of the disorders for which we were providing therapy? Was our knowledge about the content of therapy, and the relationship of that therapy to the communication disorder being treated, sufficiently explicit and extensive that it was logical to examine the efficacy of that therapy? My reaction was that there was little hard evidence available about what kind of approaches were most beneficial for what kind of communication disability.

Without some basic theories addressing these issues it was premature to give less prominence to any form of therapy. All therapies need to be given due and fair consideration, and attempted or not, depending on the needs of a particular individual at a particular time, not on untested preconceptions of what is or is not effective therapy. Therefore, I felt that to evaluate how effective treatment was in broad terms, at that stage, represented not only putting the cart before the horse, but also failing to nourish the horse.

---

[1]Note that the three studies described above were published in medical, not speech therapy journals.

Another basic reservation I had at that time was that the tools of language assessment available in the early 1980s were not ideal as diagnostic instruments, as pointers for different types of therapeutic intervention, or as pre- and post-therapy measures (Byng, Kay, Edmundson, & Scott, 1989). It seemed that we had no adequate tools either for assessment that informed therapy or for measurement of the effects of therapy.

THE ADVENT OF COGNITIVE NEUROPSYCHOLOGY

Parallel with these developments in speech and language therapy, another movement that has had a considerable impact on aphasia intervention in the U.K. was taking place. Toward the end of the 1970s, cognitive experimental psychologists were becoming interested in attempting to account for disorders of language processing in models representing normal language processing (Coltheart, Patterson, & Marshall, 1980). This methodology has developed into a new discipline called cognitive neuropsychology. The basic approach is to try to identify where, within empirically based models of language processing, the deficit underlying an aphasic person's impaired language is situated.[2]

Current models usually represent the component modules of the language processing system through box and arrow diagrams, in which the boxes represent stores of information and arrows represent processes linking them. Different kinds of models representing connectionist networks have recently begun to be considered, and attempts have been made to simulate the effects of damaging the language system by lesioning connectionist networks (e.g., Hinton & Shallice, 1991). These models offer an alternative way of thinking about the architecture and implementation of language processing. Whatever the form of the model, empirically based models of normal language functioning offer a logical, coherent framework within which a basic account of any type of language impairment can be approached. A patient's pattern of deficits can be elucidated in terms of the interaction of impaired and preserved components of the language processing system.

One of the promises that this type of approach holds is that it allows us to get below the surface symptoms to look at the underlying problems. We know that a similar surface symptomatology can often mask different underlying impairments (e.g., Berndt, 1987), and that this superficial similarity might be misleading in planning therapy. If we know more about the nature of the underlying language problem, we may be in a

[2]Texts describing this approach include Coltheart (1986), Ellis and Young (1988), Shallice (1988). For illustrations of the application of this approach see Coltheart, Sartori, and Job (1987).

better position to target therapy for the language impairment more accurately (Byng & Coltheart, 1986). A number of therapy studies have been carried out using this methodology to investigate the nature of the language impairment (e.g., Behrmann, 1987; Bruce & Howard, 1987; Byng, 1988; Coltheart & Byng, 1989; de Partz, 1986; Jones, 1986; Nickels, Byng, & Black, 1991).

One of the advantages of this approach is that it can provide some theoretically motivated predictions of the outcome of therapy. Because the models try to make explicit the relationships among different aspects of language processing, it is possible to hypothesize what should happen to one aspect of language processing when a different aspect is treated. For example, if someone is relearning letter-sound correspondences through therapy, then there is no obvious reason why repetition, for example, should improve. Models suggest that knowing how a letter sounds should not affect the processes involved in going from a spoken word to repetition of that word. On the other hand, it should improve ability to read words aloud, specifically words that can be read aloud through application of rule-governed procedures, but not words that do not conform to these procedures, that is, words with irregular spelling-to-sound correspondences (for an example of this prediction in practice see de Partz, 1986, and Seron and de Partz in Chapter 6). Thus we can be quite specific about what aspects of language processing this therapy should benefit.

Alternatively, suppose that therapy were planned for a person with a naming problem. We could hypothesize that the problem in naming pictures was a result of underspecified semantic representations. That is, given the choice of two semantically close words to match to a picture, the patient might confuse the correct name with the one similar in meaning. We could hypothesize that, in this case, one of the factors underlying the problem in naming pictures is that insufficiently specified semantic representations are accessing the phonological output system (e.g., Howard & Orchard-Lisle, 1984). Suppose that a naming therapy were instituted that was based not on encouraging naming, but on making semantic distinctions among closely related items, thereby focusing on semantic features. The therapy might not involve any naming, and yet an improvement in naming would be predicted because the therapy is aimed at the problem underlying the symptom, and therefore should alleviate the symptom (see Jones, 1989, for an example). In addition, any other tasks depending on distinguishing semantic features, such as comprehension of semantically close words, should also show an improvement.

Thus, thinking through the implications of the architecture of the language processing system can assist therapists in predicting the effects of therapy. This in turn can help to measure the effectiveness of intervention; if we can demonstrate that our therapy has affected the aspects of processing that we anticipate should be affected, but not those that we do not anticipate should be affected, we are in a stronger position to claim that our intervention has been influential in bringing about change. Alternatively, if the therapy does not produce the expected outcome, then we are in a good position to ask why it did not. It may be that there was no effect of therapy; in this case it is legitimate to ask whether it did not work because, even though the area selected for treatment was appropriate, the therapy itself was not effective, and therefore an alternative type of therapy should be attempted. On the other hand, it may be that the hypothesis about the problem was incorrect and should be reconsidered.

In addition, it is clear that pre- and post-therapy measures should include not only treated and untreated language functions, but also some untreated language functions that are related and some that are unrelated to the function being treated. The relationships among the functions must be specified, so that predicted improvements in related but untreated functions can be measured, providing yet more evidence for the efficacy of the therapy (e.g., see Byng, 1988).

This is, of course, a time-consuming procedure, but I think that most aphasia therapists would agree that therapy is not a simple matter of applying a predetermined formula, but of trial and error to find the key to the communication disability and a means to get out of it. The rational way of proceeding suggested by cognitive neuropsychological methodology offers a logical way of pursuing this trial-and-error approach.

BEYOND COGNITIVE NEUROPSYCHOLOGY: HYPOTHESIS TESTING AS A CLINICAL ROUTINE

There are limitations, however, on the "strict" application of this type of approach. A strict application would suggest that there must be clearly articulated models ready to apply to impaired language that make explicit every process involved in getting from the message to the spoken or written word and from the spoken or written word to full comprehension. We are, in reality, far from that stage. Currently, the best developed cognitive neuropsychological models are for single word processing, and even these models do not specify in detail the nature of all the processes involved. Thus, it seems that the best way for therapists to proceed is not to rely on the advent of ideal cognitive neuropsychological models of different aspects of language processing, but rather to adopt a "hypothesis testing" approach, in which keen clinical observation is informed by a range of notions from psycholinguistic and cognitive neuropsychological theories and research. Disordered language is still understood in relation to normal processing, but reliance on the provision of clearly articulated models is diminished.

This is not to suggest that clearly articulated models of language processing are not desirable—they are crucial; this development is simply a matter of expediency, not desirability. Adequate cognitive neuropsychological models often do not exist at the level of language at which a clinician may want to intervene with a particular person with aphasia. If we develop hypothesis testing as a routine clinical procedure, then we can proceed in a rational and logical way to investigate and interpret language disorders when there are no explicit, clinically applicable models to motivate that investigation. This procedure would also have the effect of highlighting relevant areas of language deficit for theoretical research. It is vital to the progression of the field that clinical relevance and insight interact with and contribute to developments in theoretical analyses of language impairments.

There are also, of course, many aspects of communication disability that transcend models. Certainly, the interaction among different aspects of the language disability and factors specific to an individual, such as personality, reaction to the disability, or individual differences arising from different experiences of language, need to be considered in a quite different way.

Howard and Hatfield (1987) suggest that,

> To plan treatment, it is not essential to demonstrate beyond all doubt what the underlying impairment is. All that is required is a hypothesis sufficiently detailed to be able to motivate therapy. A hypothesis should be able to predict the patient's response to therapy and the pattern of errors that will occur in it. Treatment is then a test of the hypothesis; if it does not run as predicted, the hypothesis will need to be changed. A therapist must know what changes he/she is trying to effect, and how; to decide what they should be requires an idea of what is wrong. (p. 130)

What would a hypothesis testing approach involve? The initial hypothesis has to come from observation of the person with aphasia. The initial hypotheses about the kinds of difficulties a person might have come from observing how the person interacts with the environment and with other people, and by noting the level of the disorder in conversational language. Assessment tasks, more accurately described as investigative procedures, are then selected or devised on the basis of these early hypotheses, the aim being to carry out hypothesis-driven assessment rather than to derive assessment-driven hypotheses (Jones & Byng, 1989). The investigative procedures will then be designed and carried out to test the hypotheses.

A caveat should be made here. This way of proceeding could be interpreted as limiting the potential for diagnosis and therapy, that is, only those problems that the therapist observes will be followed up, which might lead to the neglect of important aspects of the language disability. This would be a misinterpretation of the purpose of the hypothesis testing approach. The suggestion that the initial hypothesis should come from observation of the patient does not preclude a much wider investigation of a person's language disabilities. The progression from the initial hypothesis-driven investigations would be into both wider and deeper issues about the nature and effects of the language impairment.

Hypothesis-driven investigations do not preclude looking at all language modalities and all forms of communication. All of these would naturally be part of a full investigation, in the same way that they are part of an all-embracing standardized test. The difference is that the language would be investigated as part of a continuous process through which one investigation would suggest further aspects of the impairment to consider. These aspects would, in turn, suggest different possibilities to follow up, all from a perspective relevant to the individual person with aphasia. This process can be documented as fully and comprehensively as any standardized procedure. The materials to be used might not be standardized, but aphasia therapists use a huge variety of materials in their day-to-day work, many of which are not standardized. Impressions about a patient gathered during the course of this work would not be discounted just because they were gained by using nonstandardized materials. It is, of course, important to establish not only that any tasks given to people with aphasia can be carried out by nonaphasic people but also that there are no reasons for failure on a task that can be attributed to the specific materials used rather than to a language impairment.

Therapy itself can be integrated into the investigative procedures, and interpretation of the language deficit can continue during the process of therapy. Thus a hypothesis could be formulated about what the problem might be, and a strategy selected to overcome it (Howard & Patterson, 1989). The strategy can be modified when performance suggests that the hypothesis was either not entirely accurate or because some change had taken place. We often can learn as much about the nature of the disorder by implementing therapy and monitoring the patient's response as we can through exploratory investigations.

It becomes clear in discussion with clinicians from many different "orientations" that many of them are already applying many aspects of this kind of hypothesis-testing approach. It is my impression that, in practice, many therapists regard much of their work with people with aphasia as exploratory, as they constantly revise what they do in response to the performance of a particular individual. Therefore, what is described here represents nothing new; the only differences are, first, that this process previously has taken place implicitly and has not been communicated among therapists and, second, this process has not been adequately informed and driven by concepts and theories about language derived from psycholinguistics and cognitive neuropsychology.

FROM DEFICIT TO THERAPY

Interpreting language deficits in terms of models of normal language processing has given us a way to explore and theorize about the nature of language deficits. Having a good hypothesis about the nature of the language deficit is a prerequisite for a good program of therapy. The therapist needs to know what to treat. But there is more to a good program of therapy than knowing what aspect of the language or communication disability to attend to. Howard and Hatfield (1987) capture this:

> The problem that has dogged aphasia therapy is the relationship between a hypothesis of the form of the impairment and the actual process of therapy. Knowing what is wrong does not in any simple way determine what to do about it. (p. 130)

The communication deficit itself seems to attract the majority of the research in aphasia; much less attention has been paid to describing therapies and even less to analyzing the process of therapy, so that the therapy itself has become the "Cinderella" of the whole process of rehabilitation in aphasia. Basso (1989) made the following observation about therapy:

> It is very difficult to know what aphasia therapy is . . . What occurs under the heading of aphasia rehabilitation in one place may have nothing in common with what occurs in a different place except for the fact that a speech therapist and a patient interact with each other. (p. 17)

This seems to be an accurate reflection of the state of the art, and it highlights a number of problems: How can therapy be evaluated, developed, or communicated if we are not even clear about what it is that we are considering? A whole new set of questions needs to be asked about therapy to determine how it works and to clarify what we are trying to do through therapy.

I would want to describe the "process of therapy" as the interactive process between the therapist and the person with aphasia through which change in the communication disability is effected. I would conceptualize this process as comprising five main protagonists: the person with aphasia, the therapist, the language impairment, the focus of the therapy—either a specific aspect of the communication impairment or a strategy to circumvent it—and the task and materials. Most accounts of therapy take seriously only the role of the therapist and the task and materials. The impact of how the patient responds to what the therapist does is not described; although, in practice, therapists proceed in therapy by modifying the task, their manner of responding, or what they ask the patient to do in response to what the patient does. This is the process of therapy.

Currently, our knowledge about the process of therapy is implicit. Asking clinicians to be explicit about exactly what they are doing in therapy is a hard task, not, I believe, because they do not know what they are doing, but for two principal reasons. One was expressed by Howard and Hatfield (1987) as follows:

> Theoretically-motivated work from a variety of viewpoints has provided detailed analyses of the deficits underlying some aphasic patients' difficulties. Compared with these sophisticated analyses, many therapists' treatment techniques that are used in day-to-day practice appear too simple; they do not feel as if they do justice to the complexity of the problem. We suggest that this is because there is no explicit metatheory available that explicitly relates a deficit analysis to the process of treatment. (p. 5)

The masking of a sophisticated therapeutic process by what appears to be a simple technique has also been described by McCrae Cochrane and Milton (1984). Describing the development of their conversational prompting technique, they suggested colorfully that "the (therapy) method which evolved might be compared to so-called 'natural' childbirth in its use of a sophisticated technique that gives the impression of a natural-looking process" (p. 5).

The second reason is, I believe, that what a clinician does becomes somehow intrinsic to his or her performance. There seems to be a kind of "automatic pilot" that a good clinician develops and then switches on, which suggests how to present a task, how and when to modulate it, how to respond to a specific response by the patient, and so on. Clinicians make these decisions all the time, but on what criteria do we base these decisions? How do we judge whether we are right? How do we evaluate whether the therapy was appropriate, and if it wasn't, what part of it to modify—the task, the materials, or our interaction with the aphasic person?

Many clinicians would call whatever process takes over "clinical intuition," or the outcome of experience. The implication of these two responses is that nothing can be done to make a good aphasia therapist; you either have to "have it" or you have to be old. I do not believe that the process of therapy is just intuitive. I do believe that the process can be taken apart, to some extent, to try to understand what really goes on between patient and therapist. Having taken it apart, we can begin to get some concepts about what the dynamics and mechanics in therapy are.

As yet we have no theoretical framework for the process of therapy through which the different components of the process of therapy can be studied and related. It would seem that therapy itself needs to develop into an independent theoretical domain to enable us to develop and disseminate effective therapies for aphasia. A detailed analysis of the process of therapy combined with a theory of the deficit should then be enmeshed to provide a theory of change, which is surely what a theory of therapy should be. Caramazza (1989) described this in the following terms:

> There is the problem . . . of the unsupported (and overly simple) assumption that all one needs for motivating therapeutic intervention is a theory of normal cognitive processing and a procedure for uncovering, from patterns of impaired performance, the locus of functional lesion to the normal system. Undoubtedly, the identification of the underlying cause of an impairment is an important step in deciding on an intervention strategy. However, an informed choice cannot be made in the absence of an equally rich theory of the modifications that a damaged cognitive system may undergo as a function of different forms of intervention. This latter aspect of the rehabilitation process remains largely unexplored. (pp. 396–397)

However, we do not want to create a theory of therapy that results in the formulation of prescriptive "treatment regimes." Rather, we would want to distill sets of procedures to implement in therapy and sets of principles governing those procedures. The provision of procedures would include suggesting tasks to use in therapy, defined in detail. This detail would include not only an enumeration of the stimuli, materials, and modalities, but also a description of the therapeutic interactions, that is, how the therapist responded to the patient in relation to the type of response made by the patient.

There is no advantage in clarifying the therapy procedures unless at the same time the principles governing the therapy are also elucidated. The principles of therapy would include those aspects of the implementation that often seem to have to be learned through experience and tend to remain as implicit knowledge, because we have not, so far, attempted to be explicit about them and describe them separately from the procedures implemented. These principles would include many of the following factors that are intrinsic to the decision-making process of the therapist during the process of therapy: How the initial form of therapy is determined; under what circumstances this decision is reinforced or changed; how a specific procedure is intended to work for a specific individual with aphasia; when a procedure needs to be modified and in what ways; at what pace to take a session, when to leave the person to search and when to intervene; and when an aphasic person has derived all possible benefit from a procedure (Byng, 1992).

The procedures and principles of a particular therapy should not only be documented in detail, but, crucially, they must be related to the specific type of deficit for which they are intended and to other variables that impinge on the way that an individual might respond to therapy. Given this information, another therapist could see more clearly how the therapy relates to what he or she is doing. It may be that a therapist, on consideration of a specific aphasic person, would want to modify some of the procedures, but maintain some of the principles. Conversely, similar procedures might be implemented with a different set of principles. I would suggest that principles and procedures can be devised for any therapy for a communication impairment in aphasia, not only for specific language therapies but also for nonverbal strategies, compensatory strategies, and so forth. These sets of procedures and principles could be combined to provide a detailed analysis of the process of therapy and the foundation for developing a theory of therapy.

THE CONTEXT FOR THERAPY FOR THE LANGUAGE DEFICIT

In conclusion, I want to clarify the context for the kind of approach that I have described in this chapter. It applies only to one part of the whole process of facilitating recovery from the effects of aphasia: How we might investigate and treat the communication deficit. There are many more aspects of recovery from aphasia than I have covered here. To make this quite explicit, the following set of features describes what I take to be the scope of what aphasia therapists do when they work toward recovery with a person with aphasia:

- delineate the uses of language made by the person with aphasia prior to becoming aphasic;

- facilitate adjustment to the change in communication skills;

- investigate the nature and effects of the language deficit with respect to the whole language system;

- attempt to remediate the language deficit itself;

- increase the use of all other potential means of communication to support, facilitate, and compensate for the impaired language;

- enhance the use of the remaining language;

- provide an opportunity to use newly acquired and emerging language skills, not just in a clinical environment, but in more normal communicative situations;

- attempt to change the communication skills of those around the person with aphasia to accommodate the aphasia.

This broad scope demonstrates the variety of skills with which a therapist needs to approach each person with aphasia. The negative results of the broad-based clinical trials described earlier have tended to make many aphasia therapists relegate therapy to remediate the language deficit in aphasia to the "Cinderella" role of their work because it is difficult to prove and difficult to discuss even among themselves. It is time that an adequate apologia should be made for aphasia therapy.

Much of what I have described in this chapter is already happening in practice, but there has been no means of communicating it, of sharing knowledge, because we do not have a methodology, a terminology, or even a conceptual structure with which we can discuss what we do. Therefore, I am not advocating any new, different brand of therapy, but rather suggesting that existing therapies are probably, for the most part, appropriate but not sufficiently sharply focused or readily communicated. I think we need to heighten our awareness of what is already happening in therapy, so that we can start to be explicit about what we are doing, why we are doing it, and how we think it should change the aphasic person's method and content of communication.

ACKNOWLEDGMENT

Maria Black and Eirian Jones have contributed substantially and generously to the ideas expressed in this chapter.

REFERENCES

Basso, A. (1989). Spontaneous recovery and language rehabilitation. In X. Seron & G. Deloche (Eds.), *Cognitive approaches in neuropsychological rehabilitation* (pp. 17–37). Hillsdale, NJ: Lawrence Erlbaum.

Behrmann, M. (1987). The rites of righting writing. *Cognitive Neuropsychology, 4*(3), 365–384.

Berndt, R. S. (1987). Symptom co-occurrence and dissociation in the interpretation of agrammatism. In M. Coltheart, G. Sartori, & R. Job (Eds.), *The cognitive neuropsychology of language* (pp. 221–233). London: Lawrence Erlbaum.

Bruce, C., & Howard, D. (1987). Computer generated phonemic cues: An effective aid for naming in aphasia. *British Journal of Disorders of Communication*, 22(3), 191–201.

Butfield, E., & Zangwill, O. L. (1946). Re-education in aphasia: A review of 70 cases. *Journal of Neurology, Neurosurgery and Psychiatry*, 9, 75–79.

Byng, S. (1988). Sentence processing deficits: Theory and therapy. *Cognitive Neuropsychology*, 5, 629–676.

Byng, S. (1992). Testing the tried: Replicating therapy for sentence processing deficits in agrammatism. *Clinics in Communication Disorders: Approaches to the Treatment of Aphasia*, 1(4), 34–42.

Byng, S., & Coltheart, M. (1986). Aphasia therapy research: Methodological requirements and illustrative results. In E. Hjelmquist & L-G. Nilssen (Eds.), *Communication and handicap: Aspects of psychological handicap and technical aids* (pp. 191–213). North Holland: Elsevier.

Byng, S., Kay, J., Edmundson, A., & Scott, C. (1989). Aphasia tests reconsidered. *Aphasiology*, 4(1), 67–91.

Caramazza, A. (1989). Cognitive neuropsychology and rehabilitation: An unfulfilled promise? In X. Seron & G. Deloche (Eds.), *Cognitive approaches in neuropsychological rehabiltation* (pp. 383–398). Hillsdale, NJ: Lawrence Erlbaum.

Coltheart, M. (1986). Cognitive neuropsychology. In M. Posner & O. S. M. Marin (Eds.), *Attention and performance XI*. Hillsdale, NJ: Lawrence Erlbaum.

Coltheart, M., & Byng, S. (1989). A treatment for surface dyslexia. In X. Seron & G. Deloche (Eds.), *Cognitive approaches in neuropsychological rehabilitation* (pp. 159–174). Hillsdale, NJ: Lawrence Erlbaum.

Coltheart, M., Patterson, K. E., & Marshall, J. (1980). *Deep dyslexia*. London: Routledge & Kegan Paul.

Coltheart, M., Sartori, G., & Job, R. (1987). *The cognitive neuropsychology of language*. London: Lawrence Erlbaum.

David, R., Enderby, P., & Bainton, D. (1982). Treatment of acquired aphasia: Speech therapists and volunteers compared. *Journal of Neurology, Neurosurgery and Psychiatry*, 45, 957–961.

de Partz, M-P. (1986). Reeducation of a deep dyslexic. *Cognitive Neuropsychology*, 3(2), 149–177.

Eaton Griffiths, V. E. (1975). Volunteer scheme for dysphasia and allied problems in stroke patients. *British Medical Journal*, 3, 633.

Eaton Griffiths, V. E. (1980). Volunteer stroke scheme for dysphasic patients with stroke. *British Medical Journal*, 281, 1605–1608.

Ellis, A., & Young, A. (1988). *Human cognitive neuropsychology*. Hove: Lawrence Erlbaum.

Hinton, G. E., & Shallice, T. (1991). Lesioning an attractor network: Investigations of acquired dyslexia. *Psychological Review*, 98, 74–95.

Holland, A. L., & Wertz, R. T. (1988). Measuring aphasia treatment effects: Large-group, small-group, and single subject studies. In F. Plum (Ed.), *Language, communication and the brain* (pp. 267–273). New York: Raven Press.

Howard, D. (1986). Beyond randomised controlled trials: The case for effective studies of the effects of treatment in aphasia. *British Journal of Disorders of Communication, 21,* 89–102.

Howard, D., & Hatfield, F. M. (1987). *Aphasia therapy: Historical and contemporary issues.* Hove and London: Lawrence Erlbaum.

Howard, D., & Orchard-Lisle, V. (1984). On the origin of semantic errors in naming: Evidence from the case of a global aphasic. *Cognitive Neuropsychology, 2,* 163–190.

Howard, D., & Patterson, K. E. (1989). Models of therapy. In X. Seron & G. Deloche (Eds.), *Cognitive approaches in neuropsychological rehabilitation* (pp. 39–64). Hillsdale, NJ: Lawrence Erlbaum.

Jones, E. V. (1986). Building the foundations for sentence production in a nonfluent aphasic. *British Journal of Disorders of Communication, 21,* 63–82.

Jones, E. V. (1989). A year in the life of PC and EVJ. *Proceedings of the First Aphasia Therapy Symposium.* British Aphasiology Society.

Jones, E. V., & Byng, S. (1989). The practice of aphasia therapy: An opinion. *Bulletin of the College of Speech Therapists,* No. 449, 7–10.

Lincoln, N. B., Mulley, G. P., Jones, A. C., McGuirk, E., Lendrem, W., & Mitchell, J. R. A. (1984). Effectiveness of speech therapy for aphasic stroke patients: A randomised controlled trial. *Lancet, 1,* 1197–1200.

McCrae Cochrane, R., & Milton, S. B. (1984). Conversational prompting: A sentence building technique for severe aphasia. *Journal of Neurological Communication Disorders, 1,* 4–23.

Meikle, M., Wechsler, E., Tupper, A., Benenson, M., Butler, J., Mulhall, D., & Stern, G. (1979). Comparative trial of volunteer and professional treatments of dysphasia after stroke. *British Medical Journal, 2,* 87–89.

Nickels, L., Byng, S., & Black, M. (1991). Sentence processing deficits: A replication of treatment. *British Journal of Disorders of Communication, 26,* 175–199.

Pring, T. R. (1989). Evaluating the effects of speech therapy for aphasics and volunteers: Developing the single case methodology. *British Journal of Disorders of Communication, 21,* 103–115.

Rossiter, D., & McInally, K. (1989). Aphasia services: Provision or privation? *Bulletin of the College of Speech Therapists,* No. 449, 4–6.

Shallice, T. (1988). *From neuropsychology to mental structure.* Cambridge: Cambridge University Press.

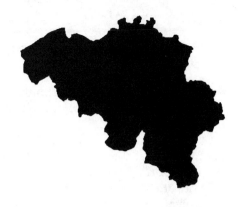

CHAPTER 6

The Re-education of Aphasics: Between Theory and Practice

XAVIER SERON
Unité de Neuropsychologie Cognitive
Faculté de Psychologie
Université de Louvain
Louvain-la-Neuve, Belgium

MARIE-PIERRE de PARTZ
Unité de Revalidation Neuropsychologique
Cliniques Universitaires Saint-Luc
Bruxelles, Belgium

Any general presentation of the rationale of aphasia re-education runs the risk of overemphasizing the theoretical and methodological principles underlying the practices of speech therapists and neuropsychologists. At the same time it risks underemphasizing what, aside from theory, the practices effectively are. This difficulty results from two main sources: The tendency to idealize in any theoretical presentation, and the tendency to neglect the institutional, sociological, medical, and economic constraints that surround effective practices in any specific re-educative setting.

This presentation cannot completely avoid these difficulties, but, in order to try to face them, it will be divided into three parts: (1) a brief description of the concrete constraints that exist in the rehabilitation of aphasic patients in our center in Belgium, as well as a short description of our patient population; (2) a presentation of our theoretical principles in re-education; and (3) a critical evaluation of our daily practices.

THE CLINICAL SETTING

The Brussels Neuropsychological Rehabilitation Unit (hereafter BNRU) is located in a general hospital (Cliniques Universitaires Saint Luc) and is directly associated with a neurological service. The patients are referred to the BNRU from the neurological service and also from other departments (physical medicine) and other institutions for either diagnosis or re-education for cognitive disorders. The BNRU is composed of two different clinical groups: one is concerned with the diagnosis and re-education of patients with focal brain lesions; the other is devoted to the diagnosis and rehabilitation of patients with diffuse brain lesions, especially Alzheimer's disease at its first stage. The BNRU does not hospitalize patients during therapy and thus offers treatment only to outpatients. A first consequence of this is that we generally work with patients who do not have severe physical disabilities despite their cognitive deficits. Disorders of our population are mostly vascular and traumatic in etiology, but a few disorders are seen with infectious or anoxic etiologies.

THE THERAPEUTIC CONTRACT

In our country, re-education is not paid for by the patient but is covered by legal insurance. (Since this is a legal obligation, everyone is insured!) Nevertheless, before starting re-education we propose that the patient sign a contract with the BRNU. We have decided to create such a contractual relationship for many reasons.

First, at least in most western societies, a contract is signed only with an individual who is considered responsible. For example, a contract is never signed with an insane person or with a minor. Therefore, signing a contract with an aphasic patient sends him or her at least two messages: The first is that you consider him or her a responsible adult person; the second emphasizes that you consider therapy a mutual endeavor. This in turn means that both therapists and patients have responsibilities in the re-educative enterprise. In fact, during therapy, the clinicians will have something to do, but so will the patient. Thus treatment cannot be viewed by the patient as a passive enterprise, because he will have to be an "actor" and not only a "patient." However, sometimes the severity of the initial disorder (e.g., global aphasia or severe comprehension deficits) renders the patient unable to understand the terms of the contract. In such cases, the contract is signed by a member of the patient's family.

Second, the re-educative contract determines a time schedule for the therapy and specifies the precise, specific objectives of the treatment. In general, any contract is signed for a 6-month period, and contains the objective of the therapy (to improve word finding, to speak more fluently, to re-learn reading a newspaper, and so on); the frequency and weekly distribution of the treatment sessions; the general content of the therapy (language training sessions, group sessions, relaxation, and so on); and finally, the names of the responsible therapists.

Third, the contract is the means by which the efficacy and the coherence of the therapy is controlled. Every contract is preceded by the establishment of baseline measurements which vary according to the objective of therapy, and at the end of a 6-month period, post-therapy measurements are also made. Moreover, because therapists may go on holiday or become ill, any new therapist who may have to abruptly intervene in ongoing therapy will know the objectives of treatment and the general outline of what is to be done.

In our country, the duration of therapy does not exceed 2 years, which are legally reimbursed. Therefore, we can only propose a maximum of four successive contracts. As we repeat the contract procedure, it is interesting to note progressive modification in the formulation of the objectives. For the first contract, the content is determined principally by the therapist, even though the objectives of therapy are the result of negotiation between the speech therapist and the patient. This is primarily because the patients do not yet understand clearly what has transpired Consequently, they are very dependent on the suggestions of the therapist and accept almost all propositions presented to them. However, in subsequent contracts, patients have had the opportunity to be confronted with the handicap that resulted from their cognitive deficits, and the objectives become progressively more personalized and more related to the difficulties encountered by the patients in daily-life situations. An extreme example is the short contract we signed with a 65-year-old retired businessman with Wernicke's aphasia, which had a very precise demand: This man wanted to be able to propose a toast at his daughter's wedding!

THE THEORETICAL BACKGROUND

Our approaches in aphasia therapy are guided by two theoretical considerations. The first is that language behavior results from the functioning of complex processing and specific subcomponents; this is the cognitive root of our therapies. The second emphasizes that language is a communicative behavior which serves a variety of functions in natural situations. This constitutes the pragmatic side of our treatment rationale.

THE COGNITIVE ORIENTATION

If one considers that aphasia disorders result from a selective breakdown in a modular and complex architecture, then one should also emphasize that it is theoretically insufficient to plan therapy on the basis of symptom-level analysis of the disorders. From this perspective, it makes no sense at a theoretical level to have ready-made programs for Wernicke's or Broca's aphasias, or even ready-made programs for anomia or agrammatic deficits, because these aphasic syndromes or symptoms are highly heterogeneous. In cognitive neuropsychology many leading researchers consider that, in order to understand the nature of the disorders, it is necessary to conduct the analysis on a single case basis (Caramazza, 1986; Shallice, 1979). We would suggest that the same reasoning applies to therapy, and that, before starting therapy, the first step is to try to understand, on an individual basis, the nature of the underlying deficit that results in an aphasic symptom. This individually based evaluation is often time consuming. In our center, the analyses by which we understand the nature of the disorder often take 1 to 2 months. After formulating a hypothesis about the location of the underlying deficit, we then try either to reorganize function or re-establish it. From a less optimistic perspective, we may limit our interventions to trying to enhance the adaptation of the patient to specific everyday situations. The term functional reorganization implies that more or less the same behavior can be produced by recruiting other processing mechanisms. Functional re-establishment refers to reteaching the defective processes or representations. At the present time there is no cognitive rationale for choosing one alternative or the other (reorganization or re-establishment). It is probable that in the future such a decision will be more dependent upon neurobiological parameters, such as brain plasticity, and severity and location of the lesion, and less dependent on a cognitive analysis.

The reorganization rationale, which is more frequently used, is an important renewal in cognitive therapy of Luria's perspective (Luria, 1970). Having identified a disorder in a cognitive architecture, we try to demonstrate that, by using the nondefective components, we can improve the patient's performance. The only psychological condition required in this approach is that such a reorganization make sense in a cognitive architecture. That is, it is necessary to be able to specify that the same output in a cognitive system may be realized through the activation of other (undamaged) processing components. The existence of alternative routes could have been established either by previous experimental research in cognitive psychology or by the observation in neuropsychological studies of double dissociations, such as the lexical and nonlexical routes in reading. Another source of inspiration is to look at the existence of other potentially interesting mechanisms which may also be deduced from studies of the development of cognitive systems.

As illustrations of re-establishment rationale, we provide two examples of therapies performed in the BRNU. The first therapy involved a patient, SP, who had a deep-dyslexia (de Partz, 1986). That is, SP had a major alteration of the phonological process of reading and a partial deficit of the lexical process. Indeed, SP was unable to read isolated letters and nonwords, that is, to use the grapheme-phoneme conversion rules. His reading of words was better but not perfect; it was influenced by certain lexical and semantic variables such as grammatical class, frequency of use, and imagery. A therapy program was developed to reteach SP to use the phonological reading procedure by using spared lexical knowledge as a relay between simple and complex graphemes and their pronunciation. That is, we taught him to use a lexical code. The therapeutic program consisted of three stages: First, the association of the letter with the verbalization of a word (e.g., M → *"maman"* ["mother"]); second, the association of the letter with the first phoneme of each relay word (e.g., M → *"m . . . amam," "m"*); and third, the automatization of the use of the phonological procedure by training the reading of nonwords and by reteaching some graphemic contextual rules (e.g., conversion rule of the letter E, usually read /oe/ but changing to /E/ in a double consonant context as in *EFFET* [effect]). After a year of intensive practice to automate this strategy, the patient was able to read slowly and correctly.

The second course of therapy was conducted with a patient with surface dysgraphia (de Partz, Seron, & van der Linden, 1992). From the pretherapeutic investigation, we concluded that the patient, LP, presented an important dissociation between phonological and lexical writing procedures. The effects of regularity of spelling and frequency of use and the production of spelling regularizations suggested that he was forced to rely on the conversion of sub-word phonological segments into orthographic segments when he failed to access spellings stored in the orthographic output lexicon. Moreover, residual reading impairments were located at two levels in the cognitive system: in access to the visual input

lexicon, often preventing the patient from judging his own written productions as correct or incorrect, and in access to the semantic level, because of homophone confusions and a general semantic deficit not limited to reading.

The writing therapy consisted of two stages. In the first stage, we tried
to reinforce the better-spared phonological procedure of spelling by teaching the patient contextual conversion rules. For example, the French rule
specifying that, in an intervocalic position, phonemes /s/and /z/ have to
be converted into SS (as in *BOISSON* [drink]) and S (as in *MAISON*
[house]) respectively. In the second stage, we proposed to reteach the
spelling of some irregular and ambiguous words by means of an original technique, a visual imagery strategy. Indeed, because of his verbal
memory deficit we had to select a treatment procedure that did not require too much of a verbal memory load, as do techniques such as those
used by Hatfield (1982) and Behrmann (1987). Hence, for each word LP
spelled incorrectly, we associated a semantically related image with the
misspelled grapheme shape of the written words (see Figure 6–1). As
illustrated by this example, we tried to discover drawings with a semantic relationship with the word *PATHOLOGIE* (pathology) that were also
capable of integrating the shape of the defective graphemes. In this case,
the letter H was lengthened and transformed into a "hospital bed,"
which has a semantic relationship with *pathologie*. Then, a training procedure was used to teach a set of written words with their respective let-
ter-embedded drawings. The therapy was consequently item specific. In
post-therapy, we observed a selective imagery training effect: The words

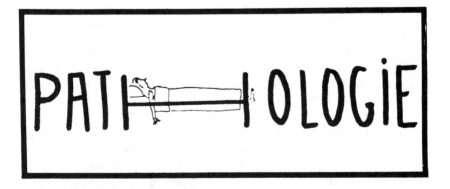

Figure 6–1. Example of drawing conceived for the imagery strategy in re-education.

trained with the visual-imagery strategy improved significantly in comparison with a classical methodology and with untrained words. Moreover, the lack of difference between words trained with drawings produced by the patient and with those produced by the therapist indicated that the patient, from a long-term functional perspective, was able to use his own drawings as effectively as those proposed by the therapist. The stability of these effects was corroborated 6 months after the end of therapy when the performance profile was not significantly different from that at the end of the therapy.

These two therapies were both aimed at re-establishing some functional behavior, but they were different with respect to the content of what was relearned. In the deep dyslexic case, the therapy consisted of re-establishing the functioning of a specific processing route in reading which permitted the transformation of graphemes into phonemes. Thus, a generalization of the improvement to material other than that used in therapy could be expected. In therapy for the surface dysgraphic patient, the objective was to reinstate missing information in a store by using imagery. Here the therapy is item specific, and one does not expect generalization to other stimuli unless the patient himself uses the imagery strategy to relearn the spelling of nontrained words.

The reorganization rationale is different and consists of the use of different processing from that used before the onset of the disorder. In some cases such a reorganization consists of reactivating a mode of processing that had existed at some earlier point in development.

Let us consider an example in number processing disorders. A patient may have specific difficulties accessing arithmetical facts (e.g., see the case DC, described by Warrington in 1982). This patient became unable to retrieve automatically the answer to simple arithmetical problems such as $3 + 5$, $6 - 7$, and so on. However, we know that during development there is an evolution of the strategy used by children to answer simple arithmetical problems: Before applying a retrieval strategy, children use counting-on or counting-all algorithms (Ashcraft, 1982). With patients who have difficulty accessing arithmetical facts, and who present no major difficulties in oral counting, it would be interesting to train them to re-utilize such a backup procedure in a more systematic way, rather than trying to re-establish automatic access to degraded or inaccessible stored knowledge. Such a reorganization rationale is, of course, possible only when at least two different procedures exist which, when correctly applied, can produce correct results and when it appears that one procedure has remained intact. We believe that a cognitive pretherapeutic examination should inform the therapist about the organization of the different cognitive architectures, to indicate if there are multiple routes, and to provide guidelines about which processing sub-components that could be used for re-education are intact.

THE LIMITS OF THE COGNITIVE APPROACH

As many authors have emphasized, at the present time our cognitive theories are about the architecture of stable cognitive systems, but they are not about cognitive change. However, what is of interest to speech therapists is promoting changes in linguistic or communicative behaviors. It can happen that, after proposing a cognitive interpretation of a disorder, one finds no cognitive theories capable of indicating how a damaged cognitive function can be restored, reorganized, or optimalized (Caramazza, 1989; Coltheart, Bates, & Castles, in press). One may thus ask about the relationships in clinical practice between cognitive theory and the elaboration of therapy (Wilson & Patterson, 1990). In our opinion the relationships are indirect, and the actual efficacy of cognitive approaches in therapy has yet to be demonstrated. The main interest in performing a detailed cognitive analysis of a disorder before the therapy is to indicate to the clinician which processing components are defective as well as which are still preserved. Then, after deciding upon one of the possible strategies (reorganization, re-establishment, optimalization, or modification of some environmental settings), the clinician must creatively develop exercises and materials which can be used to attain the therapeutic objectives. The re-educative enterprise thus remains an innovative activity, but in the selection of exercises and materials, the clinician should be guided by the pre-therapeutic cognitive analysis. That is, the clinician should be guided by what he or she knows about the patient's cognitive functioning. More precisely, for every exercise, the clinician should examine what kinds of processes are activated and ascertain whether these processes are still intact.

In some cases, such an analysis may help the clinician to organize the different steps in therapy. This was the case in the re-education of an anomic patient (Bachy & de Partz, 1989). Indeed, in the case of SP, while deep dyslexia was observed, a dissociation also appeared between oral naming, which was defective, and written naming, which was partially preserved. In some cases the patient wrote, or more often began to write, the words he was unable to produce orally (e.g., SP was unable to name the picture of a glass but said "wine" and wrote GLASS or to say "elephant" but wrote ELEPH). The naming therapy was planned to make use of the superiority of access to orthographic representation, and consisted of asking SP to visualize the form of the word (or word fragments) and to use this mental representation to induce the production of the oral counterpart. But because the written form had to be decoded before being uttered aloud, the naming therapy was subordinated to reading therapy. Naming therapy was started only after reading therapy had made possible a minimal decoding of graphemes, thus permitting SP to read the word fragments.

A major difference between cognitive and semiology-based or behavioral interventions lies in the formulation of the objectives. For example, in a semiology-based approach, the re-education of an agrammatic patient will have the objective of improving the production of complex grammatical structures. In a cognitive approach, the first step will be to try to identify the disorder responsible for the agrammatic verbal output. So if, as in studies by Byng (1988) and Nickels, Black, and Byng (1991), it seems that the verbal output deficit results from an impairment at the level of mapping thematic relations onto syntactical structures, then we should try to re-educate the patient using therapy methods that these authors proposed precisely for that difficulty. However, if it seems that the locus of the difficulty resides in the elaboration of syntactical structure, then one may prefer to use, for example, the reconstructive approach proposed by Naeser (1972). Because neuropsychological deficits may result from different subjacent disorders, we do not propose using general ready-made methods according to a semiological analysis.

The problem with our single-case cognitive approaches in re-education is, of course, that, in their present state of development, they apparently cannot be extrapolated or generalized. More specifically, we are not able to present results on groups of patients indicating that a specific method has been efficacious with a certain percentage of them. The risk of remaining anecdotal in presenting our results clearly constitutes a handicap, and we are well aware that to convince speech therapists, one has to present more consistent results. It should be noted, however, that the situation is gradually changing: Single-case oriented re-education may be replicated (Le Dorze, Jacob, & Coderre, 1991), and if the replication fails, this failure could itself be informative for designing other therapies. A clear example of this was recently offered by Nickels's (1992) attempt to replicate the de Partz deep dyslexic re-education. Initially her patient, TC, had succeeded in associating letters with "relay" words and then in associating letters with the initial phonemes of relay words. However, the patient encountered major difficulties when he was required to assemble single phonemes in the production of a word. At this point in the therapy, the de Partz procedure seemed to be inapplicable. A complementary investigation of the patient's disorders gave rise to the identification of an unnoticed disorder, the inability to blend strings of phonemes. The identification of this disorder resulted in a modification of the re-educative program, and Nickels used the relearning of letter/phoneme correspondences not to teach mechanisms for sublexical reading, as in the de Partz therapy, but to teach the patient to generate his own phonemic cues. These cues, together with an emphasis on semantic processing of words, allowed him to select a lexical entry in the phonological output lexicon. In this case, the contribution of theory occurred during the therapy. The fact that the de Partz therapy had not been efficacious with Nickels's patient cannot be used as an argument against the de Partz procedure. It simply means that the de Partz procedure is efficacious for some deep dyslexic patients; whereas the Nickels procedure is efficacious with other patients who, while also suffering from deep dyslexic reading disorders, had other subjacent deficits that caused their symptoms. The potential advantage of the cognitive approach lies in the fact that, given the detailed analysis of the patient's disorders before and during the therapy, categorizing the type of patient who might be a good candidate for a particular therapy is more fine-grained than it is for classical semiology-based approaches.

THE PRAGMATIC ORIENTATION

In addition to semiological and cognitive therapies directed at specific linguistic disorders, we propose functional rehabilitation for certain patients to improve their ability to communicate in everyday life. Among the various "functional" techniques, including role-playing activities, group therapies, and so forth (see Aten, Caligiuri, & Holland, 1982; Holland, 1982), we have chosen to apply Promoting Aphasics Communicative Effectiveness (PACE), the pragmatic approach to language rehabilitation developed by Davis (1989), and Davis and Wilcox (1981, 1985), and adapted in our Unit by Clerbaut, Coyette, Feyereisen, and Seron (1984). Based on the principle of natural and referential communication, the usual PACE setting is as follows: The clinician and the aphasic patients take turns picking up one from a stack of illustrated or written cards that are placed face down on the table between them. The basic task is to communicate the information that is depicted or written on the card without showing its face to the other participant. In contrast to role-playing activity and in accordance with learning principles, PACE treatment allows a modeling of communicative behaviors, with the clinician influencing the patient's behavior by acting appropriately in the situation. For all forms of PACE, the following principles have been established:

1. The treatment interaction consists of an exchange of new information between clinician and patient;
2. The clinician and the patient participate equally as sender and receiver of messages;
3. The patient is allowed free choice with respect to the selection of communicative channels with which to convey messages; and,
4. Feedback from the clinician is based on the patient's success in communicating a message and is characteristic of receiver feedback occurring in natural settings.

As now used in the BRNU, the PACE procedure has several unique features.

- First, at the beginning of the therapy, for psychological reasons, it is often necessary to convince patients that, even if their linguistic abilities are defective, they are still able to communicate. Thus, early in therapy, by distracting patients from the formal and linguistic aspects of their difficulties, PACE reduces anxiety and frustration, and shows patients that some communication is still possible.

- Second, insofar as the technique trains replacements for deficient linguistic abilities, it is applied only temporarily at the beginning of therapy in patients whose language improves significantly. It is used definitively in patients whose linguistic abilities remain inadequate.

- Third, the PACE procedure is usually proposed first in anosognosic patients to develop awareness that a problem exists. Indeed, in such a natural communication setting, it is easier to give concrete feedback on the lack of intelligibility of the message and/or the difficulties of comprehension.

- Fourth, the functional PACE setting can be used to train or to control the transfer of linguistic therapies. So, for example, if the clinician has retaught thematic relations to a patient with Broca's aphasia, it can be interesting to train that patient to transfer this learning to more functional speech acts which can be elicited in the PACE conversation setting.

- Fifth, the PACE procedure seems particularly indicated to treat pragmatic disabilities (difficulty maintaining a conversational topic, violation of some of the Grice conversational principles) observed in some patients with Wernicke's aphasia or with a frontal syndrome.

Despite these features, PACE has some limitations. First, centered on referential communication, the PACE setting could be inappropriate for aphasic patients who present cognitive deficits other than language disorders (e.g., difficulty in extracting relevant information from pictures). Second, restricted to referential conversation, this therapeutic technique cannot cover all the speech acts encountered by the patient in everyday life. To lessen this problem, other variants are proposed, such as describing spatial configurations to the communicative partner in such a way that the partner can produce them precisely without seeing them. Similarly, each participant can be required to ask the other questions, for the purpose of discovering the content of a picture that is placed out of sight.

If the PACE technique, like other pragmatic therapies, contributes greatly to improving communicative effectiveness, let us point out that other methods also help in achieving this objective, and are often more appropriate. Indeed, some therapists restrict their therapeutic intervention with aphasics to pragmatic therapies. We do not believe it is sufficient to place patients in natural conversational settings, in role-playing, or in group settings to resolve linguistic difficulties. Most of the pragmatic approaches aim to develop *compensations* for linguistic disturbances, not *treatments for* them. Moreover, if the relations between language and its use in context seem to be evident, we still lack knowledge about the cognitive mechanisms that control these relations. From this point of view, pragmatic therapies remain empirical.

A REALISTIC APPRAISAL

The cognitive analysis of language disorders is a complex enterprise which is time-consuming and requires a solid theoretical foundation. A speech therapist engaged in many different therapies probably does not know all of the current theoretical models of psycholinguistic functioning and does not have time to examine every patient in depth. Thus, the orientation we have described is surely unrealistic for private speech therapy interventions, and requires the collaboration of several therapists, each with his or her own specialization, in a rehabilitation center. As a result of rapid developments of these models, cognitive test batteries need to be brought up to date. Frequent changes in a battery could be prejudicial to the reliability of the test/retest procedure in the same patient.

Nevertheless, despite these limitations, we argue that an attempt systematically to connect cognitive analysis and re-educative practices seems an interesting and valuable enterprise. It is premature to affirm the effectiveness of cognitive approaches. At present it makes no sense to compare, on a quantitative basis, cognitive versus empirical approaches. In the actual state of the art, many successes or failures in therapy are dependent on the intuitions (or "trial and error") of the therapists, rather than resulting from a cognitive pre-therapeutic evaluation. However, the main reason to look at more efficacious methods for language therapy results from the feeble evidence regarding their actual efficacy. In fact, it has been suggested that, in the language domain, therapies performed by professionals are no more efficacious than therapies by informed volunteers, or naive volunteers, and it has even been suggested that patients do just as well with no treatment at all. (On this point see the controversial discussion on language intervention that has occupied speech therapists in England for over a decade: David, Enderby, & Bainton, 1982; Lincoln, et al., 1984; Meikle, et al., 1979.)

In our opinion, given the current state of development, the major question is not whether cognitive therapies are or are not more efficacious than classical therapies. The question is whether cognitive therapies are efficacious and whether they actually propose another rationale that can help to move clinical practice forward in this field. At the present time one can only bet.

REFERENCES

Ashcraft, M. H. (1982). The development of mental arithmetic: A chronometric approach. *Developmental Review, 2,* 213–236.

Aten, J., Caligiuri, M., & Holland, A. (1982). The efficacy of functional communication therapy for chronic aphasic patients. *Journal of Speech and Hearing Disorders, 47,* 93–96.

Bachy, N., & de Partz, M. P. (1989). Coordination of two reorganization therapies in a deep dyslexic patient with oral naming disorder. In X. Seron & G. Deloche (Eds.), *Cognitive approaches in neuropsychological rehabilitation* (pp. 211–247). London: Lawrence Erlbaum.

Behrmann, M. (1987). The rites of righting writing: Homophone remediation in acquired dysgraphia. *Cognitive Neuropsychology, 4*(3), 365–384.

Byng, S. (1988). Sentence processing deficits: Theory and therapy. *Cognitive Neuropsychology, 5*(6), 629–676.

Caramazza, A. (1986). On drawing inferences about the structure of normal cognitive systems from the analysis of patterns of impaired performance: The case for single-patient studies. *Brain and Cognition, 5,* 41–66.

Caramazza, A. (1989). Cognitive neuropsychology and rehabilitation: An unfulfilled promise? In X. Seron & G. Deloche (Eds.), *Cognitive approaches in neuropsychological rehabilitation* (pp. 383–398). London: Lawrence Erlbaum.

Clerbaut, N., Coyette, F., Feyereisen, P., & Seron, X. (1984). Une méthode de rééducation fonctionnelle des aphasiques: La P.A.C.E. *Rééducation Orthophonique, 22,* (138), 329–344.

Coltheart, M., Bates, A., & Castles, A. (in press). Cognitive neuropsychology and rehabilitation. In G. Humphreys & J. Riddoch (Eds.), *Cognitive neuropsychology and cognitive rehabilitation.* London: Lawrence Erlbaum.

David, D., Enderby, P., & Bainton, D. (1982). Treatment of acquired aphasia: Speech therapists and volunteers compared. *Journal of Neurology, Neurosurgery, and Psychiatry, 45,* 957–961.

Davis, G. (1989). Pragmatics and cognition in treatment of language disorders. In X. Seron & G. Deloche (Eds.), *Cognitive approaches in neuropsychological rehabilitation* (pp. 317–353). London: Lawrence Erlbaum.

Davis, G., & Wilcox, M. (1981). Incorporating parameters of natural conversation in aphasia treatment. In R. Chapey (Ed.), *Language intervention strategies in adult aphasia* (pp. 169–193). Baltimore, MD: Williams & Wilkins.

Davis, G., & Wilcox, M. (1985). *Adult aphasia rehabilitation: Applied pragmatics.* Windsor: NFER-Nelson.

de Partz, M. P. (1986). Re-education of a deep dyslexic patient: Rational of the method and results. *Cognitive Neuropsychology, 3,* 149–177.

de Partz, M. P., Seron, X., & van der Linden, M. (1992). Re-education of a surface dysgraphic patient with a visual imagery strategy. *Cognitive Neuropsychology, 9*(5), 369–401.

Hatfield, M. F. (1982). Diverses formes de désintégration du langage écrit et implication pour la rééducation. In X. Seron & C. Laterre (Eds.), *Rééduquer le cerveau* (pp. 135–156). Brussels: Mardaga.

Holland, A. (1982). Observing functional communication of aphasic adults. *Journal of Speech and Hearing Disorders, 47,* 50–56.

Le Dorze, G., Jacob, A., & Coderre, L. (1991). Aphasia rehabilitation with a case of agrammatism: A partial replication. *Aphasiology, 5*(1), 63–85.

Lincoln, N. B., Mulley, G. P., Jones, A. L., McGuirk, E., Lendrem, W., & Mitchell, J. R. A. (1984). Effectiveness of speech therapy for aphasic stroke patients: A randomised controlled trial. *The Lancet, 8388,* 1197–1200.

Luria, A. R. (1970). *Traumatic aphasia.* The Hague: Mouton.

Meikle, M., Wechsler, E., Tupper, A., Benenson, M., Butler, J., Mulhall, D., & Stern, G. (1979). Comparative trial of volunteer and professional treatments of dysphasia after stroke. *British Medical Journal, 2,* 87–89.

Naeser, M. A. (1972). A structured approach teaching aphasics basic sentence types. *British Journal of Disorders of Communication, 5,* 70–76.

Nickels, L. (1992). The autocue? Self-generated phonemic cues in the treatment of a disorder of reading and naming. *Cognitive Neuropsychology, 9,* 155–182.

Nickels, L., Black, M., & Byng, S. (1991). Les déficits du traitement de la phrase: Théorie et thérapie. In M. P. de Partz & M. Leclercq (Eds.), *La rééducation neuropsychologique de l'adulte* (pp. 99–117). Paris: Publication de la Société de Neuropsychologie de Langue Francaise.

Shallice, T. (1979). Case-study approach in neuropsychological research. *Journal of Clinical Neuropsychology, 1,* 183–211.

Warrington, E. K. (1982). The fractionation of arithmetical skills: A single case study. *Quarterly Journal of Experimental Psychology, 34A,* 31–51.

Wilson, B., & Patterson, K. E. (1990). Rehabilitation and cognitive neuropsychology: Does cognitive psychology apply? *Applied Cognitive Psychology, 4,* 247–260.

CHAPTER 7

The Concept of Holistic Rehabilitation of Persons with Aphasia

MARIA PACHALSKA

Institute and Clinic of Rehabilitation
Academy of Physical Education
Cracow, Poland

The concept of holistic rehabilitation of patients with aphasia is presented in this chapter. First, some information on the history of aphasia therapy in Poland is presented. Next, principles of assessment are discussed. Then, the theoretical framework of holistic rehabilitation is given, with emphasis on a model for aphasia therapy called the Complex Aphasia Rehabilitation Model (CARM) (Pachalska, 1986a). Methods for both individuals and groups, focused on the stimulation and training of language functions, cognitive functions, and communication in general are discussed. Finally, the efficacy of the treatment is shown. It is emphasized that the primary goal of holistic rehabilitation of an aphasic person is the restoration of his or her effective communication, as well as the fullest possible reintegration into society.

DEFINITION OF HOLISTIC REHABILITATION

One meaning of rehabilitation is restoration of efficiency. Although authors dispute the nature of rehabilitation, they agree that its basic purpose is to reintegrate persons with aphasia into society as active participants. Holistic rehabilitation provides treatment aimed toward fulfilling biological, psychological, and social needs, thus increasing the potential for good health. This in turn makes it possible to continue physical and mental activity into very old age, to eliminate some disorders, and to prevent social dependence. Holistic rehabilitation attempts to work out effective ways to help disabled persons satisfy their own needs and give them opportunities: (1) to develop effective communication and optimum social activity; (2) to reintegrate, as fully as possible, into society; and (3) to share each others' experiences.

The World Health Organization (WHO) defines rehabilitation as a complex coordinated use of medical, social, educational, and occupational means to adapt a disabled person to new ways of life, and to enable him or her to attain a maximum recovery and return to society. WHO's statement reaffirms the notion that treatment should not end when an individual acquires physical health, but should lead to the resumption of an active social life. However, it requires qualification. Because brain damage affects both private and social life,

> a notion of "disability" cannot be measured only as physical disfunction (sic), but with situational circumstances . . ., the WHO statement requires further clarification. Each man has his own image of his psychological ability and it accordingly forms his needs. The needs of a man of high intellectual abilities differ from those of a man of exceptional physical skills. Thus, "disability" means the inability to realize man's needs; individual and social aspects of self realization. (Pachalska, 1986a, p. 15)

ETIOLOGY OF APHASIA

Aphasia resulting from stroke is a serious problem in Poland. Stroke is the major cause of aphasia (76.5–81.4% of cases in Poland), followed by head injury (5.1–13.7%) and brain tumor (4.6–9.6%). A survey conducted by the Ministry of Health and Social Welfare (1989) reported that 538,000 patients (357,000 men and 181,000 women, a ratio of roughly 3:2) received some type of medical care for cerebrovascular accidents (CVAs) in 1988 in Poland. These figures do not include chronic post-stroke patients who did not seek medical care, so the actual number of patients with CVAs may be greater.

Stroke distribution with respect to age, gender, and region was studied in 1982, 1985, 1987, and 1989. Stroke was found to be more frequent in big cities than in villages, and more frequent in men than in women. An increase in the incidence of stroke, especially in men, was noted in cities during the years 1982–1989. A tendency for stroke to occur at earlier ages was noted over the study period, especially in men living in cities, with most strokes occurring between the ages of 50 and 69.

A BRIEF HISTORY OF APHASIA THERAPY IN POLAND

The first account of aphasia recovery in Poland was given in 1883 by a prominent Polish physician, Ludwik Bierkowski (1837). From then until the 1950s, the major focus of investigations (conducted mostly by neurologists and neurosurgeons) tended to be clinico-pathological correlates of aphasia. In 1969, a systematic study of aphasia in Poland was done by Jerzy Konorski, a neurologist, and Lucjan Stepien, a neurosurgeon at the Metropolitan Psychoneurological Institute in Pruszkow in collaboration with H. Kozniewska, S. Mempel, J. Szumska, and S. Zarski. They concentrated on correlating aphasia with the site of the lesion. Since Konorski's death, this neurophysiological research has been continued by his collaborators.

The early 1960s marked the beginning of psychological research in aphasia. At that time, Mariusz Maruszewski, a disciple of Luria, performed intensive studies of brain mechanisms of speech, aphasia recovery, and therapy at Warsaw University (Maruszewski, 1966). He also created "A Team of Speech Therapy" which undertook examination and therapy of aphasic patients in the Medical Academy in Warsaw. Currently, neuropsychological studies of aphasia are carried out in Warsaw (D. Kadzielawa), in Cracow (M. Pachalska), in Lublin (B. Kaczmarek, M. Klimkowski, A. Herzyk), and in Wroclaw (J. Przesmycka-Kaminska).

Treatment programs for specific higher cortical functions, using cognitive approaches, have been developed and evaluated in the Cracow Center of Aphasiology by the author and her colleagues (Kaczmarek, 1991; Pachalska, 1980). Neurolinguistic research on patients with aphasia was initiated in Cracow in 1953 by the late Janina Lopatkiewicz, a neurolinguist. Lopatkiewicz and colleagues described stability or variability in disorders of naming responses (Lopatkiewicz, 1961, 1988).

In the latter half of the 1960s a Laboratory of Brain Mechanisms of Speech was created by Witold Doroszewski at the Institute of Polish Language in the Polish Academy of Sciences. The Laboratory, now under the direction of linguist Halina Mierzejewska, explores the disintegration of the language system in aphasia. Neurolinguistic studies are also being carried out in Crakow (M. Zarebina), in Gdansk (W. Tlokinski), in Lublin (B. L. J. Kaczmarek, M. Klimkowski), in Poznan (M. Safinska-Fechner), and in Warsaw (M. Sadowska). Treatment programs for language functions were introduced by Maruszewski (1974); Szumska (1980); Kadzielawa and Romero (1978); Tlokinski (1986); and Pachalska (1986a, 1990).

Several factors resulted in the aphasia treatment currently in common practice in Poland. These factors include the advent of speech pathology as a health profession, the emergence of rehabilitation medicine as a medical specialty, the mass media explosion with resultant greater public interest in aphasia, and a climate of increased medical expectations in an age of technology. As social and attitudinal changes took place, logopedia (speech-language pathology) grew rapidly.

Logopedia was introduced in Poland by L. Kaczmarek (senior) in the early 1960s in Lublin. This discipline is concerned with all aspects of linguistic communication and, therefore, corresponds to what is sometimes called human communication studies in the United States (for more detail, see B. L. J. Kaczmarek, 1991). A number of professional associations was formed, among them the Polish Society of Logopedics, the Polish Society of Aphasiology, and the Polish Neuropsychological Society.

Present day professional training of logopedists is quite complex. Logopedists take a 2-year post-graduate program leading to a diploma in logopedics. This program is offered at four institutions: Lublin (established in 1970), Warsaw (1974), Gdansk (1980), and Cracow (1984). To be admitted to these programs, a candidate must have a master's degree in clinical psychology, pedagogy, linguistics, or physiotherapy. Also required is an internship in speech and language therapy.

Another important step was the creation of the Cracow Center of Aphasiology, started in 1980 by the author. Devoted to studies of assessment and treatment, this Center includes: the Aphasiology Research Laboratory at the Institute of Rehabilitation of the AWF; the Cracow Aphasia Rehabilitation Center "Afa-Club"; and the Aphasia Clinic, including a Laboratory of Art Therapy, in the Rehabilitation Center of the AWF in Witkowice (near Cracow). Also in 1980, the author developed a Complex Aphasia Rehabilitation Model (CARM), and later evaluated its effectiveness (Pachalska, 1986a). CARM was also successfully implemented and evaluated at the Aphasia Ward in Gdansk, headed by W. Tlokinski (1990).

A further important step was the development of rehabilitation clubs called "Afa-Clubs." These clubs are designed to provide social and community-based services for aphasic patients and to share the Cracow experience with patients in seven other regions of Poland.

Recently, public interest in aphasia problems has greatly increased, partly because of a series of articles and films about famous Polish public figures, such as the pianist Maria Lasocka and the painter Krystyna Habura, both of whom have recovered from stroke and aphasia (Pachalska & Knapik, 1988a, 1990). Special television programs have been introduced, such as "Bariery" (Barriers), which focus on disabled persons (including persons with aphasia) living in society. National journals devoted to problems encountered by disabled people, such as *Czlowiek* (The Man), part of which focuses on aphasia, are also being published. Deeper insights into aphasia are provided by personal accounts of people who have recovered from aphasia in a special annual journal of patients, *Afa-Echo*. Rehabilitation of patients with aphasia has also been influenced by the dramatic increase of strokes, especially in men who are still in their productive years, but also in young children, as well as by the increase of traffic accidents.

During the course of establishing aphasia research in Poland, a number of theories have been developed. Although theoretical differences exist, all approaches are based on clinical studies, and research is closely connected with therapy. The Polish Societies of Aphasiology and Neuropsychology coordinate and integrate the various approaches.

ASSESSMENT

Assessment of aphasic patients in Poland is conducted mainly by neurologists, neuropsychologists, logopedists, and neurolinguists. The purpose of neurological assessment is primarily to determine the nature and symptomatology of the disorder, the site of the lesion, and the response to medical treatment. The neuropsychological assessment aims at discovering the nature of cognitive, memory, and perceptual disorders, and at characterizing the linguistic disturbances in their broadest aspect. The goal of the neurolinguistic evaluation is to provide insight into the language disturbances. It does so by conducting linguistic analyses of the patient's utterances and then determining the interaction of various linguistic levels. The logopedic assessment generally addresses the phenomenon of aphasia, its structure and symptoms; differential diagnosis of aphasia and other linguistic disorders; and questions concerning the dynamic characteristics of aphasia (cognitive functions, memory, emotional, and motivational aspects, personality, etc.).

Results of these evaluations are related to how patients with aphasia communicate, and which channel of communication they are able to use effectively. It is also important to know how aphasia affects interpersonal functions. This assessment attempts to provide a prognosis and to select the most fruitful goals and areas for rehabilitation.

In most neurological and rehabilitation wards in Poland. Luria's approach is used. Some clinics, however, have begun to use the standardized Cracow Test. The standardized Cracow Test of Differential Diagnosis of Aphasia (CTDDA) (Pachalska, Kaczmarek, & Knapik, 1991) samples a wide variety of language behaviors at different levels of difficulty. It was standardized on a representative group of native Polish healthy adults, and 240 persons with aphasia. The standardized version of CTDDA is the result of a systematic revision of the experimental version (Pachalska, 1986a).

The CTDDA distinguishes four basic types of aphasia: (1) paradigmatic, (2) syntagmatic, (3) mixed, and (4) global. This neurolinguistic taxonomy of aphasia results from clinical verification and modification of Kaczmarek's theoretical classification of aphasia (1991); however, it includes two additional forms of aphasia, mixed and global. The three final indexes are Linguistic Functions Index (LFI), Aphasia Index (AI), and Brain Damage Index (BDI).

To supplement the information obtained using the standard test battery, a variety of standardized and nonstandardized tests, aimed at specific language and communication disorders, is used. They are:

The Token Test (DeRenzi & Vignolo, 1962);

Communicative Abilities in Daily Living (CADL) (Holland, 1980);

The Edinburgh Functional Communication Profile (Skinner, Wirtz, & Thompson, 1984); and

Communicative Abilities in Social Situations (Pachalska & Knapik, 1989).

The author and her colleagues have recently translated and standardized the Boston Diagnostic Aphasia Examination (BDAE) (Goodglass & Kaplan, 1983). Also during 1991, the author began translation and standardization of the Western Aphasia Battery (WAB) (Kertesz, 1982), and the Müller and Code Scale of Psychosocial Adjustment (Müller & Code, 1989). These represent important steps in international cooperation.

HOLISTIC REHABILITATION OF PATIENTS WITH APHASIA

Holistic rehabilitation in Poland focuses on therapy that is planned, organized, and provided on the basis of a detailed understanding of a patient's individual needs. Treatment is provided during acute care, home care, and posthospital rehabilitation.

STAGES OF TREATMENT

ACUTE CARE

We introduced early rehabilitation in our center, and as a result, stimulation during the coma stage begins the rehabilitation process. Cognitive retraining is the ongoing and integrated rehabilitation procedure used by the therapeutic team. Rehabilitation is focused on the patient and the effects of the illness, but once the patient leaves a hospital, the specific needs of the family are also paramount.

HOME CARE

After 6 to 8 weeks of treatment for stroke or head trauma, a patient is sent home or to a nursing home and often ceases to receive rehabilitation services. A previously effective home health program is currently not functioning because of financial problems. The Polish Society of Aphasiology is planning to implement a rehabilitation program that will provide care in rehabilitation units, patients' homes, and nursing homes.

POSTHOSPITAL REHABILITATION

Long-term rehabilitation often follows the acute care phase. Rehabilitation services are provided in day facilities, inpatient wards and clinics, "Afa-Clubs," and in social and community-based facilities. Success in rehabilitation is often related to long-term maintenance, so practitioners try to establish good relationships among the various institutions and services.

The therapeutic team is assembled according to the patient's needs and stage of rehabilitation. It includes a specialist in rehabilitation medicine, a neurologist, a neuropsychiatrist (if needed), a nurse, a physiotherapist, an occupational therapist, a neuropsychologist, a neurolinguist, a logopedist, a social worker, a vocational instructor, and an orthotics and prosthetics technician, as well as family, friends, and volunteers.

We employ a program, prepared by the author (Pachalska, 1986a), for training the therapeutic team in a multidisciplinary approach to rehabilitation. Each member of the rehabilitation team lectures to the trainees, paying special attention to teaching them how to communicate with an aphasic patient, how to use gestures, drawings, and special materials (pictograms, communication boards, itineraries, and so on). Therapists also are taught, through videotapes, to "read" facial expressions and gestures. This training is also provided to the family members and is one of three parts of counseling in CARM.

Group clinicians and family members are also trained in functional strategies during cognitive group sociotherapy. Active assistance of family members (the second part of counseling), important in group therapy, is provided to strengthen the family ties. This training also helps to solicit reinforcement and facilitate generalization, as stressed by Kearns (1986). In addition, any modality (e.g. verbal, gestural, writing, drawing), that can be used to communicate successfully is accepted, reinforced, and programmed in the group setting at home.

Studies of behavior videorecorded during group therapy (Knapik & Knapik, 1990; Pachalska, 1986c) have shown that trained therapists achieve a significantly more precise level of communication in their patients by increasing the number and complexity of gestures. Gestures are slowed down and pauses are frequent and longer for therapeutic purposes.

ATTRIBUTES OF HOLISTIC REHABILITATION

Clinical rehabilitation procedures include a series of dynamically interacting steps:

- gathering necessary information about language and communication disorders as well as related problems by means of testing and observational methods;

- framing hypotheses about the nature and course of the problem based on a critical analysis of the data gathered; and

- testing these hypotheses during therapeutic intervention.

The above steps are accounted for in the Complex Aphasia Rehabilitation Model (CARM) (Pachalska, 1986a). CARM provides for the selection of specific therapeutic procedures for the particular physical, psychological, and social needs of the aphasic individual, identified through diagnosis as well as through therapeutic observations during the rehabilitation process. CARM includes five basic therapeutic techniques for individual and group treatment (including community-based treatment). The treatment consists of physiotherapy, occupational therapy, logotherapy, psychotherapy, and sociotherapy oriented not only for standard treatment but also for stimulation and training of language functions, cognitive functions, and communication. All of these techniques have been described in detail in previous work (Pachalska, 1986a).

The main attributes of CARM originated from Dega's theory of rehabilitation. His theory was first introduced at the Poznan Rehabilitation Clinic in the early 1950s and later elaborated on by his collaborators and disciples (Dega, 1975; Dega & Milanowska, 1988; Grochmal & Zielinska-Charszewska, 1980; Pachalski, 1988; Weiss, 1961). Four aspects of rehabilitation are emphasized: universality, early intervention, complexity, and continuity. Each is described below.

Universality means that rehabilitation is an integral part of basic treatment and embraces all main disciplines in inpatient and outpatient health services. It is available to any citizen who needs it.

Early intervention means beginning rehabilitation simultaneously with basic treatment, which markedly improves the results and shortens the period of treatment.

Complexity refers to the team. Rehabilitation should include medical, occupational, and social applications.

Continuity refers to the process of therapy. The process, once begun, should continue until the patient achieves maximum psychic and physical capability, as well as the ability to work and/or to resume his or her place in society. This rehabilitation profile has been fully implemented in only six rehabilitation centers in Poland, among them, the Cracow Center.

THEORETICAL FRAMEWORK OF HOLISTIC REHABILITATION UNDER CARM

The theoretical framework of CARM assumes that complex reorganization of disturbed functional systems of the brain can take place as the result of the interaction of internal (concerned with the patient) and external (therapeutic and environmental) factors during holistic rehabilitation (Pachalska, 1986a, 1989).

The hypothesis of complex reorganization of disturbed functional systems is based on recent data on the activity and reintegration possibilities of the brain according to the theory of brain plasticity (Grochmal, 1985), reorganization of functional systems (Luria, 1963), reorganization of image processes (Pachalska, 1991b), and mechanisms of social integration (Finkelstein, 1980).

CARM is based on our theory of aphasia as well as on our Neurobehavioural Model of Communication (NMC) (for a description, see Pachalska, 1986a), which is published (in part) in English (Pachalska, 1991a). Another influence is the Neurocybernetic Model of Image Processing (NMIP) (for a description, see Pachalska, 1991b). On these bases we are able to recognize disturbed and preserved language and cognitive capabilities, organize therapeutic information, and select therapeutic procedures according to patient needs.

MODELING PERCEPTIVENESS AND EXPRESSIVENESS OF THE PATIENT

Properly organized therapeutic intervention requires the selection of the correct channel of intervention, as well as the use of an adequate proportion of nonlinguistic to linguistic material in modeling perception through intra- and intersensory stimulation and through intra- and intersystemic processing of information. Clinicians also must model patient expressiveness. Clinicians must control the information flow, and encourage patients to use any channel they can. Clinicians must make certain that patients comprehend a given message.

In stimulation and training, information may be arranged in three main ways: Selective, systematic, and mixed. These are defined as follows: (1) selective arrangement concentrates on communication without taking into account the patient's linguistic competence; (2) systematic organization of information entails combining a sequence of messages and their practical application in the Polish culture; and (3) the mixed configuration, obviously, is a combination of the two arrangements.

In our clinic we focus mainly on systematic configuration of therapeutic information because our research shows that aphasic patients understand this configuration significantly better than they do a selective or "mixed" presentation (Pachalska, 1988a). Therefore, we prefer socioculturally oriented materials such as popular poems, word games, and other types of materials such as postcards, photos, pictures, or toy animals. Such materials create social interactions, and are especially helpful in stimulating communication in real-life situations.

In our center, we are very attentive to the emotional coloring of nonlinguistic material sent through visual and acoustic channels, as well as through the haptic channel, specifically of touch. This approach increases the possibility of patients' understanding and remembering complex situations as well as integrating and generalizing them.

In holistic rehabilitation the special role of touch may be characterized in two ways. The first concerns contact with things, and the second describes contact with other people. Thus, touch allows sensuous perception of objects, which in turn makes the polymodal connections that enable the imaging of complex situations. The sense of touch also expresses the social ties of the patient with others. Contemporary aphasiologists appreciate a role for touch in the restoration of gnosis and nomination, but few acknowledge the role of touch in interhuman contacts in the process of rehabilitation. Positive ties, as is well known, are related to positive emotions, which, according to our model, improve the effectiveness of rehabilitation in general, including communication.

NEEDS-ORIENTED THERAPEUTIC INTERVENTION

Therapeutic intervention in holistic rehabilitation can be provided in either an unstructured or a structured format, according to the patient's needs.

Unstructured methodology corresponds to what others call a "stimulation approach" (Schuell, Jenkins, & Jimenez-Pabon, 1964; Wepman, 1951). This type of therapy is provided by all of the therapeutic specialists in our center. Adequate stimuli are presented to elicit target responses, which are selectively reinforced to facilitate within the brain the complex reorganization of function necessary for linguistic operations.

Stimulation methods are used in two groups of patients: Those in whom language disorders have precipitated psychogenic changes in attitude toward their own capability and toward the environment; and those in whom the disorders are a consequence of neurodynamic brain disturbances, observed in particular shortly after brain damage.

The basic approach of stimulation methods is to create therapeutic situations that facilitate language output. This is done to make patients aware that they can accomplish a given task and to give positive reinforcement for all utterances.

Structured methodologies rely heavily on information processing models to provide principles and steps used. We use a direct and indirect language-oriented approach and a cognitive approach. Two structured methods aimed at social communication have also been introduced (Knapik, 1990; Pachalska, 1988b).

LANGUAGE-ORIENTED APPROACHES

Language-oriented approaches are introduced primarily for improving language functions. Different methods are applied according to the severity and the neurolinguistic type of aphasia.

This training is direct. For the most part, direct methods are used with patients in whom some reserves in the damaged hemisphere are observed, or when there are indications that the disturbed function can be assumed by the healthy hemisphere, that is, that dominance for language is not complete. Linguistic skills are developed in two ways. The first concerns the communicative situation itself, with the situation serving as a focus for developing individual skills. This can be seen as a "top down" approach. Another way of developing skills is a "bottom up" approach in which the training of individual modalities is stressed; in this way the patient is provided with sufficient support to be able to convey messages.

Linguistic material used in language-oriented methodologies falls into two major categories: Grammatical (phonetic, prosodic, structural) and literary (lyric, epic, dramatic). Materials can be verbal, written (also Braille if needed for blind persons), or gestured (if needed, or for deaf persons).

Paradigmatic aphasia training is focused on phonology, morphology, and syntax. Therapists try to help the patient to comprehend simple words (always remembering that patients have problems understanding ambiguous and complex notions), simple and complex phrases, and finally texts. Simultaneously, the patient is asked to build utterances, beginning with saying and/or writing simple and complex words, then phrases, and finally texts. Patients are trained to participate in dialogue and conversation and to participate in discourse.

Syntagmatic aphasia training is focused on phonology, lexicon, and semantics. Therapists attempt to stimulate imagery as a way to help patients express themselves, providing examples of the correct pronunciation of a given text (word, phrase). Subsequently, the patient practices vocal and graphic expression. Materials and techniques are designed to develop the ability to "see" appropriate objects in the case of words, and simple or complex situations, in the case of phrases or more complex texts.

In mixed aphasia, training is focused on reception as well as expression, with proportions of attention to each depending on the nature of the disturbances. If the patient manifests more paradigmatic than syntagmatic disturbances, the therapy program includes more exercises in reception than expression. If the patient's problems are more syntagmatic, expression is trained first. Indirect methods, as described for global aphasia below, are introduced if necessary.

In global aphasia, because the structures concerned with linguistic communication are completely destroyed and the patient must acquire language skills in a new way, we initially introduce indirect (minor hemisphere) methods of therapy. Nonlinguistic stimulation and training are given through visual, auditory, and kinesthetic channels. Several different types of stimuli and methods are used. For the visual channel, we use a modification of Visual Action Therapy (VAT) (Helm-Estabrooks, Fitzpatrick, & Baresi, 1982). For the acoustic channel, a modification of the nonverbal version of Intonation Therapy (TMR) is introduced (Van Eeckhout, Hornado, Bhatt, & Ceblais, 1983). The kinesthetic channel is accessed through Kinaesthetic Therapy for Apraxia (KTA) (Pachalska, 1983). Stimulation might also include the senses of smell and taste, if appropriate. Thus, functioning is rebuilt by using the abilities that are preserved.

When the profile of a recovering patient with global aphasia seems to be similar to severe paradigmatic, severe syntagmatic, or severe mixed aphasia, additional direct language training is introduced. Such patients are trained in comprehension and production of spoken and written (and sometimes gestured) texts.

COGNITIVE APPROACHES

Cognitive approaches aim at improving specific cortical functions. Programs using this approach are based on cognitive neuropsychology and information processing models. The main goal of therapy is to isolate the mental processes that can be regarded as functionally modular, and to specify the mechanism of each, as well as the interrelationships among particular processes. The use of this approach, therefore, allows clinicians to make inferences about the specific processes that might be impaired in a given patient, which in turn provides a rationale for planning step-by-step rehabilitation procedures.

Using highly structured cognitive programs we train memory (Knapik, 1989) and thinking processes (Pachalska, 1982). We also attempt to reduce depression and anxiety (Pachalska & Knapik, 1988b). However, our center also employs less structured programs of art therapy combining direct (Kuzak [Pachalska], 1978) and indirect (Pachalska, 1988a) language-oriented methodologies with cognitive training. One such program is a "newcomer" to the range of therapeutic procedures incorporated in CARM: Language Oriented Art Therapy (LOAT) offered in individual and group sessions (see Pachalska, 1988c, 1990).

LOAT consists of two subprograms: The first, Objective-Practical Therapy, is for all patients; the second, Symbolic Thought Therapy, is mainly for patients who exhibit artistic skills.

Objective-Practical Therapy includes diagnosis and therapy. Diagnosis includes evaluation of disturbances in drawings; creative abilities, including the capability of decoding and encoding appropriate symbols, and the ability to perceive and create artistic forms; and the need for artistic expression. The therapy begins with stimulation to create. Selected drawings, pictures, pieces of music, poetry, and so forth are used as stimuli. The patients are required to present their impressions through drawing, painting, and/or modeling (a) essential elements, (b) the main topic, (c) mood, and (d) the creation of the final work.

The team discusses ideas for creation of the final work. This is especially useful when patients produce a joint work of art. Extra stimulation (e.g., a piece of music presented for interpretation in drawing) might be presented to encourage patients to assess the critical relationship between the work's theme and the artistic product.

In Symbolic Thought Therapy, patients who exhibit artistic skills or those who were practicing artists learn to "read" works of art in order to be able to create. In this program we develop symbols and symbolic work. Patients are trained to perceive and express their impressions. An example of the success of this program is provided by Figure 7–1, a picture by the famous painter Krystyna Habura, who recovered symbolic thought when engaged in LOAT following a stroke.

The procedures used in both artistic and linguistic activities correspond to the stages used in the first program. A wide range of artistic activities is employed, including drawing with pencil, charcoal, chalk, crayon, or ink; painting with oil and water colors; producing graphics; engraving plastic and wood; modeling, and making cut-outs. Additional activities are introduced, if necessary, to improve knowledge of the semantics of colors and forms.

During LOAT we use polymodal (nonlinguistic and linguistic) stimuli, and patients are encouraged to express themselves through any usable channel. LOAT is conducted jointly by a professional artist trained in the

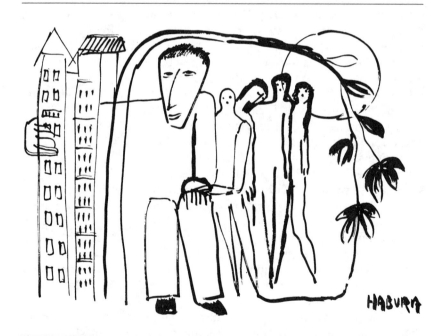

Figure 7–1. Picture of self-reintegration by an aphasic painter, assisted by other patients and the therapist (by courtesy of Krystyna Habura, 1991).

principles of communication and a logopedist, with the cooperation and supervision of a neuropsychologist, a neurolinguist, and a neuroanthropologist as well as of prominent art, music, and theater critics.

The most spectacular effects with art therapy have been achieved in artists who suffered from aphasia. One example is Maria Lasocka, a prominent Polish pianist with deep syntagmatic (motor) aphasia and right hand hemiparesis. She participated in art therapy aimed at restoring the skills required for playing the piano. In addition to CARM, therapy was designed to help the pianist to reorganize rhythmic structures, learn to write, read, and play musical notes with the right hand supported by the left, retrieve known and unknown melodies, and to compose. Some indirect stimulation techniques were also used, such as painting, drawing, and modeling. After three years of therapy, aphasia and hemiparesis have been remediated, and the artist has returned to her work as a pianist in the Higher Drama School at Cracow.

COMMUNICATIVE APPROACHES

Communicative approaches are directed toward practical application of the skills necessary for communication in real-life situations. This final aim of holistic rehabilitation was also emphasized by Sarno (1965). The specific therapeutic interventions at our center include both functional communication approaches and social communication oriented treatment.

Functional Communication Approaches

When an aphasic patient is unable to participate in social activities, even if he or she has regained adequate use of language, we introduce compensatory techniques focusing on relatively intact communicative strengths and functional communication approaches including PACE (Davis & Wilcox, 1981), Functional Communication Treatment (Aten, 1986), and Social Communication Oriented Treatment (SCOT) (Pachalska, 1986c). Treatment involves the use of socioculturally and emotionally relevant materials designed to facilitate specific abilities, such as the use of gesture. Several sets of material are introduced to stimulate panel discussions or natural conversations. These include postcards, famous legends, and stories from the Crakow region. One of the patients' favorite sets is a group of 20 postcards of Crakow and 10 popular illustrated legends ("Wanda," "Krak," "Wawel dragon," etc.). Patients, their families, and therapists carry on a panel discussion. Tasks are structured (from the simplest to the more difficult) so that all group members can participate.

Social Communication Oriented Treatment

We introduce SCOT when a patient with aphasia is frustrated by the inability to communicate effectively to those in his or her environment. SCOT serves as indirect language training, combined with stimulation aimed at the general reorganization of the personal and social aspects of communication. It is mainly community-based treatment, provided in physical therapy, occupational therapy, psychotherapy, sociotherapy, and speech therapy, and it includes planned outings called "therapeutic tours" and group meetings.

Therapeutic tours are introduced to remedy withdrawal from active community life. It is not only the patient who isolates himself. Isolation results from the inability to communicate with others, and is often intensified by a physical handicap. One such tour is the "Afa-Rally," organized by a social worker together with the Disabled Drivers Club. During the rally, the patients with aphasia communicate with drivers. Special symbols are used to show the situation on the road and stimulate language processes at the same time. The rally takes a whole day, and participants must complete a number of tasks that require communicative and/or motor skills at "control points." Communication occurs also during lunch and dinner as well as during "stop points" (various famous buildings such as museums and castles). At the end, awards are given to the winners and their families during an official dinner (Pachalska, Czarnocka, Knapik, Ladecki, & Rafalski, 1985).

During therapeutic tours patients, families, therapists, and other members of a particular tour engage in real-life situations designed to provide many possibilities for communication. Therapeutic tours are also aimed at stimulation of communication in various surroundings (grocery stores, restaurants, movies, theatres, museums, etc.). Social situations create conditions for practicing conversations with familiar persons and strangers. Therapists can observe how each individual acts and communicates in real-life situations, which enables them to provide appropriate help with such interactions.

Group meetings are related to the theme of a particular tour, with discussion aimed at reintegration of various personal communicative abilities, such as orientation in communicative conditions, planning what to say, and choosing the form and content of expression acceptable in a particular environment. SCOT tasks are directed toward using language in natural contexts, participation in two-person conversation, and communication in groups.

Using two therapeutic approaches and family support, we help the patient discover his or her personal style of communication. The two approaches are: *minimalization*, or the elimination or reduction of socially inappropriate phrases and behavior that sometimes occur after stroke, and *optimalization,* or the improvement of speech and communication style in conjunction with stimulation of the ability to engage in proper and pleasant ways to communicate. To improve communication, self-cuing techniques also are used. Patients can practice cuing techniques during spontaneous communication. With the help of the family, clinicians can identify failure to use self-cuing techniques, and remedial steps can be taken to rectify inappropriate use of cuing strategies during group sessions. Self-cuing techniques may provide an important means of reducing anxiety before attempting to communicate, and therefore permit the patient to approach the premorbid style of communication.

However, the therapeutic team must support the patient with the proper material. Therefore, we introduce several aids, helpful in practicing self-cuing techniques. For example a "lexicon of persons with aphasia" and a "dictionary of emotions," enabling the expression of one's feelings and emotional needs (See Figures 7–2 and 7–3), were prepared with the help of families and patients who had recovered from aphasia.

In holistic rehabilitation, program flexibility is ensured by selecting techniques that fit the patient's medical and neurolinguistic needs. Family support is provided according to the particular situation through the Therapeutic Program for Family and Patients (TPFP) (Knapik, 1986).

HOLISTIC TREATMENT FOR GLOBAL APHASIA

When a patient with global aphasia recovers consciousness after a stroke, he tries to communicate his needs to other people. If the reactions of those in the environment are appropriate, they help to stimulate communication. At this stage most patients perceive only nonverbal messages. The patient may understand some gestures, such as stretching out the hand to greet others or to part from them. The patient may smile to greet someone and look sad when he leaves.

Despite the loss of linguistic communication, the patient is able to interpret the behavior of other people, and to distinguish whether they are angry or indifferent. The patient understands the paralinguistic context which includes speech prosody (i.e., melody, accent, rhythm, tone, strength, duration of voice), as well as gestures, and facial expressions.

In the CARM rehabilitation process, the author recorded the changes that occurred in global aphasia, and observed that aphasic patients rely at first on situational context, then begin to understand verbal-graphic or verbal-gestural instructions, and last begin to understand the questions they are asked. They also respond to their family name and the name of their hometown. The evolution of communication from non-

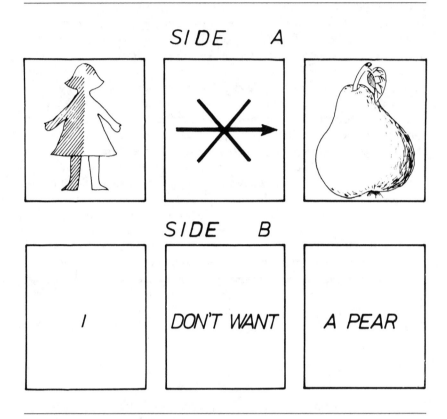

Figure 7–2. An entry in the "Lexicon of Persons with Aphasia." A pictographic illustration of sentence. Side A—pictograms, Side B—their linguistic counterparts.

linguistic to linguistic in patients with global aphasia is presented in Figure 7–4.

The early stage of recovery is the signal appeal stage. At first a patient with global aphasia nods or shakes his head in agreement or disagreement, shrugs his shoulders or spreads his arms (meaning "I don't know"), or stretches out his hand (meaning "give me"). The patient uses utterances consisting of several sounds to communicate, for example, *Oy-ey-yey, pa . . pa . . pa,* and so on. The utterances are differentiated by melody and a limited number of expressions and gestures.

Some language signals such as vocatives can appear after a stroke. Later, stable situational semantic signals appear as gesture or sound. Thus, the patient asks *"to . . . to?"* using a rising intonation (meaning "Is it good?"), he shakes his head saying *"to"* (meaning no), and says *"to . . . to . . . to?"* taking a therapist's microphone in his hand and examining it. It is noteworthy that the number of syllables is often the same as in the corresponding word or sentence and the modulation of voice is also appropriate.

In the next stage motivated (nonarbitrary) language symbols occur, for example, *s . . . s . . . s* (imitating a sound of a snake presented in a pic-

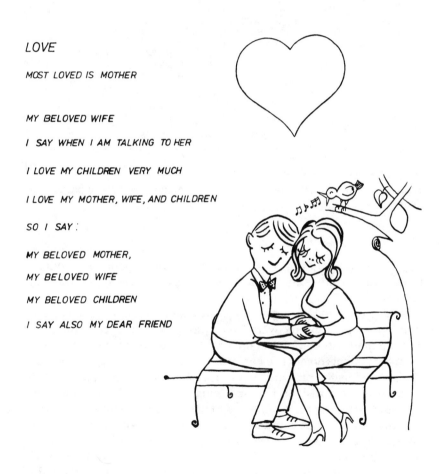

LOVE

MOST LOVED IS MOTHER

MY BELOVED WIFE

I SAY WHEN I AM TALKING TO HER

I LOVE MY CHILDREN VERY MUCH

I LOVE MY MOTHER, WIFE, AND CHILDREN

SO I SAY :

MY BELOVED MOTHER,

MY BELOVED WIFE

MY BELOVED CHILDREN

I SAY ALSO MY DEAR FRIEND

Figure 7–3. An entry in the "Dictionary of Emotions."

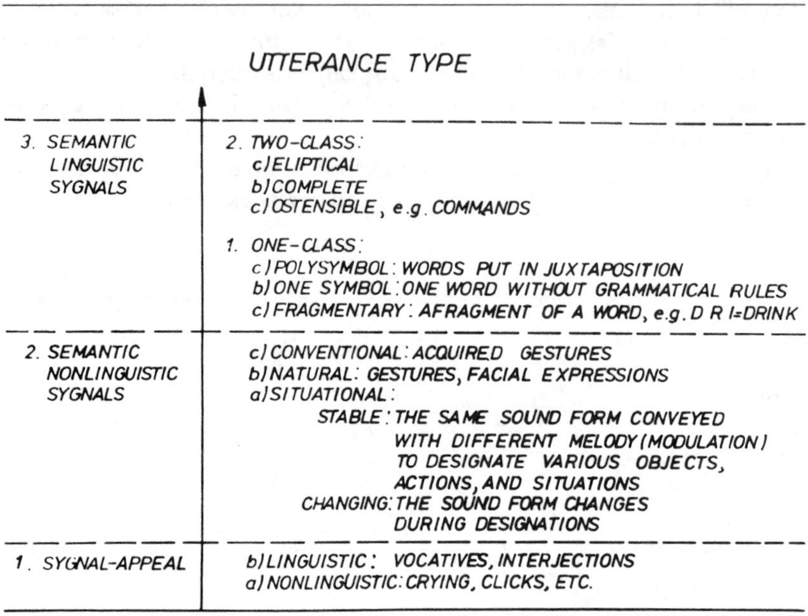

UTTERANCE TYPE

3. SEMANTIC LINGUISTIC SYGNALS	2. TWO-CLASS: c) ELIPTICAL b) COMPLETE c) OSTENSIBLE , e.g. COMMANDS
	1. ONE-CLASS: c) POLYSYMBOL: WORDS PUT IN JUXTAPOSITION b) ONE SYMBOL: ONE WORD WITHOUT GRAMMATICAL RULES c) FRAGMENTARY: A FRAGMENT OF A WORD, e.g. D R I=DRINK
2. SEMANTIC NONLINGUISTIC SYGNALS	c) CONVENTIONAL: ACQUIRED GESTURES b) NATURAL: GESTURES, FACIAL EXPRESSIONS a) SITUATIONAL: STABLE: THE SAME SOUND FORM CONVEYED WITH DIFFERENT MELODY (MODULATION) TO DESIGNATE VARIOUS OBJECTS, ACTIONS, AND SITUATIONS CHANGING: THE SOUND FORM CHANGES DURING DESIGNATIONS
1. SYGNAL-APPEAL	b) LINGUISTIC : VOCATIVES, INTERJECTIONS a) NONLINGUISTIC: CRYING, CLICKS, ETC.

Figure 7–4. The evolution of utterances from nonlinguistic to linguistic in patients with global aphasia (from Pachalska, 1989).

ture) or *cucoo* (imitating a cuckoo). On the whole patients do not like to use these sounds, perhaps because they know it is the way children speak.

Next is the one-class signal stage. Despite its similarities to language development, during recovery from aphasia there are fewer questions, and the modulation of voice, mimicry, and gestures is less rich. Moreover, the patients do not use diminutives. For example, the first one-class signals used by the patient DA (41 years old) were fractional ones, *afa*—kava (meaning coffee) and *py*—pit (meaning to drink), and then a complete symbol, *nie* (no). A tendency to use nuclear syllables of a word is also noted. The most common distortions observed during a naming task are: reduplications; elision, or of an initial syllable; elision and reduplication; augmentation; deformation; metathesis with deformation; and contamination with elision. Utterances are often accompanied by rich facial expressions and gestures. Some elements of pantomime can also be observed.

The two-class signal stage follows. Only one patient, EM (43 years old, group E), in a study described below, was able to construct simple sentences after a 10-month period although some structural deviations still occurred (e.g., ... *water* ... *drink* ... *milk* ... *milke* ... *no* ... *drinks* ... *mil* ... *no* ... *a lady and drinks milky* ... *coffee with milk* ... *yes* ... *oh* ... *Lady drink coffee with milk*).

Other patients limit themselves to much shorter utterances (e.g., *baty da* [*herbaty daj*—give tea] by the patient TS, 64 years old, group E; *mam Tito* [*mam Tito*—I have a dog called Tito] by the patient FL, 54 years old, group E; *bywe tam* [*bewem tam*—I was there] by MW, 54 years old, group E).

IMPROVEMENT OF LINGUISTIC FUNCTIONS

We studied the therapeutic value of CARM in different neurolinguistic types of aphasia using the Cracow Test of Differential Diagnosis of Aphasia (CTDDA). Two groups of patients were evaluated, total CARM (group E) and a control group given traditional therapy (group C). The test was administered four times: pretreatment; after 1 month of treatment; after 3 months of treatment; and 3 months post-treatment.

The analysis of mean value of LFI (see Figure 7–5) reveals that in paradigmatic aphasia, both groups (E and C) scored below the mean (group C = 37.63, group E = 38.07). Their scores did not differ significantly before treatment. At the next evaluations the means of LFI reached 62.83 in group C and 82.53 points in group E. The differences between the two groups after 3 months of treatment were large and statistically significant. At the fourth examination (after 3 months without treatment), a slight decrease in the index was observed in both groups.

Patients with syntagmatic aphasia in both groups were low and the difference was not significant. At the next examination the index increased, reaching 42.08 points in group C and 58.05 in group E; the difference was large and statistically significant. The increase of the index in group C was 19.48 and in group E was 35.24 points. At the next examinations, after finishing the treatment and after 3 months of staying at home, only a slight increase in the index was noted.

In the case of mixed aphasia the pretreatment indices were below the mean in both groups and did not differ significantly. A significant increase, however, was noted at the next examination, and at the third examination the index reached 47.22 points in group C and 64.25 for group E. This difference was statistically significant. After 3 months without treatment, a slight decrease of the index in both groups was noted.

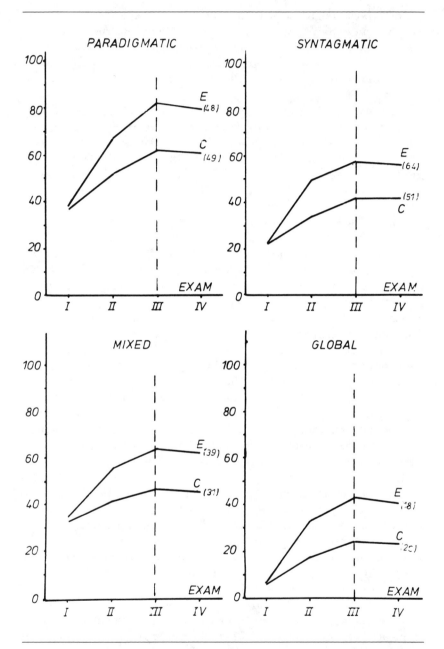

Figure 7–5. Mean value of Language Functions Index (LFI) at examinations 1, 2, 3, and 4. **A.** CARM group. **B.** control group. Numbers in brackets indicate number of patients.

In the groups of patients with a global aphasia the initial index level was very low in both groups (group C = 5.13, group E = 5.29). At the next examination, a notable increase in the indices of both groups took place. By the third examination, the increase for group C was 19.35 and for group E was 38.52 points. The mean value of the index was 24.48 points in group C and 43.81 points in group E, and this difference between the groups was statistically significant. In the last examination (3 months after treatment was terminated), an insignificant decrease of the index value was observed.

The above data confirmed the efficacy of CARM for reintegration of linguistic functions, with the magnitude of differences related to the type of aphasia. (For more detail, see Pachalska & Knapik, 1991.)

We separately documented the therapeutic value of Art Therapy for reintegration of language functions using 30 patients with severe "chronic" aphasia, hemiplegia, or hemiparesis. The experimental group treated with LOAT consisted of 18 patients (group E) and a control group treated with a traditional art therapy program (group C). Groups were matched for a similar proportion of patients who showed artistic skills and severity of manual dysfunction. The examinations were administered three times: before treatment, after 44 weeks, and after 88 weeks of treatment. To assess language functions we chose eight subtests from the Set of Neuropsycholinguistic Tests (Pachalska, 1986a). Mean value (percentages) of points gained by the patients are presented in Figure 7–6.

The data show that, at the first examination, patients from both groups showed only minimal performance on some tests. At the second examination an increase was noted; the increase was especially pronounced in group E, with increases three times greater. The biggest increases were observed in calculation, writing, reading, and naming. Lower scores were obtained on spontaneous speech, telling a story, and sense of humor. On the third examination a further increase in test performance was observed, which was two-, three-, and even fourfold greater in group E than in group C. The most significant increases (from 25–35%) took place in naming, comprehension, reading, writing, and calculation.

EVALUATION OF COMMUNICATION

Changes in communication were recorded in various social situations during 10 months of therapy in patients with global aphasia treated with two different programs. An analysis of 304 five-minute videotaped situations showed a significantly greater increase in positive communicative acts (monologue, dialogue, and group interactions) by patients who

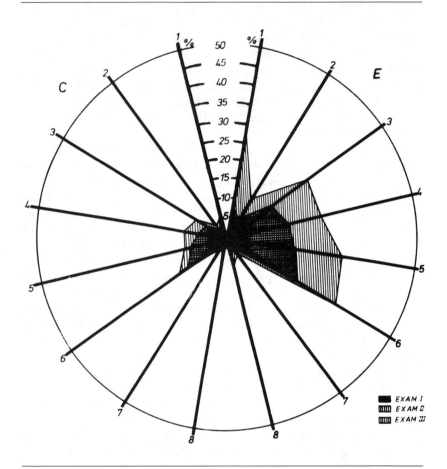

Figure 7-6. Mean value (percentage) of points scored by patients from groups C and E on examinations 1, 2, and 3 on eight linguistic tests: 1—naming, 2—spontaneous speech, 3—comprehension, 4—reading, 5—writing, 6—calculation, 7—storytelling, 8—sense of humor.

were given CARM (18 patients) compared to those who were given standard therapy.

Evaluation of improvement in aphasia is not complete without documenting improvement in the personal communication style of individual patients. The instrument we use for this evaluation is the Test of Communicative Abilities in Social Situations discussed previously. However, because we have not yet accumulated enough patients who have completed the Social Communication Oriented Approach, we are unable to report definitive results concerning the efficacy of this program.

More than 10 years of carefully designed and documented studies (Kaczmarek & Pachalska, 1987; Kuzak [Pachalska], 1978; Pachalska, 1986a; Pachalska, 1989; Tlokinski, 1990) during which CARM has been compared with other standard programs of aphasia therapy, as well as years of clinical experience, have confirmed the efficacy of the CARM program.

CONCLUSIONS

Research conducted according to the holistic approach helps to clarify a theory of aphasia based on a neurolinguistic approach. This research also helps us to discover the neural mechanisms of language recovery in aphasia through elaboration of NMIP and evaluation of CARM.

Once we have determined specific needs, both short- and long-term goals are specified, and activities for the patient are planned and, when possible, recorded. Our goal is to determine whether the patient has improved, remained the same, or deteriorated, and to prevent acceptance of status quo, which itself often leads to depression and other maladaptive reactions. As the result of our data collection, we also are able to modify the goals and strategies of intervention and thus maximize recovery.

It should be noted that recovery from aphasia to premorbid levels is rarely achieved, because linguistic deficits are closely interwoven with other disturbances of cognitive function. Therefore, treatment programs must address the patient's social as well as biological and psychological needs.

We believe that holistic rehabilitation can be accomplished only through a better understanding of the aphasic patient's problems, that is, recognizing the complex interrelationship of emotions and the learning process. It is important to have a comprehensive view of the patient's life experiences and to evaluate the impact of these factors on the patient's ability to respond to training. Thus, therapists must be able to guide therapy using a holistic approach.

It is worth noting that most aphasiologists concentrate on linguistic skills or functional communication, omitting myth, science, and art. These activities pertain to communication, which entails encoding and decoding appropriate symbols. However, we still do not know much about symbolic processing, about its cerebral organization, or about personal style in selecting particular symbols. Therefore, future treatment programs should focus on these areas.

Art Therapy, which requires the use of cognitive processes, is also very important. We have to learn to "read" works, to name symbols of art in order to be able to appreciate and to express them. Art Therapy provides good opportunities for modeling the perceptiveness and expressiveness of the patients, and for modeling a personal style of selecting appropriate symbols and a personal style of communication. Therefore, Art Therapy for patients with aphasia necessarily entails a far more encompassing perspective.

Communicative adequacy and personal style of communication are other foci of modern rehabilitative aphasiology. Social communication oriented approaches (e.g., SCOT) are directed toward communication in real-life situations, and provide the opportunity to learn more about communicative adequacy and restoration of a personal style of communication acceptable in the patient's environment.

One final caution is needed regarding methods of rehabilitation of patients with aphasia in the future. If the primary goal of rehabilitation is not only the restoration of patients' communicative skills, but also their reintegration within society, then efforts must be made to enable them to get jobs or to otherwise regain the sense of having a meaningful life. Unless this occurs, optimal reintegration of patients within society will not be achieved. So we must select the more difficult, but potentially more rewarding, ways which lead to intensive research in diagnosis and rehabilitation of patients with aphasia.

A holistic approach to rehabilitation is an important direction for future work with aphasic patients because it concentrates on:

1. internal factors (recognition of biological, psychological, and social aspects of the brain damage and aphasia, and also mechanisms of recovery); and
2. external factors (verification of existing methods, elaboration of new effective methods of diagnosis and therapy, and the composition and educational level of therapeutic team).

Choosing to pursue holistic rehabilitation research is difficult. However, it is possible to overcome this problem by even more specific work on the taxonomy of goals and methods used in therapy.

Future directions for aphasia therapy depend on whether aphasiologists can overcome differences in opinion about essential subject matter, such as the definition of the subject of research, its structure and function, and methodological problems. These differences are not simply the result of different world and scientific views held by researchers and clinicians. They also represent differences in opinion about subject matter and errors in research methodology.

Therefore, we must concentrate on more detailed analysis of rehabilitation problems and the exchange of findings at the international level, including both positive and negative results of specific therapeutic techniques. Research efforts that arise from interdisciplinary teams involved in therapy should have a practical aspect, that is, provide answers to the question of how to help the person with aphasia to find the sense of life.

REFERENCES

Aten, J. L. (1986). Functional communication treatment. In R. Chapey (Ed.), *Intervention strategies in adult aphasia* (2nd ed., pp. 266–276). Baltimore, MD: Williams & Wilkins.

Bierkowski, L. (1837). *Kilka uwag o waznosci i potrzebie stosowania gimnastyki leczniczej.* Cracow: Wyd. Univ. Jagiellonski.

Davis, G. A., & Wilcox, M. J. (1981). Incorporating parameters of natural conversation in aphasia treatment. In R. Chapey (Ed.), *Language intervention strategies in adult aphasia* (pp. 169–193). Baltimore, MD: Williams & Wilkins.

Dega, W. (1975). Rehabilitacja—polska specjalnosc. *Problemy, 7,* 16–17.

Dega, W., & Milanowska, K. (1988). Model of medical rehabilitation in Poland. In M. Pachalska (Ed.), *Contemporary problems in rehabilitation of persons with aphasia* (pp. 37–41). Cracow: AWF.

DeRenzi, E., & Vignolo, L. A. (1962). The Token Test: A sensitive test to detect receptive disturbances in aphasia. *Brain, 85,* 665–678.

Finkelstein, V. (1980). *Attitudes and disabled people* (p. 33). New York: World Rehabilitation Foundation.

Goodglass, H., & Kaplan, E. (1983). *The assessment of aphasia and related disorders. Boston Diagnostic Aphasia Examination.* Philadelphia: Lea & Febiger.

Grochmal, S. (1985). Neurofizjologiczne mechanizmy w kompensacji zaburzen ukladu nerwowego. In W. Dega (Ed.), *Zdolnosci kompensacyjne i mozliwosci ich wykorzystania u osob z ogniskowym uszkodzeniem osrodkowego ukladu nerwowego* (pp. 30–35). Warszawa: PZWL.

Grochmal, S., & Zielinska-Charszewska, S. (1980). *Rehabilitacja w chorobach ukladu nerwowego.* Warszawa: PZWL.

Helm-Estabrooks, N., Fitzpatrick, P. M., & Baresi, B. (1982). Visual action therapy for global aphasia. *Journal of Speech and Hearing Disorders, 47* 385–389.

Holland, A. L. (1980). *Communicative abilities in daily living.* Baltimore: University Park Press.

Kaczmarek, B. L. J., (1991). *The communicative brain: A neurolinguistic outlook.* Unpublished manuscript.

Kaczmarek, B. L. J., & Pachalska, M. (1987). Polymodal approach to rehabilitation of aphasics. Proceedings of the Third Pan-Hellenic Symposium of Speech Disorders. Athens.

Kadzielawa, D., & Romero, B. (1978). Metody rehabilitacji chorych z zaburzeniami rozumienia mowy. In M. T. Nowakowska (Ed.), *Rehabilitacja chorych z afazja* (pp. 67–93). Ossolineum, Wroclaw, Warszawa, Krakow, Gdansk.

Kearns, K. P. (1986). Group therapy for aphasia: Theoretical and practical considerations. In R. Chapey (Ed.), *Language intervention strategies in adult aphasia* (2nd ed., pp. 304–318). Baltimore: Williams & Wilkins.

Kertesz, A. (1982). *The Western Aphasia Battery*. New York: Grune & Stratton.

Knapik, H. (1986). *The therapeutic program for family and patient (TPFP)*. Unpublished manuscript (in Polish).

Knapik, H. (1989). *Therapy of memory*. Paper presented at the Third National Conference on Aphasiology, Jastrzebia Gora, Poland.

Knapik, H. (1990). *Community based treatment for aphasics*. Cracow: TWK (in Polish).

Knapik, H., & Knapik, K. (1990). *Theoretical and practical considerations in aphasia group therapy*. Paper presented at the Fourth National Conference of Aphasiology, Cracow, Poland.

Konorski, J. (1969). *Integracyjna dzialalnosc mozgu*. Warszawa: PWN.

Kuzak (Pachalska), M. (1978). Group art therapy for aphasic patients. In *Proceedings of the II Polish Symposium on Rehabilitation* (pp. 79–86). Krakow: AWF.

Luria, A. R. (1963). *Restoration of function after brain injury*. New York: Macmillan.

Lopatkiewicz, J. (1961). Analiza zaburzen nominacji w afazji. Rozpr. *Wydz. Nauk Med. PAN,* 6(2), 129–144.

Lopatkiewicz, J. (1988). Studies in the variabilty of naming disorders in aphasia. In M. Pachalska (Ed.), *Contemporary problems in the rehabilitation of persons with aphasia* (pp. 195–202). Cracow: AWF.

Maruszewski, M. (1966). *Speech and brain, neuropsychological problems*. Warszawa: PWN (in Polish).

Maruszewski, M. (1974). *The patient with aphasia and his therapy*. Warszawa: Nasza Ksiegarnia (in Polish).

Müller, D. J., & Code, C. (1989). Interpersonal perception of psychosocial adjustment to aphasia. In C. Code & D. Müller (Eds.), *Aphasia therapy* (2nd ed.). London: Cole & Whurr.

Pachalska, M. (1980). *Cognitive approach to aphasia rehabilitation*. Cracow: TWK (in Polish).

Pachalska, M. (1982). *Therapy of thinking processes*. Cracow: TWK (in Polish).

Pachalska, M. (1983). *Kinaesthetic therapy of apraxia (KTA)*. Cracow: TWK.

Pachalska, M. (1986a). *A complex model of rehabilitation of the persons with aphasia*. Cracow: AWF (in Polish).

Pachalska, M. (1986c). The evaluation of speech therapy of global aphasic persons treated by therapeutic teams trained and untrained in nonlingual communication. In *Logopedics and phoniatrics issues for future research, Proceedings of the XXth IALP Congress* (pp. 118–119). Tokyo: Publ. Organizing Committee of the Congress.

Pachalska, M. (1988a, November). *Selective or rather systematic configuration of the therapeutic information given to the patient with aphasia*. Paper presented at the Second Polish Conference of Aphasiology, Cracow, Poland.

Pachalska, M. (1988b). Social communication oriented treatment (SCOT). Cracow: TWK (in Polish).

Pachalska, M. (1988c). Art therapy in aphasia. In M. Pachalska (Ed.), *Contemporary problems in the rehabilitation of persons with aphasia* (pp. 365–371). Cracow: AWF.

Pachalska, M. (1989). Complex aphasia rehabilitation model (CARM) (in press).

Pachalska, M. (1990, September). *Language oriented art therapy.* Poster presentation at the Fourth International Aphasia Rehabilitation Congress, Edinburgh, Scotland.

Pachalska, M. (1991a). Group therapy: A way of reintegrating patients with aphasia. *Aphasiology, 6*, 541–554.

Pachalska, M. (1991b). Recovery of a pianist with aphasia (in Polish, in press).

Pachalska, M. (in press). The efficacy of modeling in PACE—therapy.

Pachalska, M., Czarnocka, I., Knapik, H., Ladecki, B., & Rafalski, L. (1985). "Apha-Ralies"—modern form of rehabilitation of patients with aphasia. In *Proceedings of the Fifth Symposium of Rehabilitation.* Cracow: TWK (in Polish).

Pachalska, M., Kaczmarek, B. L. J., & Knapik, H. (1991). Cracow test of differential diagnosis of aphasia (CTDDA) (in Polish, in press).

Pachalska, M., & Knapik, H. (1988a, June). *Recovery of piano playing skills in aphasic pianist.* Videotape presented at the Third International Aphasia Rehabilitation Congress, Florence, Italy.

Pachalska, M., & Knapik, H. (1988b). Method of nonlinguistic psychotherapy for persons with aphasia. In M. Pachalska (Ed.), *Contemporary problems in the rehabilitation of persons with aphasia* (pp. 233–236). Cracow: AWF.

Pachalska, M., & Knapik, H. (1989). *Communicative abilities in social situations.* Unpublished manuscript.

Pachalska, M., & Knapik, H. (1990). *A fascinating world of artistic creation after stroke.* Videotape presented at the Second Polish Congress on Rehabilitation, Cracow, Poland.

Pachalska, M., & Knapik, H. (1991). An evaluation of CARM for reintegration of linguistic functions in patients with aphasia (in press).

Pachalski, A. (1988). The Polish concept of rehabilitation. In M. Pachalska (Ed.), *Contemporary problems in the rehabiltation of persons with aphasia: Proceedings of the First International Aphasia Rehabilitation Congress* (pp. 48–51). Cracow: AWF.

Sarno, M. T. (1965). A measurement of functional communication in aphasia. *Archives of Physical Medicine Rehabilitation, 46*, 101–107.

Schuell, H., Jenkins, J. J., & Jimenez-Pabon, E. (1964). *Aphasia in adults: Diagnosis, prognosis, and treatment.* New York: Harper & Row.

Skinner, C., Wirtz, S., & Thompson, J. (1984). The Edinburgh functional communicative profile. Buckingham: Winslow.

Szumska, J. (1980). *Metody rehabilitacji afazji.* Warszawa: PZWL.

Tlokinski, W. (1986). *Mowa. Przeglad problematyki dla psychologw.* Warszawa: PWN.

Tlokinski, W. (1990). *Efficacy of CARM for language functions.* Paper presented at the Second Polish Congress on Rehabilitation.

Van Eeckhout, P., Honrado, C., Bhatt, P., & Ceblais, J. C. (1983). De la TMR et de sa practique. *Rééducation Orthophonique, 21*(132), 305–316.

Weiss, M. (1961). Podstawy rehabilitacji leczniczej. *Zdrowie Publiczne, 4–5.*

Wepman, J. M. (1951). *Recovery from aphasia.* New York: Ronald Press.

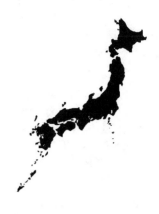

CHAPTER 8

Aphasia Treatment in Japan

SUMIKO SASANUMA
Tokyo Metropolitan Institute of Gerontology
Toyko, Japan

HISTORY AND BACKGROUND

The dawn of scientific investigation of aphasia in Japan dates back almost one hundred years. Until the end of the 1950s, however, studies focused largely on clinico-pathological correlates of aphasia, and were conducted mostly by physicians with a theoretical background in European psychiatry or neuropsychiatry. In the early 1960s a more empirical/pragmatic approach to the problem of aphasia was first introduced to this country through a new discipline called speech and language pathology (or logopedics in some European countries). Since that time, there has been an increasing interest in the therapeutic aspects of language and communication disorders in aphasia, with substantial expansion of the field as a whole. The past two decades have witnessed significant development in the level of both theoretical and technical sophistication in clinical aphasiology.

The first clinic in Japan devoted exclusively to the treatment and rehabilitation of aphasic patients was established in Kageyu Rehabilitation
Hospital in the spring of 1965 with three speech and language clinicians
as staff members and myself as a supervisor. This was two years after the
inauguration of the Japanese Association of Rehabilitation Medicine and
about one year after the visit to the same hospital by Martha Taylor, then
chief of Speech Pathology Services, Institute of Physical Medicine and
Rehabilitation, New York University Medical Center. In May, 1965, one
month after its inauguration, the clinic was honored with a visit by Hildred Schuell, who happened to be visiting the Kyushu University as a
member of the Minnesota University team for the Kyushu-Minnesota
collaborative research project on stroke. The visits by these figures undoubtedly had a great impact on the future development of this new
field in this country. Many other hospitals began to follow the example
of Kageyu Hospital, which resulted in a sharp increase in the number of
aphasia clinics in Japan over the next three decades. At the present time,
more than 500 clinics are estimated to exist throughout the country (Survey Committee on Aphasia Rehabilitation in Japan, 1989). Along with
this increase in the number of aphasia clinics, there has been an increasing awareness among various sectors (including the medical, socio-
welfare, and educational sectors) of the importance of rehabilitation
services for aphasic individuals. Clinical as well as basic research on the
evaluation and treatment of aphasia has begun to gain a firmer status in
aphasiology. In 1977, two academic organizations directly involved in
scientific study of aphasia and related issues, the Japanese Society of
Aphasiology and the Neuropsychology Association of Japan, were inau-
gurated. Each of these organizations has a membership of over a thous-
and at the present time.

We do not have reliable data on the incidence/prevalence of patients
with aphasia. This is partially due to the lack of qualified speech and language clinicians to diagnose and identify aphasic patients. According to
an estimate derived from several sources, however, we have a rough total of at least 100,000 stroke-induced aphasic patients plus 10,000 more
patients who have aphasia with other etiologies, who are candidates for
clinical intervention of some sort (Sasanuma, 1989).

Table 8–1 shows the age distribution of aphasic patients based on the
series of four surveys referred to above (Survey Committee on Aphasia
Rehabilitation in Japan, 1979, 1983, 1986, 1989).[1] It can be seen that the

[1] These surveys were conducted by the Japanese Society of Aphasiology as part of its project, with the primary objective of obtaining an overview of clinico-social conditions of
aphasic patients in this country. In each survey, a questionnaire was mailed to a large number of hospitals and institutions throughout the country (from 862 in 1978 to 1,455 in 1988)
with a response rate of 31% in 1978 and 44% in 1988. Items on the questionnaires included (1) the demography (the total number of aphasic patients served, etiologies of aphasia,

Table 8-1. Percentage age distribution of aphasic patients based on the four nationwide survey series

Patient Age (in years)	Years of Survey			
	1978 (N = 4,809)	1982 (N = 9,579)	1985 (N = 12,990)	1988 (N = 11,605)
<39	12.2	6.5	7.6	9.0
40–49	18.8	14.6	17.4	13.9
50–59	26.7	25.1	28.9	27.4
60–69	29.1	31.9	30.5	29.1
70 +	12.2	21.4	15.2	20.2
Unknown	1.0	0.4	0.4	0.5

prevalence of aphasia has been at a peak in people in their 60s for the past 10 years, and that patients aged 60 and over comprised between 41.3 and 55.7% of the total, making up almost half of the aphasic population. This distribution reflects a change in the age distribution for aphasic patients from two earlier surveys conducted in the latter half of the 1960s (Sasanuma, 1972a, 1972b) that showed the greatest prevalence of aphasia in the 50s age bracket, with only 31 and 34 % of patients, respectively, in their 60s or over. In one of these surveys, which included 269 stroke-induced aphasic patients consecutively admitted to a large rehabilitation hospital from 1965–1969, patients in their 50s constituted the largest group (38%), followed by those in their 60s (27%), and 40s (22%) (Sasanuma, 1972a). A similar age distribution was found in another survey of 348 aphasic patients admitted to two different rehabilitation hospitals from 1964–1970 (Sasanuma, 1972b). This drastic change in the age distribution of aphasic patients over the past two decades in this country has raised manifold issues in the rehabilitation of elderly aphasic individuals, which will be discussed later in a separate section.

age, and gender); (2)content of rehabilitation services offered to these patients (e.g., availability of systematic therapy programs, the number of speech and language clinicians engaged in these programs, training background of the clinicians), therapy schedules (frequency and length of therapy sessions), types of therapy sessions offered (proportions of individual therapy, group therapy, counseling, and guidance services, etc.), types of facilities available (individual therapy rooms, audio-visual equipment, etc.); and (3) opportunities for returning to paid jobs for the treated patients, among others. Analyses and comparisons of data obtained in the four surveys over the decade indicate that there has been a steady increase in (1) the number of hospitals and institutions offering aphasia therapy, (2) the number of aphasic patients served, and (3) the number of speech-language clinicians engaged in aphasia therapy. On the other hand, the principal causes of aphasia, as well as age and gender distributions of aphasic patients, tend to remain relatively unchanged.

A RAPID RISE OF CLINICAL APHASIOLOGY

A surprising fact about speech pathology in Japan is that an officially recognized certification system for speech and language clinicians has yet to be established. However, according to the above mentioned series of nationwide surveys on aphasia rehabilitation services conducted in 1978, 1982, 1985, and 1988, there has been a steady increase not only in the number of hospitals and institutions with clinics or services offering aphasia therapy (212 clinics in 1978 as compared to 365 in 1988), but also in the number of speech and language clinicians engaged in the evaluation and treatment of aphasic patients in these clinics (236 in 1978 versus 584 in 1988). The number of aphasic patients receiving therapy also has increased considerably (5,027 in 1978 versus 11,605 in 1988).

The majority of the clinicians are graduates of a 1-year graduate-level training course in speech and language pathology offered by a nonuniversity government-supported training school, the College for Speech-Language-Hearing Therapists,[2] the National Rehabilitation Center for the Disabled. However, some clinicians have attended shorter courses. Only a handful of clinicians have had 2 or more years of graduate level professional training in speech-language pathology, most of them in the United States. The quality of services offered in clinics, therefore, may vary considerably, depending not only on the number of clinicians available, but also on the level and nature of professional training of the individual clinicians.

In spite of all these adverse circumstances, Japanese clinical aphasiologists, on the whole, have been highly enthusiastic about upgrading their training, trying to absorb all of the available information on aphasiology and related areas coming from different parts of the world, and integrating it into their own clinical practice and research. Therapeutic approaches currently in use in this country, therefore, are not much different from those prevalent among our colleagues in other parts of the world, although we do have some specific issues and problems of our own. In the following sections, I present an overview of the state-of-the-

---

[2]This nonuniversity training school was established by the Ministry of Health and Welfare in 1971 to alleviate the situation. It is 1 year in length and admits 20 to 30 students who have completed 4 years of college study. The curriculum consists of courses in basic areas (speech science, linguistics, anatomy and physiology, medical areas, and psychology) and those dealing with speech, voice, language, and hearing disorders, to bring the total for all areas to 80 semester hours. Additionally about 400 hours of practical experiences are provided. Thus, as far as the content of the program is concerned, it is essentially similar to that of the typical program accredited by the American Speech-Language-Hearing Association in the United States. However, our program has some definite shortcomings. First, it is a 1-year course with an inordinately high concentration of coursework hours. Second, it has no clinical fellowship year. Furthermore, because the majority of the teaching staff are lecturers from outside institutions, the courses tend to be less efficiently organized and integrated than would be ideal.

art aphasia treatment approaches currently in use in Japan as well as some efficacy data, and then move on to the statement and description of some important issues facing aphasiologists in Japan.

MAJOR TYPES OF TREATMENT APPROACHES

The wide variety of intervention strategies currently in use in Japan can be classified into three broad categories or types of approaches: (a) language therapy approaches, (b) cognitive neuropsychological approaches, and (c) functional communication approaches, which are reciprocally interrelated in aphasia rehabilitation.

The goal common to all of these approaches is to establish the most effective means of communication for individual patients so that they can relate meaningfully to those around them. The basic clinical procedures used to accomplish this goal comprise a series of dynamically interacting steps: (1) Gathering necessary information about language and communication disorders as well as the related problems by means of testing and observation, (2) framing hypotheses about the nature and cause of the problem based on the critical analysis of the data gathered in step 1, and (3) testing these hypotheses through therapeutic intervention. Procedures in Steps 1 and 2 amount to assessment or evaluational diagnostic work-up, which is crucially important for the adequate planning and execution of the treatment and rehabilitation procedures in Step 3.

LANGUAGE THERAPY APPROACHES

The first category of approaches represents traditional language therapy for aphasia, characterized by highly structured, direct intervention aiming at the modification of multi-modality language functions.

A large variety of therapeutic approaches has been developed under this category, depending on the theoretical stance of the clinician. The two major methodologies which have been widely used are the "stimulation approach" (Schuell, Jenkins, & Jimenez-Pabon, 1964; Wepman, 1951) and the "programmed instruction approach" (Holland, 1970). The stimulation approach is characterized by an organized presentation of controlled, intensive, and adequate stimuli to the patient for the purpose of eliciting target responses. These responses are selectively reinforced, to facilitate the reorganization of functions within the brain necessary for linguistic operations. The deblocking method described by Weigl (1961) may also be incorporated as a variant of the stimulation approach. The programmed instruction approach, on the other hand, rigorously applies operant conditioning principles derived from learning theory and draws heavily on psycholinguistic data to guide the content and order of presentation of the linguistic materials presented to the patient. Between these two, there is a wide spectrum of approaches which differ mainly in the relative amount of structure employed. Common to all of these approaches, however, is the use of stimulus conditions designed to elicit optimum responses from the individual patients and to determine contingencies of reinforcement.

The components or levels of language which can be selected for direct application of the specific methodologies include auditory discrimination, retention and comprehension of various units of speech, word retrieval or lexical processing, syntactic comprehension and production of sentences of various types and complexities, articulation and prosody, and reading and writing, among others. To guarantee the specificity and effectiveness of the therapy programs used, it is imperative that target areas be selected on the basis of critical analyses of symptom patterns of individual patients in such a way that an appropriate hypothesis about the nature of underlying neuropsychological mechanism(s) can be formulated.

The usual procedure followed to meet this requirement is the administration of a comprehensive, standardized language test. Three language tests of this type are currently in use in Japan: the Standard Language Test of Aphasia, or SLTA (Hasegawa, 1975), the Roken (a Japanese abbreviation for Tokyo Metropolitan Institute of Gerontology) Test for Differential Diagnosis of Aphasia, or RTDDA (Sasanuma, Itoh, Watamori, Fukusako, & Monoi, 1978), and the Japanese version of the Western Aphasia Battery (Sugishita, 1988). The RTDDA can be thought of as a hybrid of the Minnesota Test for Differential Diagnosis of Aphasia (MTDDA) and the Boston Diagnostic Aphasia Examination (BDAE). Its rationale and overall structure are comparable. Of course, the nature and type of specific subtests in the RTDDA are uniquely Japanese. An example is the inclusion of a fair number of subtests for processing *kana* (phonetic symbols for syllables) and *kanji* (morphographic symbols of Chinese origin) in the battery, because the relative performance levels in *kana* and *kanji* processing provide important information for diagnosis and treatment of Japanese aphasic patients.

In some clinics, the findings obtained from these standard test batteries are supplemented by the administration of additional tests for the in-depth assessment of specific areas of dysfunction. Some examples of these tests include (1) the Japanese version of a short form of the Token Test (Spellacy & Spreen, 1969), (2) the Syntax Test of Aphasia (Fujita, Miyake, & Nakanishi, 1983) for systematic evaluation of sentence comprehension and production abilities, and (3) Kana/Kanji reading Tests (Sasanuma, 1980a), developed for detailed examination of oral reading and comprehension of kana and kanji words controlled for relevant variables. Tests for nonlinguistic cognitive abilities including orientation, various aspects of memory, visuo-spatial and constructional abilities (Sasanuma et al., 1985) are also given to selected patients to gain a more complete picture of their mental status (Benton, 1982).

The candidates for the traditional stimulation approaches include the majority of patients with mild to moderately severe aphasic involvement. With patients whose aphasia is very mild, it is often necessary to devise a highly individualized advanced-level program focusing on specific requirements or problems that might arise in the process of their vocational and/or social rehabilitation and adjustment. For severely impaired patients, the majority of intervention activities can focus on enhancing functional communication abilities (see the third type of approach below).

COGNITIVE NEUROPSYCHOLOGY APPROACHES

As an adjunct to the multi-modality treatment approaches just described, a variety of programs aimed at specific components or processes of language, such as word retrieval (e.g., confrontation naming), written word processing (e.g., reading and writing kana and kanji words), and syntactic processing (e.g., sentence comprehension and production) have been developed, and their effectiveness evaluated (Fujita, 1976; Kashiwagi & Kashiwagi, 1978; Monoi, 1976; Sasanuma, 1980a, 1986). These treatment programs are usually based on recently developed methodology which makes use of cognitive neuropsychology and information processing modeling to work on specific components of language (Lesser, 1987, 1989; Seron & Deloche, 1987). The essence of this approach is to isolate the mental processes which can be regarded as functionally modular, and to specify the mechanism of each as well as the interrelationships among subprocesses. The use of this approach, therefore, allows the clinician to make inferences about the specific loci or stage(s) of functional deficits in a given patient, which in turn provides a rationale for planning step-by-step retraining procedures (Sasanuma, 1986, 1988a). In the following, I briefly describe one such program that focuses on the impairment of kana processing, a problem often exhibited by Japanese aphasic patients of various types, especially those with Broca's aphasia.

PROGRAMS FOR KANA PROCESSING

In Japanese orthography, two types of nonalphabetic characters, kanji and kana, are used in combination. They are distinct from each other as well as from alphabetic writing systems, such as English, in the way each encodes spoken language. Kanji maps onto lexical morphemes of spoken Japanese, whereas each kana character represents a speech unit known as "mora" which is roughly equivalent to a syllable. The orthography-to-phonology relationships for kanji and kana are also quite different: Each kanji has several alternative readings depending on its context, whereas each kana character virtually always represents one and the same mora of spoken Japanese with no context sensitivity. As a result of this dual nature of Japanese orthography, various types and degrees of functional dissociations between kana and kanji processing tend to take place in our patients (Sasanuma, 1980b, 1985, 1986). Impairment of kana processing poses a major problem for patients. This is because the ability to process kanji, which is often preserved relatively well, cannot fully compensate for the deficit of kana processing, because function words and predicate inflections as well as many content words of Japanese origin are represented in kana. Furthermore, a relatively large proportion of aphasic patients exhibits various types and degrees of impairment in kana relative to kanji processing. Thus, a number of programs focused on a variety of kana processing deficits have been developed to meet these patients' needs.

The standard approach to kana retraining uses some variants of the process models for reading and writing kana and kanji to assess and interpret impaired performances in a given patient and to develop a retraining program accordingly. Monoi (1990) has hypothesized three functionally independent levels of kana processing: The moraic segmentation level (segmentation of a spoken word into its component mora-sized units), the moraic identification level (identification of each mora-sized component unit of a spoken word), and the mora-kana correspondence level. Each of these three levels can be impaired selectively in individual patients, although the second and third levels tend to be impaired to a similar degree in the majority of patients. The step-by-step treatment procedures for kana impairment at different levels of processing have been described and the recovery processes in selected patients have been reported (Kashiwagi & Kashiwagi, 1978; Monoi, 1976, 1990; Suzuki, Monoi, & Fukusako, 1990; for the theoretical background see Sasanuma, 1980a).

The following is an example of a kana writing and reading program specifically developed for patients with impairment at the level of kana-mora correspondence rules for individual kana characters (Kashiwagi & Kashiwagi, 1978). The goal of the program was to teach the patient a compensatory strategy of using a kanji as a key word to form an associative link or a detour to facilitate kana-mora correspondences. Reorganization of the patient's ability to write and read individual kana characters was the first goal, and the functional use of this skill in reading and writing words and sentences in various communicative situations was the final goal.

Program for Kana Writing

The 46 kana characters without diacritical marks constitute the targets in the first stage of retraining. For each kana, a key word kanji is selected to form the kana-kanji link. The criteria for selection of the key words are: (1) The initial syllable of the key word is identical to the pronunciation of the target kana character; (2) the key word should be familiar to the patient so that he can read and write it easily and can retrieve its phonological form (or can say the word as a whole) on hearing the first syllable of the word.

For each kana character, the patient is helped to go through the five steps as shown in Table 8–2. In *Step 1*, the patient says the key word (in this example *kaki* or "persimmon," which is a high frequency word in Japanese) on hearing the initial syllable of the word, presented by the therapist. In *Step 2*, he writes the key word kanji (柿), and in *Step 3*, he writes the target kana linked with this key word kanji (か). *Step 4* is the stage for gradual phasing-out of the strategy of using kanji key words as intermediary steps until this is done internally or omitted altogether, and *Step 5*, the last step, is devoted to expansion of the ability to write each kana character not only individually but also in words and sentences.

Program for Kana Reading

The program for kana reading also consists of five steps as shown in Table 8–3. In *Step 1*, the patient writes the key word kanji after the written presentation of the target kana (か - 柿).

In *Step 2*, he reads the key word out loud [kaki], and in *Step 3*, he separates the initial syllable of the key word and says it by itself. *Steps 4 and 5* are phasing out and expansion stages, just as they are in the program for writing kana.

In sum, the gist of these programs is to exploit the better preserved kanji processing ability in the patient and to use the meaning or seman-

---

Table 8–2. Five-step treatment program for writing kana characters

Step 1. Say the key word ([kaki] or "persimmon") on hearing the initial syllable of the word([ka] → [kaki])

Step 2. Write the key word kanji (柿)

Step 3. Write the target kana (か) linked with the key word

Step 4. Gradually phase out the strategy of using the kanji key word

Step 5. Expand the ability to write the target kana in words and sentences

Table 8-3. Five-step treatment program for reading kana characters

Step 1. Write the key word kanji after the presentation of the target kana
（　か　→　柿　）

Step 2. Read the key word out loud [kaki]

Step 3. Separate the initial syllable of the key word and say it by itself
([kaki] → [ka])

Step 4. The same as in kana writing

Step 5. The same as in kana writing

tic representation of kanji as an intermediary to reorganize the kana-mora linkage.

Three patients, two with Broca's and one with amnestic aphasia, were given these programs. The linguistic examination prior to the initiation of the program revealed that spontaneous speech was severely impaired in all patients; the patients with Broca's aphasia produced one- or two-word utterances, and the patient with amnestic aphasia produced so-called "empty" speech. Both auditory and reading comprehension were functional for daily communication in all three patients. Writing and oral reading of kana were severely impaired in all patients in contrast to substantial preservation of their ability to read and write kanji. Each patient was given four or five 45-minute therapy sessions per week for a period of from 6 to 14 months.

The results of pre- and post-treatment evaluations of kana processing showed that all patients significantly improved their writing and reading, not only of individual kana characters, but also of kana words, indicating that these programs were indeed effective.

Suzuki, Monoi, and Fukusako, (1990) introduced a partial modification of the kana writing and reading programs described above, based on their observation that the patients often had difficulty recalling the key word in Step 1 as well as isolating the initial mora (*ka*) from the rest of the multi-mora key word (*kaki*) in Step 3. To bypass these problems, they proposed the use of a one-mora kanji key word (e.g., 蚊 "mosquito" pronounced as *ka*) coupled with a cue word (e.g., 蚊取線香 "mosquito-repellent incense" which is closely associated with the key word) to facilitate the retrieval of the key word. This modified program has proved to be beneficial for severe aphasic patients who showed only limited improvement, or no improvement at all, with those programs using multi-mora key words.

In the above, we have had only a glimpse of cognitive neuropsychological approaches to language impairment in aphasia. Granted that they leave much to be desired in terms of both theoretical and technical elaboration and refinement, they appear to offer a major breakthrough in the treatment of aphasia.

FUNCTIONAL COMMUNICATION APPROACHES

The third type of aphasia treatment focuses on the patients' functional communication abilities rather than their linguistic accuracy or language functions per se, and uses a variety of approaches that encourage and reinforce conversational exchange of information in natural contexts.

There seem to be at least two lines of evidence that have enhanced our current enthusiasm for developing communication-oriented pragmatic approaches. The first has to do with accumulation of data indicating that recovery from aphasia to the premorbid level of linguistic function is rarely achieved. The second is concerned with the series of studies in the past decade reporting marked preservation of discourse and pragmatic abilities in many aphasic patients relative to their linguistic abilities per se (Ulatowska, Friedman-Stern, Weiss-Doyle, Macaluso-Haynes, & North, 1983; Ulatowska, North, & Macaluso-Haynes, 1981, among others). These findings corroborate our frequent observations of aphasic patients whose communication behaviors in real-life situations are quite functional, in contrast to their severely impaired linguistic functions.

The concept of measuring functional communication abilities in aphasia was first discussed in a paper by Taylor (1965), the outgrowth of which was the development of a rating scale called the Functional Communication Profile, or FCP (Sarno, 1969). A more recent functional communication assessment tool is Holland's (1980) Communicative Abilities in Daily Living, or CADL. Our Test for Functional Communication Abilities (Watamori et al., 1990) might be considered a modified version of CADL adapted to Japanese patients. The test consists of 34 subtests incorporating everyday communication activities. In the testing situation, these subtests are sequenced in such a way as to simulate a natural life situation in order to maximize extralinguistic contexts. A 5-point scale is used to assess the degree of communicative adequacy of the patients' responses. Results yield information about the functional communication skills of individual patients that is not adequately provided by the traditional aphasia test batteries.

Comparisons between functional communication abilities as measured by this test and linguistic functions as measured by the traditional aphasia tests disclosed that performance levels measured by the two tests were not necessarily correlated in individual patients. Some patients performed better on the former than the latter, and others vice versa, indicating relative independence of functional communication abilities from linguistic functions, and hence the need for planning and implementation of specific intervention strategies for each patient.

The development of specifically designed communication-oriented programs and their implementation for individual patients are currently at the experimental stage. Various programs for fostering the patients' language use and their ability to convey and receive messages effectively in everyday life situations are now in the process of being developed, implemented, and evaluated for their efficacy on an individual basis. In doing so we borrow ideas from some relevant methods including PACE (Promoting Aphasics' Communication Effectiveness), developed by Davis and Wilcox (1985), functional communication treatment proposed by Aten (1986), and more recent techniques such as the system of Conversational Coaching, a program of behavioral training in requesting and cognitive counseling developed by Holland (1991), among others.

The limited data that we have collected through working on communication-oriented approaches with our patients (Watamori, 1991) appear to be promising as well as ecologically valid. We believe that these pragmatic approaches should be integrated with standard language therapy and/or cognitive neuropsychological approaches for aphasic patients from the outset of treatment, because the primary objective of aphasia treatment is to help each individual achieve maximal recovery of communication abilities in real-life situations.

THE EFFICACY OF TREATMENT

Standard procedures to document the effect of multi-modality language therapy programs consist of administering a comprehensive formal test, pre- and post-treatment, and comparing the two evaluations. In general, re-evaluation procedures using the comprehensive battery take place once every 3 months. Parallel to these procedures, somewhat less formal procedures to monitor progress are used in daily clinical sessions by maintaining careful records of the patient's responses to treatment tasks to identify subtle changes in performance.

It is not an easy task, however, to provide comprehensive, definitive data showing that a given treatment approach has brought about a significant change in the language behavior of the patient beyond what is expected to occur as a result of spontaneous recovery. This is chiefly because of the large number and complexity of the variables involved (e.g., etiologies, types, severities, and duration of aphasia; sites and extent of lesions; age, health, and psycho-social background of patients; types, intensity, and duration of treatment programs, etc.). Nevertheless, an increasing number of studies in recent years has succeeded in controlling some of the important variables, and more quantitative information on the behavioral change has been obtained. Some of these are large group studies without control (nontreatment) groups; others are so called single-subject-time-series (subject-as-his-own-control) studies. An example of group studies appears below.

Fukusako and Monoi (1984b) investigated the recovery processes of 303 predominantly stroke-induced aphasic patients examined and treated between 1972 and 1981 at Tokyo Metropolitan Geriatric Hospital. The age of the patients ranged from 18 years to 87 years (a mean of 59.7 years), with 53% over 60 years old (geriatric aphasics) and 47% under 59 years old (adult aphasics). The time elapsed since the onset of aphasia for the majority of the patients was between 1 and 18 months. In terms of types of aphasia exhibited by these patients there was a striking difference between the geriatric and the adult groups. In the geriatric group, the incidence of global aphasia was significantly higher, whereas the incidence of Broca's aphasia was significantly lower as compared to the adult group. All patients received language therapy, essentially of a stimulation approach type, two to six sessions per week, for at least 2 months. Improvement was defined in terms of the percent increase in the total score on the Roken Test for Differential Diagnosis of Aphasia (RTDDA) (Sasanuma et al., 1978) administered pre- and post-treatment. A patient was judged "improved" if his gain after therapy was over 20% when his initial score was lower than 50% on the RTDDA. When his initial score was over 50%, 10% was the minimum gain judged "improved."

The results indicated that 46% of the patients improved, and improvement was related to the following variables:

1. *The type and severity of aphasia:* Improvement was greater for conduction aphasia and mild Broca's aphasia (with minimal comprehension deficits), followed by amnesic aphasia, moderate to severe Broca's aphasia (with comprehension deficits), Wernicke's aphasia, and global aphasia.
2. *The age of the patients:* Only 35% of the geriatric aphasics showed improvement as compared to 58% of the adult aphasics. Furthermore, the final level of post-treatment performance was significantly lower in the geriatric aphasics than in the adult aphasics. Fewer than 25% of the geriatric patients reached the level of 80% or better on the RTDDA (80% is considered the minimum level of functional language) as compared to 50% of the adult aphasics.
3. *Time elapsed since onset:* Incidence of improvement was significantly higher for patients with early initiation of therapy (within 3 months post-onset) than for patients with a later start, apparently indicating the effect of spontaneous recovery.

Evaluation of improvement in aphasia is not complete without documenting improvement in functional communication abilities of individual patients. However, we have not yet accumulated enough patients who have completed one of the specifically designed communication-oriented intervention programs, and therefore we are unable to report any definitive results concerning the efficacy of these programs at the present time.

VOCATIONAL AND SOCIAL REHABILITATION AND ADJUSTMENT

According to the previously mentioned series of four surveys (Survey Committee on Aphasia Rehabilitation in Japan, 1979, 1983, 1986, 1989), the percentage of treated aphasic patients returning to paid jobs (including returning to previous jobs, transfer to another section within the same company, or changing jobs) ranged from 12.4 to 16.2% of the whole group. For the remainder, the percentage of return to home was largest (49.4–56.8%) followed by transfer to other hospitals or institutions (9.9–23.4%). Similar percentages of return to paid jobs for treated aphasic patients were reported by Sasanuma (1972b) and Fukusako and Monoi (1984b), that is 18.0% (62 patients out of 348) and 18.1% (52 patients out of 303), respectively. (The latter authors also reported the percentage of return to paid jobs only for patients who were working just before the onset of aphasia [N = 192] as being 28.1%.) Among the factors found to influence the prospect of returning to paid jobs were: (1) Age of the patients (the younger the better); (2) severity of aphasia both at the beginning and at the termination of therapy (the milder the better); and (3) time post-onset when language therapy was begun (the shorter the better)(Fukusako & Monoi, 1984b; Sasanuma, 1972b). Undoubtedly, many other factors (including characteristics of the employer and the community) interact in a complex manner to influence the vocational rehabilitation of each individual.

Closely related to the topic of vocational rehabilitation are social readjustment, reintegration, and quality of life of aphasic persons after discharge. Partly because of the shortage of speech and language clinicians, only a limited attempt has been made at direct intervention into, or management of, this aspect of rehabilitation by clinicians. A few years ago, however, chronic aphasic patients and their spouses started to organize community-based groups in different parts of the country. A primary objective of these groups, usually called "Aphasia Peer Circles," is to promote "reintegration and self-development through identification with the aphasic community and peer support" (Sarno, 1986). Typical activities of these groups include: (1) Having regular meetings with social programs and information exchange, and (2) issuing circulars with short articles on a variety of topics of immediate interest and concern to the members of the groups. Sometimes, speech and language clinicians are invited as guests to these meetings or are asked to give informal talks. The number of these circles has increased at a rapid pace during the past few years, with a total of 102 local groups at the present time (Association of Aphasia Peer Circles, 1992).

ISSUES AND SUGGESTIONS

A number of issues and problems in aphasia rehabilitation face us in Japan. A few of these issues with high priority are discussed briefly in the following sections.

APHASIA IN THE ELDERLY

The elderly population in Japan during the past quarter of the century has increased to a degree unprecedented in the experience of any other country in history. This rapid increase is expected to continue at an even greater rate over the next three decades; by the year 2020, elderly individuals (65 years old and over) will constitute a quarter of the population of Japan (Ministry of Health, 1991). Consequently, Japan faces an increased incidence of age-related diseases involving higher cortical functions, including aphasia and dementia. This increase in life-expectancy in recent years is world-wide, of course, having had its share of effects on the aphasic population. Accumulated data indicate that aphasia is qualitatively different in the elderly than in younger age groups. Patients with Wernicke's aphasia tend to be older than patients with Broca's aphasia (Fukusako & Monoi, 1984a; Harasymiw, Halper, & Sutherland, 1981; Holland & Bartlett, 1985; Kertesz & Sheppard, 1981). The incidence of severe/global aphasia as well as of aphasia complicated by concomitant nonlinguistic cognitive deficits of various types and/or other communication deficits such as spastic dysarthria also increases significantly in older patients (Fukusako & Monoi, 1984b; Monoi, 1991; Watamori, Fukusako, Monoi, & Sasanuma, 1990), whereas improvement decreases significantly with age (Fukusako & Monoi, 1984b; Holland & Bartlett, 1985; Takeuchi, Kawachi, & Ishii, 1975, among others). We are highly cognizant of the results reported by Sarno (1980), indicating that age per se does not have significant negative effects on severity or recovery of aphasia, when all relevant variables are rigorously controlled. In fact, however, it is rather rare to encounter elderly aphasic patients for whom all the relevant variables other than age are identical to those for younger aphasic patients.

Taken together these findings suggest the need for more systematic investigation into the nature of interactive variables operating in aphasia in old age. Such investigation will require a comprehensive evaluation of language as well as other cognitive functions (Benton, 1982) not only in aphasic patients but also in the normal elderly. To obtain such data, we have constructed a battery of 20 tests probing four major cognitive domains: Orientation, memory, language, and visuo-spatial-constructional abilities (Sasanuma et al., 1985). Thus far, we have administered this battery to a group of healthy normal subjects ($N = 121$) between the ages of 50 and 89 years (who were recruited from senior citizen organizations in Tokyo), as well as to a group of patients with mild to moderate dementia of various types ($N = 102$) (Sasanuma, 1988c; Sasanuma et al., 1987). We believe that cognitive neuropsychological data such as these, obtained from healthy elderly subjects as well as from patients with dementia, are invaluable for gaining proper perspective and insight into the nature of aphasia in the elderly (Sasanuma, 1988b). Of particular importance from the clinical viewpoint is the need for differential diagnosis between aphasic patients with concomitant nonlinguistic cognitive deficits and those without them. According to Fukusako and Monoi (1984a), the percentage of post-stroke patients whose aphasia is accompanied by general cognitive impairment or dementia increases significantly with age, affecting 30.4% of patients in their 70s as compared to 7.8% of patients under 39 years old. It will not be an easy task to develop a diagnostic system for differentiating between patients with aphasia only and those with aphasia plus dementia. A first step toward this goal appears to be to elucidate the distinctive features of linguistic and nonlinguistic cognitive abilities and disabilities manifested by aphasic patients (without dementia) and patients with a diagnosis of dementia.

We have given the battery of 20 neuropsychological tests, described above, (Sasanuma et al., 1985) to a group of 93 aphasic patients (Fukusako, Watamori, Monoi, & Sasanuma, 1992) in order to compare their performance patterns with corresponding patterns of 91 patients with mild to moderate dementia. The aphasic patients were selected from the clinical population of the Speech Pathology Service, the Tokyo Metropolitan Geriatric Hospital, on the basis of the following criteria: (1) right-handed, (2) brain lesion confined to the left hemisphere, (3) no history of cognitive decline, and (4) no concomitant communication disorder other than aphasia. The mean time post-onset of aphasia was 10.7 months. In terms of clinical types of aphasia, 26 patients had Broca's aphasia, 20 Wernicke's aphasia, 20 anomic aphasia, 9 global aphasia, and 5 conduction aphasia; the remaining 22 were unclassifiable. The 91 patients with dementia were drawn from a pool of 102 patients with mild to moderate dementia studied by Sasanuma et al. (1987). Of these 91 patients, 52 were diagnosed as having dementia of the Alzheimer type and the remaining 39 as having vascular dementia. All 91 patients were right-handed, had adequate visual and hearing acuity to perform the required tasks, and all had at least 6 years of education.

Because the two groups of patients were significantly different in terms of age (59.2 vs. 72.8 years) and years of education (12.0 vs. 9.0 years), an analysis of covariance with these two variables as covariates was performed on each test to compare the performance of the two groups. In Figure 8–1, the means of each test for each group were plotted against the performance of the group of 93 normal elderly subjects matched for age with the group of demented patients. The shaded area represents the range of -1 SD performance on each test for the normal subjects. The solid line represents the performance profile of the aphasic patients, and the dotted line represents that of the demented patients. The open triangle in front of a given test indicates that the aphasic patients performed significantly better than the demented patients ($p < .05$) on that test, whereas the solid diamond indicates that the aphasic patients performed significantly worse than the demented patients ($p < .05$) on that test. As shown in Figure 8–1, the test profiles of the two groups are distinctly different. The aphasic patients performed significantly better than the demented patients on the test of orientation to time and space, and on all the tests of visuo-spatial abilities. In fact, their mean scores on all of the visuo-spatial tests were well within the normal range, which was in sharp contrast to the clear-cut impairment on these test in the demented patients. On the other hand, performance of the aphasic patients on six of the nine tests in the language domain was significantly worse than that of the demented patients. Among these six were sentence repetition and oral reading (of words), on which the demented patients as a group performed within, or almost within, the normal range. These are the tasks that tap the phonological rather than semantic aspects of language, which tend to be resistant to dementing illness at least in its early stage (Sasanuma, 1988b), but which are definitely vulnerable to various types of aphasia. In the domain of memory, performance of the aphasic group was significantly below that of the demented group on the two digit span tasks, but on each of the remaining two tasks, immediate and delayed story recall, the performance of the two groups was not significantly different. However, when the amount of information retained (AIR) during the delay interval (30 minutes) was examined for each group (by comparing the percentage of information units retrieved in the delayed recall condition to that in the immediate recall condition), the AIR in the aphasic group was more than

◇ 1. Orientation

♦ 2. Digit Repetition Span
♦ 3. Digit Pointing Scan
    4. Story Recall, Immediate
    5. Story Recall, Delayed

♦ 6. Sentence Repetition
    7. Following Commands
♦ 8. Naming
♦ 9. Word Fluency, Phonological
    10. Word Fluency, Semantic
♦ 11. Picture Description
♦ 12. Oral Reading
♦ 13. Reading Comprehension
    14. Writing Sentences

◇ 15. Facial Recognition
◇ 16. Clock Face
◇ 17. Clock Setting
◇ 18. Block Construction
◇ 19. Line Orientation
◇ 20. Tactile Form Perception

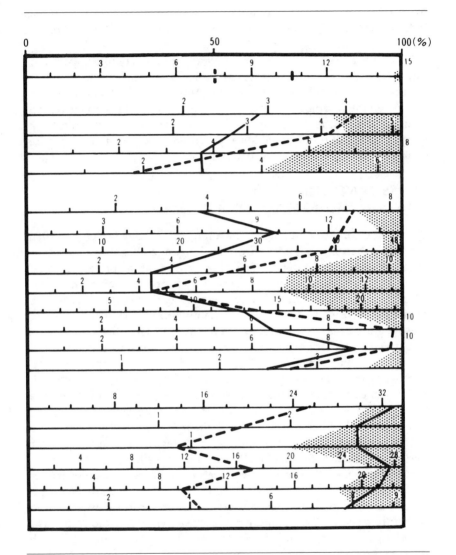

Figure 8–1. The mean performance profile on a battery of 20 neuropsychological tests for the group of 93 aphasic patients (solid line) and for the group of 91 demented patients (dotted line) plotted against the 100% baseline representing the mean performance of 93 normal healthy elderly subjects in their 60's through 80's (*M* = 83.1 years). The shaded area represents the range of −1 SD performance on each test for the normal elderly subjects. Open diamonds (◊) in front of some tests on the vertical axis indicate that the aphasic group performed significantly better than the demented group (*p* < .05) on these tests; solid diamonds (♦) in front of other tests indicate that the aphasic group performed significantly worse than the demented group (*p* < .05) on these tests.

twice as large as that in the demented group (79% vs. 37%, $p < .01$). This indicates that the AIR serves as a sensitive measure for the differential diagnosis of the two groups of patients.

Further analyses of the data are currently under way to compare performance patterns of different types of aphasia versus dementia of different etiologies (viz., Alzheimer type dementia and vascular type dementia). When the findings of these analyses become available to us, we will be in a better position to arrive at differential diagnosis of the elderly patients, which will in turn enable us to plan more adequate intervention strategies for each individual patient.

CROSS-LANGUAGE COMPARATIVE STUDIES OF APHASIA

The number of different languages in the world today is close to 3,000, yet only a handful of Indo-European languages has been the major source of documentation for aphasiology. For the study of aphasia to become a truly universal science, descriptions of aphasic deficits manifested in a broader spectrum of languages are clearly necessary, as are explanatory theories and treatment/rehabilitation procedures based on these theories (Sasanuma, 1986). As a matter of fact, there is evidence that structural variations of individual languages constitute an important variable exerting differential effects on the patterns of aphasic symptoms. A cross-language comparative study of agrammatic narratives in 14 languages (Chinese, Dutch, English, Finnish, French, German, Hebrew, Hindi, Icelandic, Italian, Japanese, Polish, Serbo-Croatian, and Swedish) has been conducted over the past few years (Menn & Obler, 1988). Some of the results obtained from Japanese aphasic patients (Sasanuma, Kamio, & Kubota, 1990) in this cross-language study indicate that so-called "representative" features of agrammatic speech are not as representative as had been thought, and in fact, some language-specific features do exist that have crucial implications for aphasia theory. Future research into other areas of aphasic symptomatology in a wider variety of languages may well uncover more such features. It is only through the integration of language-specific and language-universal data that we can construct a truly comprehensive theory of aphasia, which in turn will help us develop more effective treatment procedures.

PROFESSIONAL TRAINING OF SPEECH AND LANGUAGE CLINICIANS

Last but not least is the issue of professional training of qualified speech and language clinicians capable of treating aphasia and related problems.

We have had a long-standing dispute in Japan about the nature and level of professional training for speech and language clinicians among several groups concerned (including the responsible governmental offices, associations of speech-language-hearing therapists, a group of school teachers, and the medical associations representing rehabilitation medicine, otolaryngology, neurology, and neuropsychology, among others), but no consensus has been reached thus far. In 1988 a conference of the 26 major medical associations was held for promoting early establishment of the certificate system for medically related speech-language-hearing clinicians. Currently, joint meetings are being held regularly to discuss the matter, although we have yet to see any tangible outcome. It is extremely unfortunate that this had to happen in our field in this country, and that we have such a long way to go before we can arrive at a system which is satisfactory for all of us concerned, above all for the patients with aphasia.

REFERENCES

Association of Aphasia Peer Circles. (1992). Personal communication with Mr. Toshio Tamura, the president of the association.

Aten, J. L. (1986). Functional communication treatment. In R. Chapey (Ed.), *Language intervention strategies in adult aphasia* (2nd ed., pp. 266–276). Baltimore, MD: Williams & Wilkins.

Benton, A. L. (1982). Significance of nonverbal cognitive abilities in aphasic patients. *Japanese Journal of Stroke, 4*, 153–161.

Davis, G. A., & Wilcox, M. J. (1985). *Adult aphasia rehabilitation*. San Diego, CA: College-Hill Press.

Fujita, I. (1976). *Recovery patterns of syntactic performance in aphasic patients* (pp. 51–80), (Research Bulletin 1976). National Center of the Speech and Hearing Disorders. Tokyo.

Fujita, I., Miyake, T., & Nakanishi, Y. (1983). *Syntax test of aphasia: Experimental version II*. Committee for the Development of Aphasia Test Batteries. Tokyo.

Fukusako, Y., & Monoi, H. (1984a). The influence of age and sex on the type and severity of aphasia. *Japan Journal of Logopedics and Phoniatrics, 25*, 1–12 (in Japanese).

Fukusako, Y., & Monoi, H. (1984b). The recovery pattern in treated aphasic patients I. *Japan Journal of Logopedics and Phoniatrics, 25*, 295–307 (in Japanese).

Fukusako, Y., Watamori, T. S., Monoi, H., & Sasanuma, S. (1992). Comparison of aphasic patients and demented patients using a series of neuropsychological tests. *Japanese Journal of Rehabilitation Medicine, 29*, 556–567.

Harasymiw, S. J., Halper, A., & Sutherland, B. (1981). Sex, age, and aphasia type. *Brain and Language, 12*, 190–198.

Hasegawa, T. (1975). *Manual for Standard Language Test of Aphasia*. Tokyo: Homeido (in Japanese).

Holland, A. L. (1970). Case studies in aphasia rehabilitation using programmed instruction. *Journal of Speech and Hearing Research, 35,* 377–390.

Holland, A. L. (1980). *Communicative abilities in daily living.* Baltimore, MD: University Park Press.

Holland, A. L. (1991). Pragmatic aspects of intervention in aphasia. *Journal of Neurolinguistics, 6,* 197–211.

Holland, A. L., & Bartlett, C. L. (1985). Some differential effects of age on stroke-produced aphasia. In H. Ulatowska (Ed.), *The aging brain* (pp. 141–155). San Diego, CA: College-Hill Press.

Kashiwagi, A., & Kashiwagi, T. (1978). Kana training for the aphasics utilizing kanji as a key word. *Japan Journal of Logopedics and Phoniatrics, 19,* 193–202 (in Japanese).

Kertesz, A., & Sheppard, A. (1981). The epidemiology of aphasic and cognitive impairment in stroke: Age, sex, aphasia type and laterality differences. *Brain, 104,* 117–128.

Lesser, R. (1987). Cognitive neuropsychological influence on aphasia therapy. *Aphasiology, 1,* 189–200.

Lesser, R. (1989). Some issues in the neuropsychological rehabilitation of anomia. In X. Seron & G. Deloche (Eds.), *Cognitive approaches in neuropsychological rehabilitation.* Hillsdale, NJ: Lawrence Erlbaum.

Menn, L., & Obler, L. K. (1988). Findings of the cross-language aphasia study, phase I: Agrammatic narratives. *Aphasiology, 2,* 347–350.

Ministry of Health and Welfare Institute of Population Problems. (1991). *Population projections for Japan.* Tokyo: Health and Welfare Statistics Association (in Japanese).

Monoi, H. (1976). A kana training program for a patient with Broca's aphasia: A case report. *Communication Disorder Research, 5,* 105–117 (in Japanese).

Monoi, H. (1990). Therapy for kana writing impairment in aphasic patients. *Japanese Journal of Neuropsychology, 6,* 33–40 (in Japanese).

Monoi, H. (1991). Communication disorders in the elderly: From the clinical viewpoint. *Japan Journal of Logopedics and Phoniatrics, 32,* 227–234 (in Japanese).

Sarno, M. T. (1969). *The functional communication profile: Manual of direction.* New York: New York University Medical Center, Institute of Rehabilitation Medicine.

Sarno, M. T. (1980). Language rehabilitation outcome in the elderly aphasic patient. In L. K. Obler & M. L. Albert (Eds.), *Language and communication in the elderly* (pp. 191–204). Lexington, MA: D.C. Health.

Sarno, M. T. (1986). *The silent minority: The patient with aphasia.* The Fifth Annual James C. Hemphill Lecture, The Rehabilitation Institute of Chicago.

Sasanuma, S. (1972a). A factorial study of language impairment of 269 post-stroke aphasic patients: Part I. *Japanese Journal of Rehabilitation Medicine, 9,* 20–33.

Sasanuma, S. (1972b). Issues in rehabilitation of aphasic patients: Prognosis of vocational adjustment in treated aphasic patients. *Japan Journal of Logopedics and Phoniatrics, 13,* 26–34.

Sasanuma, S. (1980a). A therapy program for impairment of the use of the kana-syllabary of Japanese aphasic patients. In M. T. Sarno & O. Hook (Eds.), *Aphasia: Assessment and treatment* (pp. 170–180). Stockholm: Almqvist & Wiksell.

Sasanuma, S. (1980b). Acquired dyslexia in Japanese: Clinical features and underlying mechanisms. In M. Coltheart, K. Patterson, & J. C. Marshall (Eds.), *Deep dyslexia* (pp. 48–90). London: Routledge & Kegan Paul.

Sasanuma, S. (1985). Surface dyslexia and dysgraphia: How are they manifested in Japanese? In K. E. Patterson, J. C. Marshall, & M. Coltheart (Eds.), *Surface dyslexia: Neuropsychological and cognitive analysis of phonological reading* (pp. 227–251). London: Lawrence Erlbaum.

Sasanuma, S. (1986). Universal and language-specific symptomatology and treatment of aphasia. *Folia Phoniatrica, 38,* 121–175.

Sasanuma, S. (1988a). Cognitive neuropsychology approach to the study of aphasia: A case of reading impairment. *Aphasiology, 2,* 395–400.

Sasanuma, S. (1988b). Studies of dementia: In search of the linguistic/cognitive interaction underlying communication. *Aphasiology, 2,* 191–193.

Sasanuma, S. (1988c). Patterns of cognitive abilities on Higher Brain Function Test in the normal elderly and patients with mild to moderate dementia. *Geriatric Psychiatry, 5,* 503–516 (in Japanese).

Sasanuma, S. (1989). Aphasia rehabilitation in Japan. In M. T.Sarno & D. E. Woods (Eds.), *Aphasia rehabilitation in Asia and the Pacific region: Japan, China, India, Australia and New Zealand.* (Monograph #45, pp. 13–43). World Rehabilitation Fund.

Sasanuma, S., Itoh, M., Watamori, T., Fukusako, Y., & Monoi, H. (1978). *Treatment of aphasia.* Tokyo: Igaku-Shoin (in Japanese).

Sasanuma, S., Itoh, M., Watamori, T., Fukuzawa, K., Sakuma, N., Fukusako, Y., & Monoi, H. (1985). Linguistic and nonlinguistic abilities of the Japanese elderly and patients with dementia. In H. Ulatowska (Ed.), *The aging brain* (pp 175–200). San Diego, CA: College-Hill Press.

Sasanuma, S., Itoh, M., Watamori, T., Fukuzawa, K., Sakuma, N., Fukusako, Y., Monoi, H., & Tatsumi, I. (1987). Neuropsychological investigation of dementia: Heterogeneity of cognitive impairment. *Japanese Journal of Neuropsychology, 3,* 216–225 (in Japanese).

Sasanuma S., Kamio, A., & Kubota, M. (1990). Agrammatism in Japanese: Two case studies. In L. Menn & L. K. Obler (Eds.), *Agrammatic aphasia: A cross-language narrative sourcebook* (pp. 1225–1307). Amsterdam: John Benjamins.

Schuell, H., Jenkins, J. J., & Jimenez-Pabon, E. (1964). *Aphasia in adults: Diagnosis, prognosis, and treatment.* New York: Harper & Row.

Seron, X., & Deloche, G. (1987). *Cognitive approaches in neuropsychological rehabilitation.* Hillsdale, NJ: Lawrence Erlbaum.

Spellacy, F. J., & Spreen, O. (1969). A short form of the token test. *Cortex, 5,* 390–397.

Sugishita, M. (1988). *WAB aphasia test in Japanese.* Tokyo: Igaku Shoin.

Survey Committee on Aphasia Rehabilitation in Japan. (1979). Report on aphasia rehabilitation in 1978. *Japan Journal of Logopedics and Phoniatrics, 20,* 160–172 (in Japanese).

Survey Committee on Aphasia Rehabilitation in Japan. (1983). Report on aphasia rehabilitation in 1982. *Higher Brain Function Research, 3,* 425–432 (in Japanese).

Survey Committee on Aphasia Rehabilitation in Japan. (1986). Report on aphasia rehabilitation in 1985. *Higher Brain Function Research, 6,* 998–1007 (in Japanese).

Survey Committee on Aphasia Rehabilitation in Japan. (1989). Report on aphasia rehabilitation in 1988. *Higher Brain Function Research, 9,* 134–144 (in Japanese).

Suzuki, T., Monoi, H., & Fukusako, Y. (1990). Development of a kana training program for aphasic patients: Using a key one-syllable word and a cue to retrieve its meaning. *Japan Journal of Logopedics and Phoniatrics, 31,* 159–171 (in Japanese).

Takeuchi, A., Kawachi, J., & Ishii, Y. (1975). Language rehabilitation in aphasia: Some factors related to the improvement of language functions. *Kanagawa-ken Rehabilitation Center Bulletin, 2,* 46–68 (in Japanese).

Taylor, S. M. (1965). A measurement of functional communication in aphasia. *Archives of Physical Medicine Rehabilitation, 46,* 101–107.

Ulatowska, H. K., Friedman-Stern, R. F., Weiss-Doyle, A. W., Macaluso-Haynes, S. M., & North, A. J. (1983). Production of narrative discourse in aphasia. *Brain and Language, 19,* 317–334.

Ulatowska, H. K., North, A. J., & Macaluso-Haynes, S. (1981). Production of narrative and procedural discourse in aphasia. *Brain and Language, 13,* 345– 371.

Watamori, T. (1991). Rehabilitation of aged aphasic patients: A communication-oriented approach. *Japan Journal of Logopedics and Phoniatrics, 32,* 235–244 (in Japanese).

Watamori, T., Fukusako, Y., Monoi, H., & Sasanuma, S. (1990). Interactive effects of age and aphasia: With special emphasis on nonlinguistic cognitive abilities. *Japanese Journal of Rehabilitation Medicine, 27,* 379–387 (in Japanese).

Watamori, T., Takeuchi, A., Itoh, M., Fukusako, Y., Suzuki, T., Endo, K., Takahashi, M., & Sasanuma, S. (1990). *Test for functional communication abilities — CADL Test.* Tokyo: Ishiyaku (in Japanese).

Weigl, E. (1961). The phenomenon of temporary deblocking in aphasia. *Zeitschrift fur Phonetic, Sprachwissenschaft unt Kommunikations Forschung, 14,* 337–364.

Wepman, J. M. (1951). *Recovery from aphasia.* New York: Ronald Press.

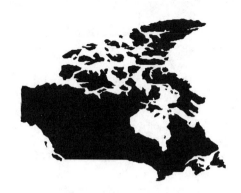

CHAPTER 9

Functional Is Not Enough: Training Conversation Partners for Aphasic Adults

AURA KAGAN
GILLIAN F. GAILEY
Aphasia Centre–North York
Ontario, Canada

Visit with us at a local community center program. Nothing particularly dramatic is occurring — just small groups of four or five people sitting around tables, chatting. Most participants are seniors; some are in wheelchairs. One of the group members seems to be doing more of the talking and, at times, there are longer periods of silence than you might expect. Laughter emanates from many of the groups, while others seem involved in serious discussion. You see newspapers on the tables, along with blank cards, paper, pencils, and markers. Photographs, maps, magnetic alphabet boards, and calendars are easily accessible to all.

Observe Peter expounding on the health care system, angry and frustrated about the way that drugs were prescribed for him; Doris expressing her strong conviction that Canadians should be free to shop wherever things are cheaper; and Shirley, Lois, and Dianne (average age 50 years) blushing and laughing about the idea of visiting a male strip club.

The lively conversations just described seem natural enough to be oc-curring at any social club. Surprisingly, though, the participants in this program are aphasic, and more than two thirds have moderate to severe language impairment. In the normal course of events, who would imag-ine it possible to discuss complex issues with someone discharged from therapy with a label of "global aphasia?"

Implicit in the above question is the idea that such a severe disability precludes the possibility of such conversations for most aphasic adults. Conversely, it is expected that individuals with more functional or effec-tive communication skills will find social conversation correspondingly easier. Our long-term involvement with aphasic adults at the Aphasia Cen-tre–North York has led us to re-evaluate the implied equivalence of func-tional communication and conversation, and, in particular, our profession-al mandate with respect to rehabilitation of individuals with aphasia.

The approach we describe has, as its core, the idea that conversation is a basic and unique form of communication, essential for maintaining psychosocial well-being. From this perspective, the consequences of re-duced ability and/or opportunity to engage in conversation are viewed as a distinct handicap for the aphasic individual. The program developed at the Aphasia Centre is specifically directed at reducing this handicap by providing aphasic participants with opportunities for conversation with skilled partners. The rationale for training volunteers as conversa-tion facilitators, and the role of the speech-language pathologist, are de-scribed within the context of the Centre.

We emphasize that the approach presented originates directly from our observation of interactions of chronic aphasic individuals and train-ed volunteers who participate in the Centre's programs. Shifts in profes-sional focus are, therefore, as much the result of lessons aphasic adults and volunteers have taught us as they are of changing perspectives in the field of speech-language pathology. Current theory and research in the area of conversation provide an explanatory framework for a process that has developed spontaneously.

BACKGROUND OF THE
APHASIA CENTRE–NORTH YORK

The Aphasia Centre–North York, previously known as The Speech and Stroke Centre, was founded in 1979 by Pat Arato. As the spouse of a relatively young aphasic person, Pat was acutely aware of the need for community-based support for aphasic people who had been discharged from therapy. The original inspiration for the Centre was a presentation made in 1978 by Valerie Eaton Griffiths and the actress Patricia Neal that focused on the potential for using volunteers to provide support for people with aphasia.

After meeting other families desperate for any post-therapy service, Pat and a dedicated group of volunteers started a communication program specifically for aphasic individuals who were no longer receiving therapy. In Pat's words, she wanted "to give aphasic people hope; to help them to talk; to let them know that life had not come to an end and that there was somewhere for them to go."

Thirteen years later, community volunteers are still an integral part of the program. Currently, there are 96 volunteers working at the Centre in various capacities. The majority attend once a week and work in conversation groups with three to five aphasic adults. Others are involved in recreational activities, a newsletter, development of program materials, administrative functions, and special events such as aphasia awareness campaigns. The Centre employs a coordinator of volunteers who is responsible for recruitment and, together with the speech-language pathologists, for ongoing monitoring of volunteers. Our volunteers, mostly women, range in age from the late teens to octogenarians. They come from diverse vocational and educational backgrounds. Being a successful volunteer does not seem to be related to any one factor, and for this reason, the Centre does not target any one group of people (e.g., university graduates or retired teachers) for recruitment.

The daily schedule balances time in preassigned discussion groups with opportunity for general socialization during breaks (see Appendix A). Additional opportunities for conversation are provided by various recreational activities such as art, ceramics, and music, again facilitated by trained volunteers. The Centre also provides individual and group counselling for members and their families by staff speech-language pathologists and a social worker.

The program fosters a working partnership among members, their families, volunteers, and professional and administrative staff. The use of normalizing terminology, whereby aphasic participants are referred to as "members" rather than as patients or clients, reinforces goals of increased independence and community reintegration. The physical location of the Centre in a noninstitutional setting is another important normalizing factor, one which enables contact with people from the community.

In acknowledgment of the chronic nature of aphasia, the Centre has developed a policy of long-term support: Individuals are given the choice of retaining lifelong membership, with the level of support dependent on individual need. A core of 100 to 125 members participates in conversation groups, attending twice weekly. This number is low enough to maintain an intimate atmosphere and to enable professional staff to follow members closely. At the same time, it is large enough to provide the critical mass and range of interests necessary for natural friendships to develop. The core group of members participating in conversation groups may also attend recreational activities. Individuals who no longer require the level of communicative support provided by the small conversation groups attend only the recreational activities and/or self-directed groups that meet regularly for discussions, lectures, or outings. Although these groups all involve volunteers trained as conversation partners, the ratio of members to volunteers is much larger; there is also greatly decreased professional input. The common denominator underlying all activities is the opportunity for conversation.

THE HANDICAP OF APHASIA: REDUCED OPPORTUNITIES FOR CONVERSATION

Most of the members attending the Centre are, as Penn (1987) describes, "experienced." They have had time to adjust to the chronicity of their language impairment and have usually developed their own repertoires of compensatory strategies. Yet, our extended involvement with more than 200 members has made us increasingly aware that the devastating psychosocial effects of chronic aphasia do not necessarily lessen with the passage of time, or as a function of severity of aphasia. In contrast to what one might expect, for example, members with mild aphasia are as deeply committed to attending conversation groups at the Centre as those with more severe impairment.

The high prevalence of depression in persons who have sustained a stroke is well documented (Robinson, Lipsey, & Price, 1985). Our members and their families consistently cite loss of established relationships and social isolation as the major negative changes in their lives. Typically, they attribute the precipitous decline in social interactions to communicative impairment and their own general reluctance to make social contact. As with 500 aphasic individuals surveyed by the National Aphasia Association (1988), our members often perceive that unimpaired people reject them because of their inability to communicate normally.

Friends who initially attempt to socialize are often discouraged by the frustration and embarrassment of struggling to communicate with the aphasic individual and may eventually allow the relationship to lapse. For families and caregivers, the communication barrier frequently results in limiting interactions to those mainly focused on specific physical wants or needs. It is the discrepancy between this type of interaction, usually structured in a question-answer format, and the more flexible social conversation used in everyday life, that prompted us to examine our approach to chronic aphasia.

CONVERSATION AND COMMUNICATION

Schiffrin (1988) describes conversation as "a basic form of communication." Although both conversation and communication involve a sender and receiver, the communicative partnership of conversation accomplishes much more than effective transmission and receipt of information. The totality, complexity, and diffuse nature of conversation is captured by Le Guin (1989) who wrote:

> We don't, we never did, go about making statements of fact to other people, or in our internal discourse with ourselves. We talk about what may be, or what we'd like to do, or what you ought to do, or what might have happened: warnings, suppositions, propositions, invitations, ambiguities, analogies, hints, lists, anxieties, hearsay, old wives' tales, leaps, and crosslinks and spiderwebs between here and there, between then and now, between now and sometime, a continual weaving and restructuring of the remembered and the perceived and the imagined. (p. 44)

The use of conversation in everyday life is so automatic, however, that its functional purpose may not be fully appreciated until the process is disrupted. In all spheres of living — family, work, social, and societal — conversation, in its broadest, interactional sense, is the common currency that enables people to function normally. Schegloff (1990) described the scope of conversation as follows: "In dealing with talk and interaction, we are dealing with the primordial site of human life. This is where the work of society gets done." Conversation is the process whereby one resolves a conflict, makes social arrangements, argues with the family, or confides in a friend; it is, in essence, integral to participating in the complete range of human interactions.

THE DUALITY OF CONVERSATION

Schiffrin (1988) noted that while conversation entails talk or verbal activity, it is at the same time "a vehicle through which selves, relationships and situations are socially constructed" (p. 272). For the aphasic adult, the dual nature of conversation as verbal language and as social interaction (Schiffrin, 1988) has very real implications: Compromising the ability to engage in conversation simultaneously affects the ability to engage in social life. From a psychosocial perspective, reduced ability to participate in social interactions results in the loss of a powerful means of defining oneself, achieving self-esteem, and maintaining relationships with others.

COMMUNICATIVE ACCESSIBILITY

Bearing in mind the centrality of conversation in accessing virtually every sphere of social activity, the consequences of aphasia are especially profound. In contrast to disabled persons whose communication is unimpaired, aphasic individuals do not have access to the psychosocial support networks which might facilitate more effective functioning. The potential benefits of self-help groups and generic social and recreational programs often are denied to the person with aphasia simply because conversation is a prerequisite to satisfying participation. For the aphasic population, there is nothing analogous to the wheelchair ramps that facilitate access for those with physical impairment; without "communication ramps," aphasic individuals are excluded from participation in the social life of the community.

THE HANDICAP OF APHASIA

It is within the context of this shrinking social environment that the real nature of the handicap of aphasia can be appreciated. We use "handicap" in accordance with the scheme developed by the World Health Organization (1980). Within this conceptual framework, a handicap exists if an individual is unable to fulfill a desired age-appropriate role, as a result of disability. We strongly support the view that "The mission of a rehabilitation program is to reduce handicap" (Willer, Guastaferro, Zankiw, & Duran, 1990, p. 4).

For the person with aphasia, reduced ability to engage in mutually satisfying conversations constitutes a handicap that is acutely experienced in virtually every aspect of daily living. This handicap has especially poignant psychosocial consequences with respect to the use of conversation as a means of validating one's own existence. Schiffrin (1988), in a review of Goffman's (1967) book, noted that "whatever it is that one attempts to mean through one's individual efforts of expression cannot alone create a self; those expressive meanings have to be understood and acted upon by the one to whom they are directed" (p. 266).

Given the need for reciprocal involvement in conversation, we specifically focus on the training of conversation partners. Without this specific intervention, aphasic individuals do not normally have many opportunities to engage in mutually satisfying conversations. The term "conversation partner" is adapted from Lyon's work on "communicative partners" for aphasic adults (Lyon, in press). We use these terms interchangeably.

ADDRESSING THE HANDICAP OF APHASIA BY TRAINING CONVERSATION PARTNERS: AN EXTENDED ROLE FOR THE SPEECH-LANGUAGE PATHOLOGIST

The communication program at the Aphasia Centre–North York provides training which enables volunteers to give aphasic adults the opportunity to engage in natural conversation. This reflects our belief that functional communication skills are not the end-point on the speech-language treatment continuum. We have not, however, always viewed our professional role as extending to the psychosocial well-being of our members.

Initially, the Centre was staffed almost exclusively by volunteers, with only minimal involvement of speech-language pathologists. Volunteers had two separate goals. The first was to work on improving members' talking, reading (aloud), and writing. Typical activities included repetition, recitation of automatic sequences, and extensive use of workbook material. The second goal was to provide social and emotional support. Socializing that occurred between "work" sessions was seen as an important part of the program.

TRACING A SHIFT IN PROFESSIONAL FOCUS

Speech-language pathology involvement at the Centre gradually increased over time, from advice given on a voluntary basis to the present situation where there is paid professional staff. In line with developments in the field in the 1980s, the focus of the communication program shifted from a focus on "talking" to a focus on "communicating." Volunteers were encouraged to perceive themselves as communication facilitators, rather than as teachers. They worked on strategies to help improve the functional communication skills of the members and to evaluate each activity in terms of the question: "Is this going to make a difference to his or her ability to communicate in the 'real' world"? Activities that did not promote generalization were not encouraged. On an informal basis, success was evaluated in terms of independence. Typical examples included members going shopping, choosing purchases on their own, and being able to indicate what they wanted to order in a restaurant.

In the process of formal evaluation of the program we began to question our role as speech-language pathologists. Evaluation had become increasingly important on a professional level and, from a practical perspective, essential in substantiating requests for funding. A small pilot study was conducted to assess change in functional communication (Kagan & Gailey, 1990). We experimented with Lomas et al.'s (1989) Communicative Effectiveness Index (CETI) and compared it to results obtained on the Western Aphasia Battery (WAB) (Kertesz, 1982). Part of the study involved administration of the above measures to eight people with chronic aphasia who attended the Centre. Results of pre- and post-testing over a 4-month period provided evidence of significant change in several of the 16 communicative situations assessed on the CETI; as expected, there was no change on the WAB.

Despite the demonstration of change in perceived communicative effectiveness, we were not convinced that we had captured the more dramatic psychosocial changes in members observed by families, volunteers, and ourselves. These changes typically involved increased motivation, communicative confidence, and social interaction, parameters that went beyond both language ability and functional communication skills.

If the most dramatic changes were psychosocial, obvious and discomforting questions arose. Were we running a purely social/recreational program? Was there a professional role for the speech-language pathologist in this setting, and if so, what exactly was it? Finally, what should we be evaluating?

We had been attributing improvements in psychosocial functioning of our aphasic members to the general positive atmosphere of the Centre, personal qualities of staff and volunteers, and the socialization that occurred between the work sessions. Contact with Jon Lyon (1989b) led us to examine the validity of using speech-language pathology skills to achieve psychosocial goals. Within this framework, we became increasingly aware that social interaction, always acknowledged as important, was not occurring outside of the communication program, but because of it. Through training by professionals, our volunteers had acquired skills that enabled natural and spontaneous interactions to occur. It was use of these skills for the purpose of socialization that resulted in the psychosocial change. Our volunteers were functioning as a "communication ramp" to normal social interaction.

Our difficulty in interpreting what was happening can be understood in terms of the history of aphasia therapy and the training we received as speech-language pathology students. The profession generally has focused on a particular role for speech-language pathologists, namely that of a "fixer" of communication deficits. The shift in focus from language usage to functional communication, although striking in its impact on therapy goals, procedures, and criteria of evaluation has not essentially altered this role; the perceived goal is still improvement in communication skill. We ourselves focused for many years on functional communication activities, such as being able to choose items independently from a restaurant menu.

The initial discomfort caused by using speech-language pathology expertise to provide aphasic adults with the opportunity for mutually satisfying conversation is related to the move away from the traditional fixer role. In offering conversational opportunities, there is a deliberate attempt to reduce the level of frustration, with the aim of allowing the aphasic participant to "forget" about the aphasia to the extent possible. We asked ourselves whether it was appropriate to use our training in this way.

Our conclusion that a shift in focus is both appropriate and necessary has come, in part, through a reconsideration of functional activities within a real life context, for example, going out to a restaurant. For most of us, a visit to a restaurant is a social occasion, an opportunity to chat with friends while enjoying a meal. Although success, in functional terms, might be defined in terms of the ability to independently order from the menu, few of us would consider this to be the real purpose of eating out. We now have a greater appreciation of the importance of providing opportunities for the restaurant conversation that is missing from the lives of many aphasic adults.

ACKNOWLEDGING THE PROFESSIONAL EXPERTISE REQUIRED TO FACILITATE CONVERSATIONS WITH APHASIC ADULTS

Considerable skill and expertise are required to facilitate natural conversations with aphasic adults. We recognize that many people, including some speech-language pathologists, do not acknowledge this. However, if exposure and motivation were all that were required, family members would automatically be excellent communication partners. At the Centre, we observe that inexperienced or untrained communication partners are initially ill-at-ease in the situation and tend to focus on didactic or task-oriented interactions.

WHY SHOULD THE TRAINING OF COMMUNICATION PARTNERS SPECIFICALLY INVOLVE A SPEECH-LANGUAGE PATHOLOGIST?

As discussed previously, conversation concurrently achieves two goals: Verbal exchange of content and psychosocial benefits. The speech-language pathologist possesses knowledge and expertise essential in helping to compensate for the verbal restrictions characteristic of aphasia. As the only professionals specifically trained in this area, we have a crucial role to play in offering aphasic adults an opportunity to simultaneously derive linguistic and psychosocial benefits from conversation. This role needs to be formally acknowledged by both speech-language pathology and other health-care professions.

The additional role that we are proposing for speech-language pathologists emanates directly from our expertise in treating and helping to compensate for language disorders. This must be distinguished from the psychosocial role that we have played for many years in providing support and counselling.

TANGIBLE RESULTS OF THE SHIFT IN FOCUS

In formulating and clarifying the shift in focus for ourselves, we have become better able to communicate our goals to the volunteer communication partners. The reaction of most volunteers has been very positive. In the words of one — "It feels right!" Improved training and the recent creation of materials specifically for the purpose of conversation have had a dramatic effect on the range and complexity of potential topics for discussion.

We have also found that family members respond positively to the explanation of the handicap of aphasia in terms of reduced ability to engage in conversation. It is an activity that has meaning for them, whereas the word "communication" is so broad that it is not always useful. Our shift in focus is reflected in the way that techniques are now presented to family members. For example, the use of yes/no questions is demonstrated in a conversational context rather than in establishing a want or need. As an aside, it seems to us that the lists of Helpful Hints, with which we are all so familiar, are frequently presented to families and nursing staff as a way of obtaining information related to physical need rather than for the purpose of social conversation.

The new perspective has been formally included in the mission statement of the Aphasia Centre (see Appendix B).

IMPLICATIONS

Although generalization of communication skill remains an end goal for many of us, we have paid a price in tending to ignore or downplay activities that do not lead us there, but may well serve important psychosocial goals. For example, we often ask ourselves the questions: "Is this functional? Will the individual be able to use it spontaneously outside of the therapy situation?" It is equally valid to question whether there are psychosocial benefits to be derived from communication activities.

The Centre's emphasis on both functional communication and psychosocial well-being requires an expansion of our repertoire of evaluative tools to include those focusing on quality of life. We have found the concept of "communicative confidence" to be useful in evaluating progress because it straddles both communicative effectiveness and psychosocial functioning.

RATIONALE FOR USING VOLUNTEERS AS COMMUNICATION PARTNERS

The use of community volunteers, who are specifically interested in talking to people with aphasia and helping them with their communication, is a crucial aspect of the program. As Lyon (1989b) has pointed out, wanting to interact with aphasic individuals, even if on a working basis, is entirely different from having to interact with them. Family members and caregivers may well want to communicate, but they also, in a sense, are obligated to do so. Although training volunteer communication partners does not replace the need to train family members, from the point of view of the person with aphasia, the fact that there is no obligation for the volunteer to participate is important.

We agree with Feyereisen (1991, p. 328) who stated that "communicative effectiveness of aphasic subjects sometimes depend (sic) on support by an attentive healthy listener," but suggested that ultimately it is conversation in its broad sense and not just communicative effectiveness or functional communication that is the critical beneficiary.

It is worth noting that the participation of volunteers ensures a relatively low ratio of professionals to aphasic individuals, making this an economical approach for treating chronic aphasia.

MAXIMIZING OPPORTUNITIES FOR CONVERSATION: OUR EXPERIENCE AT THE APHASIA CENTRE–NORTH YORK

With all types and levels of severity of aphasia, maximizing opportunities for mutually satisfying conversation is dependent on several factors. In creating the potential for conversation, we consider:

- Communicative skill of the aphasic adult
- Communicative skill of the communication partner
- Appropriate material

It may be helpful to think of these combined variables as part of an equation in which differential weighting of each variable is likely. Good results can be achieved in different ways. For example, an aphasic adult with poor communicative skills may still be able to engage in conversation when interacting with a highly skilled communication partner; conversely, an aphasic adult with excellent conversational strategies may function well with a less experienced communication partner.

COMMUNICATIVE SKILL OF THE APHASIC ADULT

Motivation and Good Pragmatics

Carol Prutting (personal communication) once commented that the person with good pragmatics is the person you would choose to sit beside. Aphasic adults who clearly indicate their desire to interact through eye contact, smiling, gesture, and body language often succeed beyond expectations in engaging communication partners in conversation. Lack of motivation in the aphasic adult, on the other hand, can prove to be more of a challenge than level of severity for a communication partner attempting to maintain a conversation.

Although many members initially appear detached or uninterested, it is important not to make a premature decision regarding motivational state. We have found that it may take as long as a year before change is consistently observed by volunteers, staff, and family members. Typically, the behaviors commented on in the Centre include increased spontaneous greetings, choosing to socialize during coffee breaks, smiling, increased participation, and steady attendance.

Severity Level and Type of Aphasia

Level of severity, at either end of the continuum, is not, in itself, reason for exclusion from the program. Aphasic individuals with co-existing psychiatric illness, degenerative neurologic disorders, behavioral, and cognitive problems may be unable to participate, depending on the severity of the condition.

Based on our experience with severe aphasia, aphasic adults' potential for successful involvement in conversations is closely tied to two of the eligibility criteria outlined by Lyon (1988) for participation in interactive drawing therapy, namely:

- Ability to indicate yes/no accurately in some way most of the time.

- Ability to understand simple questions and statements in some form (spoken, written, drawn, gestured, pointing responses, or combinations of these).

When in doubt about whether an aphasic adult is eligible, observation over a trial period is used to assess more accurately his or her ability to participate in a conversational group. We have found, for example, that some members referred to as "global" have far exceeded what would have been predicted on the basis of the label. A trial period is also necessary for new members who are initially disoriented by the large number of people, background noise, and uncertain expectations when they first begin attending the program.

At the other end of the continuum are those who are relatively independent in terms of everyday functional communication. They can, for example, order food in a restaurant, communicate with a maintenance person, and handle banking or shopping. One might question the potential benefits of the program for these individuals. However, their regular attendance at the Aphasia Centre attests to the fact that simply being functional is not good enough.

Although many aphasic individuals have some degree of receptive difficulty, most of our members have predominantly expressive disabilities. Those with predominantly receptive disabilities and fluent speech require special attention in terms of grouping and volunteer training. Groups should be limited in size and should not comprise exclusively receptively impaired individuals.

Role of the Aphasic Adult in Maintaining the Flow of Conversation

Each aphasic individual enters the program with a unique profile of communicative strengths and weaknesses. Although the pragmatic underpinnings essential to conversation remain relatively intact, the actual repertoire of compensatory behaviors varies widely among individuals. In addition to techniques that have been specifically reinforced in therapy, other strategies may develop through experience (Penn 1987).

Even when aphasia is severe, members can contribute to the conversational partnership by:

- Indicating a general willingness or interest in participating in conversation through, for example, maintaining eye contact and adopting appropriate body posture.

- Using cues to assist the communication partner(s) in formulating appropriate questions to pursue a topic. Examples could include, gesture, pantomime, drawing, pointing to resource materials, trying to write or say a keyword. These cues, however minimal, serve to help establish a frame of reference to initiate or continue a conversation.

- Indicating receptive difficulties so that the communication partner is aware of the need to reformulate, repeat or slow down.

Role of the Speech-Language Pathologist

The speech-language pathologist's role with the aphasic adult is to ensure that he or she is functioning at full potential in terms of speech and language skills, as well as in ways of compensating for the linguistic disability.

COMMUNICATIVE SKILL OF
THE COMMUNICATION PARTNER

Conceptual Difficulties Encountered in Volunteer Training

Speech-language pathologists should not fall into the trap of underestimating the difficulty of explaining the nature of aphasia to volunteers (and families of members). We tend to take for granted the breadth and depth of knowledge that goes into our professional understanding. Notions such as receptive problems being manifested expressively; the difference between speech and language; the delicate interrelationship between thought and language are extremely difficult to grasp without an appropriate theoretical background. We find, for example, that despite our input, some volunteers still comment with surprise about the intelligence of a member, with statements such as "He's really quite sharp!"

Discussing Conversation

Volunteer training reflects the philosophy of the Aphasia Centre–North York. Therefore, in addition to providing basic neurologic and linguistic descriptions of aphasia and techniques for improving functional communication, training sessions also focus on the psychosocial handicap. Issues discussed include the central role of conversation in normal life and how this is affected in aphasia. We emphasize that a primary goal for volunteer communication facilitators is to promote the feel and flow of conversation for their aphasic group members. We stress that there is no single way for volunteers to achieve this goal and that individual variations in communicative style are a part of the natural environment. Volunteers are encouraged to facilitate the spontaneous course of conversation whenever possible.

Framework for Incorporating Techniques to Facilitate Conversation

As with the explanation of aphasia, speech-language pathologists also have a frame of reference within which to incorporate techniques or strategies. For many of us, this frame of reference is so internalized that we have difficulty believing that others without our training might have difficulty with it.

The simple framework outlined in Table 9–1 was developed to help volunteers incorporate techniques for facilitating conversation, including:

Table 9–1. Examples of techniques used by volunteer communication partners to facilitate conversation

TECHNIQUE	"GETTING IN" (facilitating members' understanding)	"GETTING OUT" (facilitating members' expressive communication, to the volunteer or to another member)
Selecting appropriate resource material	Volunteers use a basic, multi-purpose resource kit, as well as material specifically created for discussion of a particular topic.	The same written and graphic material is used to facilitate a means of response for the members. Appropriate resource material is essential when asking open-ended questions.
Closed-ended and yes/no questions	Progressing sequentially from general to more specific questions in order to pursue a topic.	Modeling thumbs up or down. Encouraging pointing to yes/no cards, pictures of happy/ sad faces, or $+/-$ signs before asking questions. *Note:* For both closed and open-ended questions, volunteers are encouraged to anticipate members' potential response modes.
Gesture and pantomime	Use of slightly exaggerated gesture, combined with talk; pantomime of scenarios when appropriate.	Modeling of gesture and pantomime to encourage their use by the aphasic partner.
Interactive drawing (after Lyon, 1988; Lyon & Sims, 1986	Drawing, as the volunteer talks, helps with input and also makes members and volunteers more equal partners.	Volunteers encourage members to use drawing to give cues about topic. The drawing is interactive, with both member and volunteer using the process to facilitate conventional exchange.
Responding to receptive problems	Volunteers need to monitor group members carefully for indications of receptive difficulty. Appropriate modifications may include repetition, slowing down, more gesture, or drawing.	

continued

Table 9-1. (*continued*)

TECHNIQUE	"GETTING IN" (*facilitating members' understanding*)	"GETTING OUT" (*facilitating members' expressive communication, to the volunteer or to another member*)
Alerting to topic initiation and change	Primarily through the use of spontaneously written cue cards, relevant pictures, and gesture.	Written/graphic material used in a conversation should remain accessible for future reference.
Giving adequate processing time	Volunteers need to learn to tolerate "silences" while a member is processing information and trying to respond.	
Simultaneous multi-modal input	Volunteers working with members who have receptive difficulty are encouraged to develop the habit of constantly accompanying talk with gesture, drawing, or writing.	
Expansion and reflection of messages		Volunteers provide opportunities for members to correct or confirm, by expanding and reflecting (verbally and nonverbally) members' incomplete messages.

MAINTAINING THE FEEL AND FLOW˜OF CONVERSATION:

- All of the above techniques are used to facilitate the feel of natural conversation.

- Humor serves as a powerful means of encouraging social interaction. Shared humor also reinforces the ideal of equal partnership.

- Verbal confirmation or interpretation of members' communication.

- Verbally linking one member with another.

- Using strategies to move a conversation along when there has been an inappropriately long response time.

- Ensuring that the message gets *in* (to the aphasic adult).

- Ensuring that the aphasic adult has a mechanism for getting the message *out*.

- Maintaining the feel and flow of conversation.

Practicing Techniques to Facilitate Conversation.

Most techniques that we use as practice for communication occur within the framework of what is termed the Barrier Game (Muma, 1978). The principles involved in Barrier Games are primarily the same as those used by Davis and Wilcox (1985) in their description of Promoting Aphasics' Communicative Effectiveness (PACE).

PACE represents a significant break with earlier traditions in that it focuses on improving communicative effectiveness and simulates aspects of conversation. Although PACE is limited by a restricted range of speech acts, there is strong potential for modifying the traditional format. Pulvermuller and Roth (1991), for example, have presented creative ideas for extending the range of speech acts. We have found PACE to be an extremely useful and flexible clinical tool: It is easily adapted for different levels of severity, works well in a group, and can be presented in formats diverse enough to maintain interest and motivation. Davis and Wilcox (1985) intended that PACE would provide a structured format "resembling" natural conversation (p. 89). In our view, however, it is only by providing opportunities for real conversation that strategies such as PACE are given a meaningful context.

In addition to the use of drawn or written cards, as described by Davis and Wilcox (1985), versions of Barrier Games that we most often use include:

The game "20 Questions": One group member is given information and the others have to find out what it is. Volunteers always enter into these activities as one of the group members rather than as a group leader.

A reverse of the above game: A group member has to describe something well enough so that the others can guess what it is.

Use of videotaped material: Aphasic members first watch a video. Depending on the level of severity of the group, some "conversational coaching" (Holland, 1991) may also occur, usually by one or more of the speech-language pathologists. Naive listeners (volunteers) then come in, and aphasic group members attempt to convey the content of the videos. The advantage of videos is that they can be replayed, first for practice, and second for the purpose of confirmation. We have successfully experimented with bits of news clips, strong advertisements with humor or real drama, and "home-made" videos featuring staff at the Centre in various embarrassing situations (entitled "Accidents of Daily Living").

Conversational coaching (Holland, 1991) is also used in a debate format, where speech-language pathologists and volunteers work with aphasic members to prepare them for participation in an ac-tual debate.

Other practice techniques include role-playing and charades.

Examples of Issues Discussed with Volunteers

Distinguishing between practicing techniques to facilitate conversation and pro-viding conversational opportunity. It is essential for volunteers to grasp this distinction. The following analogy is often used to illustrate the point. A technique is compared to a tool such as a computer. Practicing tech-niques is analogous to getting to know how to work the computer. There are various ways of improving computer skills, such as going to a course or using a computer program designed for practice of specific skills. Pro-viding conversational opportunity is analogous to using the computer for what one really wants to do, for example, writing a letter. See Table 9–2 for the features that distinguish these activities.

Table 9–2. Practicing techniques to facilitate conversation versus offering op-portunities for conversation

Practicing Techniques to Facilitate Conversation	Offering Opportunities for Conversation
Activity specifically structured to practice techniques	Opportunity for use (and reinforcement of techniques) in a spontaneous, natural context
Deliberately introduce a level of challenge/frustration (e.g., barrier in PACE activities)	Attempt to reduce the level of frustration
Although content should be as interesting as possible, it is not the sole focus of the activity	Content of the conversation is an end in itself
The goal is improved functional communication skill	The goal is improved psychosocial well-being

Need to be aware of severity level of group members, as well as individual differences in ability to use compensatory techniques. Groups are organized on the basis of level of severity of aphasia and psychosocial variables. An understanding of level of severity helps the volunteer know what to expect of the members. This makes it easier to select appropriate techniques.

"Facilitator" rather than "teacher." It must be acknowledged that the role of facilitator is often more difficult than that of teacher. Many volunteers appear to derive personal satisfaction from activities such as getting members to repeat or copy words. We have to work hard to communicate the importance of the facilitative role.

"Talking for two." The volunteer's verbal activity is an essential ingredient in allowing aphasic group members to feel a part of the rhythm and flow of normal conversation. "Talk" keeps things flowing, but the type of talk is all important, as illustrated in the following example.

Sharon is part of a group of severely aphasic individuals. They are discussing relaxation and the way in which they choose to relax. Sharon moves her head in a way that prompts the conversation partner to say "Oh, you like to listen to music?" Sharon nods enthusiastically. The partner continues, "Mary, do you like to listen to music too?" In this way, Sharon is helped to feel part of a real conversation. The communication partner could respond in many other ways, for example, by saying "Oh . . . music . . . Can you say 'music'?" This response would not give the feel of conversation. In the previous example, the communication partner acted on Sharon's behalf: She verbalized Sharon's message and then used it to connect her with another group member.

Volunteers often express concern about how much they talk in the group. This may be due, in part, to our frequent emphasis on the goal of sharing the communication load. In groups where there are severe limitations on the expressive ability of the members, volunteers necessarily do much of the talking. What we emphasize for volunteers is the difference between talk that is mostly a reflection of the volunteer's feelings and opinions and talk that includes genuine interpretation of the members' nonverbal communication in order to create the feel and flow of conversation.

Training Procedure

Before starting to work as a communication facilitator, volunteers do at least 12 hours of observation. At this stage, they are provided with training manuals and have a formal orientation with a speech-language pathologist and the coordinator of volunteers. They begin a training period where they work independently with groups but are closely supervised. If evaluation by the speech-language pathologist and self-evaluation by the volunteer are satisfactory, the formal training period ends.

Preparatory and wrap-up meetings for volunteers are held daily (see Appendix B). The purpose is to continually reinforce the philosophy of the program, demonstrate techniques, give ideas for discussion, help volunteers with areas of difficulty, and maintain high motivation levels. Hands-on demonstration for volunteers occurs in the context of actual group work. We agree with Green's (1982) comments regarding training people in the aphasic individual's environment, that "to attempt this on a purely academic level would probably not achieve maximum results."

APPROPRIATE RESOURCES

Good resource material is crucial in ensuring that aphasic individuals have an optimal opportunity to engage in conversation. Although volunteers are provided with written suggestions for discussion topics and other activities related to a particular theme, spontaneity is encouraged. Theme sheets should not be regarded as "blueprints" for conversation. In addition to this type of material which is always available for use by volunteers and members, other resources have been specifically developed for use with groups where members experience moderate to severe expressive and/or receptive difficulty.

BASIC RESOURCE KIT

This kit contains basic resource materials such as photographs and personal information relevant to individual members, calendar, alphabet and number board, material for telling time, maps, color chart, pictures of staff, and pictographs of places. These are always available regardless of the topic for discussion. Other materials that are always available include pencil and paper, blank cards, and one or two daily newspapers.

RESOURCE PACKAGES FOR SPECIFIC TOPICS

Specially created resource packages are provided to enable members to participate fully in conversations on complex topics. These packages are prepared by professional staff and volunteers, and consist primarily of pictographs, accompanied by minimal text. Arranging this pictured and textual material for easy reference by aphasic members greatly increases the potential range and complexity of conversations; optimal levels of discussion occur when these resources are used by skilled volunteers and members who have been previously exposed to this method.

The pictographic material in our resource packages closely resembles that used by Bertoni, Stoffel, and Weniger (1991) in a therapy program for individuals with severe aphasia. Whereas the material they describe is used to facilitate exchange of information about practical subjects, such as transportation, weather, and daily needs, we extend the use of this type of material to provide access to in-depth conversations. The Centre's pictograph packages give members the opportunity to express their feelings and opinions on broad, complex topics including, for example, discussions on aphasia, current political crises, personal problems, and issues to be voted on at the Centre's next Annual General Meeting. Packaged material relating to aphasia, in particular, has been invaluable in facilitating discussions with our members (see Appendix C).

Initially, these packages were designed to facilitate conversations for members with severe aphasia. We have observed that members with moderate to mild aphasia also appreciate this style of resource, particularly when used as an adjunct to complex written material.

CONCLUSIONS

As Sarno (1986) indicated, knowledge of the psychosocial devastation of aphasia is not new to the speech-language pathologist. In general, however, attempts to alleviate these problems have been confined to providing support and counselling, using skills from other disciplines, such as social work. Our perception of the handicap of aphasia has given us a rationale for using speech-language pathology expertise to address these issues from a communicative perspective.

The paradigm shift we have described is tied to the pragmatic concept of the social use of language (Prutting 1982), but extends beyond it. In addition to "fixing" or compensating for the language disorder, we have a professional obligation to provide aphasic adults with the opportunity to derive psychosocial benefits from human interaction. We consider conversation the critical medium for this process. Although work is beginning to emerge in the area of conversational discourse (Mentis & Thompson, 1991; Wambaugh, Thomson, Doyle, & Camarata, 1991), aphasiologists have not yet explored the potential of compensating for the linguistic disorder within the context of natural conversation.

Speech-language pathologists in traditional settings might not realize that they are, to some extent, using their professional expertise in the manner we have described by engaging in conversations with their clients and/ or facilitating conversations between their clients and others. Too often, though, conversation is viewed as being appropriate only as the introduction or conclusion to a session of "real speech-language therapy."

In initiating a re-thinking of our role, Lyon (1989a) has pioneered development of the concept of "communicative partners," whereby aphasic adults are given an opportunity to become involved in the community, doing what they would most like to be doing. We see many other exciting applications in the training of conversation facilitators for aphasic adults. The facilitators or partners may include family members and friends, volunteers, and/or speech-language pathologists. Applications include acting as interpreters for aphasic individuals so that they can represent themselves and participate more fully in their community; training people in the community such as a specific bank teller or hairdresser; and using some of the above methods to provide access to all-important counselling services by either training professionals such as social workers or by participating as an interpreter.

Initial forays into the topic of conversation and conversational analysis reveal overwhelming complexity. The study of normal conversation will enable us to better understand these issues within the context of aphasia. There is already a relevant body of research from the fields of sociology, anthropology, philosophy, and linguistics (e.g., Goffman 1959, 1971, 1974; Grice, 1975; Gumperz, 1964; Labov, 1972; and Schiffrin, (1988). We anticipate that the study of conversation will become as necessary a part of the speech-language pathology curriculum as the study of language is today.

ACKNOWLEDGMENTS

The authors express their appreciation for the support and contributions of colleagues at the Aphasia Centre–North York, the York–Durham Aphasia Centre, and the Aphasia Centre of Ottawa–Carleton.

Picture Communication Symbols used with permission of Mayer-Johnson Co., P.O. Box 1579, Solana Beach, CA 92075, U.S.A., Phone (619) 481-2489.

REFERENCES

Bertoni, B., Stoffel, A-M., & Weniger, D. (1991). Communicating with pictographs: A graphic approach to the improvement of communicative interactions. *Aphasiology, 5*(4, 5), 341–353.)

Davis, G. A., & Wilcox, M. J. (1985). *Adult aphasia rehabilitation.* San Diego, CA: College-Hill Press.

Eaton Griffiths, V., & Neal, P. (1978). *An evening with Patricia Neal. Presentation by the Stroke Recovery Association,* Toronto, Canada.

Feyereisen, P. (1991). Communicative behaviour in aphasia. *Aphasiology, 5*(4, 5), 323–333.

Goffman, E. (1959). *The presentation of self in everyday life.* New York: Anchor Books.

Goffman, E. (Ed.). (1967). The nature of deference and demeanor. In *Interaction ritual: Essays on face-to-face behavior*. New York: Anchor Books.

Goffman, E. (1971). *Relations in public*. New York: Harper and Row.

Goffman, E. (1974). *Frame analysis*. New York: Harper and Row.

Green, G. (1982). Assessment and treatment of the adult with severe aphasia: Aiming for functional generalization. *Australian Journal of Human Communication Disorders, 10,* 11–23.

Grice, H. P. (1975). Logic and conversation. In P. Cole & J. Morgan (Eds.), *Speech Acts: Syntax and semantics* (Vol. 3). New York: Academic Press.

Gumperz, J. J. (1964). Linguistic and social interaction in two communities. *American Anthropologist, 6,* 137–153.

Holland, A. (1991). Pragmatic aspects of interaction in aphasia. *Journal of Neurolinguistics, 6,* 197–211.

Kagan, A., & Gailey, G. (1990, November). *A long-term, community-based treatment model for chronic aphasia*. Paper presented at the American Speech-Language-Hearing Association Convention. Seattle, WA.

Kertesz, A. (1982). *The Western aphasia battery*. Orlando, FL: Grune & Stratton.

Labov, W. (Ed.). (1972). The transformation of experience in narrative syntax. In *Language in the inner city: Studies in the black English vernacular*. Philadelphia: University of Pennsylvania Press.

Le Guin, U. (1989). *Dancing at the edge of the world: Thoughts on words, women, places*. New York: Harper and Row.

Lomas, J., Pickard, L., Bester, S., Elbard, H., Finlayson, A., & Zoghaib, C. (1989). The communicative effectiveness index: Development and psychometric evaluation of a functional communication measure for adult aphasia. *Journal of Speech and Hearing Disorders, 54,* 113–124.

Lyon, J. G. (1988). The use of interactive drawing to re-establish communication with expressively restricted aphasic adults: Purpose and techniques. *Seminar presented at The Speech & Stroke Centre–North York*, Ontario, Canada.

Lyon, J. G. (1989a). Communicative partners: Their value in re-establishing communication with aphasic adults. In T. Prescott (Ed.), *Clinical aphasiology conference proceedings*. San Diego, CA: College-Hill Press.

Lyon, J. G. (1989b). Generalization: Going beyond the communication task. *Session II, Seminar (The challenge of generalization: Perspective on planning, intervention and evaluation) presented at The Speech & Stroke Centre–North York*, Ontario, Canada.

Lyon, J. G. (in press). Optimizing communication and participation in life for aphasic adults and their prime caregivers in natural settings: A use model for treatment. In G. Wallace (Ed.), *Adult aphasia: Clinical management for the practicing clinician*. Baltimore, MD: Andover Medical Publishing.

Lyon, J. G., & Sims, E. (1986). *Drawing: Evaluation of its use as a communicative aid with aphasic and normal adults*. Paper presented at Second International Aphasia Rehabilitation Congress, Goteborg, Sweden.

Mayer-Johnson, R. (1981). *Picture communication symbols*. Solana Beach, CA: [Available from Mayer-Johnson Co., P.O. Box 1579, Solana Beach, CA, 92075. (619) 481-2429.]

Mentis, M., & Thompson, S. A. (1991). Discourse: A means for understanding normal and disordered language. In T. M. Gallagher (Ed.), *Pragmatics of language: Clinical practice issues.* San Diego, CA: Singular Publishing Group.

Muma, J. R. (1978). *Language handbook: Concepts, assessment and intervention.* Englewood Cliffs, NJ: Prentice-Hall.

National Aphasia Association. (1988). *Special report.* [Available from author, P.O. Box 1887, Murray Hill Street, New York, N.Y. 1056-0611.]

Penn, C. (1987). Compensation and language recovery in the chronic aphasic patient. *Aphasiology, 1,* 235–245.

Prutting, C. (1982). Pragmatics as social competence. *Journal of Speech and Hearing Disorders, 47,* 123–133.

Pulvermuller, F., & Roth, V. M. (1991). Communicative aphasia treatment as a further development of PACE therapy. *Aphasiology, 5*(1), 39–50.

Robinson, R. G., Lipsey, J. R., & Price, T. R. (1985). Diagnosis and clinical management of post-stroke depression. *Psychosomatics, 26*(10), 769–778.

Sarno, M. T. (1986). The silent minority: The patient with aphasia. *The 1986 Hemphill Lecture,* Rehabilitation Institute of Chicago.

Schegloff, E. (1990). *Born talking: Episode IV.* T.V. Series written and presented by Dr. Jonathan Miller. Produced by John McGreevy Productions and Primedia Productions Ltd. in association with the BBC and TV Ontario.

Schiffrin, D. (1988). Conversation analysis. In F. L. Neumayer (Ed.), *Linguistics: The Cambridge survey IV. Language: The sociocultural context.* Cambridge: Cambridge University Press.

Wambaugh, J. L., Thomson, C. K., Doyle, P. J., & Camarata, S. (1991). Conversational discourse of aphasic and normal adults: An analysis of communicative functions. In T. E. Prescott (Ed.), *Clinical aphasiology.* Austin, TX: Pro-Ed.

Willer, B. S., Guastaferro, J. R., Zankiw, I., & Duran, R. (1990). Rehabilitation and functional assessment in residential programs for individuals with disabilities. In J. W. Jacobson, S. N. Burchard, & P. J. Carling (Eds.), *Clinical services, social adjustment, and work life in community living.* Baltimore, MD: Johns Hopkins University Press.

World Health Organization. (1980). *International classification of impairments, disabilities and handicaps.* Geneva: World Health Organization.

APPENDIX A

MISSION STATEMENT OF THE APHASIA CENTRE–NORTH YORK

The Aphasia Centre–North York seeks to improve quality of life and maximize independence for aphasic adults and their families. We do this by providing long-term, community-based, professionally supervised communication and psychosocial programs as well as through education and research.

GOALS AND OBJECTIVES

To train volunteers and family members to communicate effectively with aphasic adults by teaching strategies that enhance the exchange of information, opinions and feelings.

To provide opportunities for natural conversation.

To lessen the handicap of aphasia by providing increased access to social life within the community.

To provide a network of emotional and social support for aphasic members and their families on a formal and informal basis, through individual counselling and group interaction.

To provide a model of organization which fosters a partnership among aphasic members, their families, volunteers and staff.

To encourage innovative programming and research.

To increase the awareness of aphasia and to provide ongoing education for students, professionals and the public.

APPENDIX B

TIME	DAILY COMMUNICATION PROGRAM SCHEDULE
A.M.	
8:30	Members start arriving at the Centre. Time for socializing and reading newspaper. Coffee/tea available — members serve themselves.
9:00	S-LP meets with volunteers to prepare for the morning's activities: • review theme materials for conversation. • discuss/demonstrate techniques and strategies. • identify potentially sensitive areas and discuss appropriate management.
9:30	Volunteers and members go to pre-assigned conversation groups (typically, 1 volunteer: 3–5 members). Group composition determined by S-LP, based on level of aphasia severity, functional communication skills, personality, and social factors. Group conversations begin; S-LP circulates among groups to observe, demonstrate, and help as required.
10:30	Volunteers and members socialize during a nutrition break. Volunteers have an opportunity to meet with S-LP to discuss problems and provide feedback.
11:00	Groups resume.
11:45	Wrap-up meeting for volunteers with S-LP to evaluate theme and the morning's activities. Another opportunity for feedback regarding individual members, group composition, what worked or did not.

APPENDIX C

PICTURE COMMUNICATION SYMBOLS

WHO?	understands me	talks to me
friends		
neighbors		
family		
we, us / volunteers		
nobody		

Picture Communication Symbols © 1981-1985 Mayer-Johnson Co.

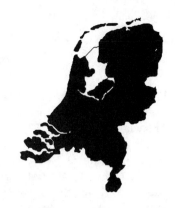

CHAPTER 10

A Multidisciplinary Approach to Aphasia Therapy

EVY G. VISCH-BRINK
FRANS van HARSKAMP
Department of Neurology
University Hospital
Rotterdam-Dijkzigt, The Netherlands

NEL M. van AMERONGEN
Department of Internal Medicine and Geriatric Medicine
University Hospital
Rotterdam-Dijkzigt, The Netherlands

SANDRA M. WIELAERT
MIEKE E. van de SANDT-KOENDERMEN
Rotterdam Aphasia Foundation
Erasmus University
Rotterdam, The Netherlands

The approach described here is based on our experience with aphasic patients referred to the Stichting Afasie Rotterdam (SAR, Rotterdam Aphasia Foundation). This organization is a cooperative effort of all nursing homes in the area and the department of Neuropsychology of the Institute of Neurology, Academic Hospital Rotterdam-Dijkzigt. Patients are investigated for their clinical complexity, for theoretical interest, but mostly to assess prognosis for therapy. The patients described here are among 267 patients with stroke-induced aphasia who were under the care of this Foundation during its first 5 years.

The effectiveness of aphasia therapy is a concern in most countries in the western world. Public health authorities are concerned about whether to provide financial support for rehabilitation of aphasic patients, and those in the field are also concerned, as evidenced by numerous publications on the topic (Basso, Capitani, & Vignolo, 1979; Lincoln et al., 1984; Wertz et al., 1981, 1986). Group studies and single case studies are used to study effectiveness. With respect to group studies, Howard and Hatfield (1987) caution that, because aphasic patients are heterogeneous, grouping them, even within aphasic syndromes, poses a hazard. They also raise the more serious objection that therapy methods and goals are often not clearly outlined or even described. Finally, they note that patient selection and patient attrition are a concern, as illustrated in studies by Wertz et al. (1986) and Lincoln et al. (1984).

The other approach is to study single cases or small patient groups. Often these patients are good candidates for therapy; young, vital, without concomitant neuropsychological disturbances and highly motivated for treatment (Bachy-Langedock & de Partz, 1989; Nettleton & Lesser, 1991). Not only are such patients a minority, but even some of them fail to progress in communication and language.

The experiences of speech therapists in the Netherlands are seldom published or evaluated. Prins (1987) conducted three studies to evaluate the effect of a language comprehension program on the recovery of aphasic patients. The results varied from no effect to a statistically insignificant trend toward amelioration with amount of therapy emerging as an important variable. Prins's equivocal findings served to increase the skepticism of health authorities.

ROUTES TO APHASIA THERAPY IN HOLLAND

Previously hospitalized aphasic stroke patients come to therapy through various routes. At discharge from hospital the patient is sent home or admitted to a nursing home or rehabilitation center. At home, neurological rehabilitation can take place in a day-treatment center annex, a nursing home, or a rehabilitation department. A neurologist is responsible for medical follow-up related to the stroke.

The general practitioner is informed about most events and transfers to other institutions; unfortunately, language diagnosis and therapy is not always mentioned. To enhance communication among speech therapists, a systematic method was recently developed to structure the information flow necessary to plan and carry out a therapeutic regime. This model, the "case-project" ("Casus-project") (Alderse Baes, Leipoldt, Dharmaperwira-Prins, & Verschaeve, 1991), systematically describes the patient's clinical picture, diagnostic information, and the course of speech language therapy.

Patients are placed largely on the basis of age and degree of motor handicap. Patients over 65 are admitted to nursing homes for rehabilitation or they spend several days a week in a day-treatment center. Patients under 65 usually go to a rehabilitation center, with a maximum stay of 6 months. Outpatient therapy is also available in rehabilitation centers or outpatient clinics.

Most nursing homes in the Netherlands use nursing and paramedical personnel for rehabilitation, and try to discharge patients either to personal care homes or to their own homes.

Unless they have concomitant neurological disturbances that interfere with daily life, aphasic patients are not referred to day-treatment centers. Instead, they are referred to speech therapists in private practice.

Recently the Dutch Consensus on stroke treatment (van Crevel, 1991) concluded: "The use of health care facilities by a stroke patient is incorrectly determined by factors such as age and motor handicap rather than type and severity of cognitive impairment and the presence of behavioral disturbances." This suggests that some changes might occur in delivery of service.

Once treatment has ended, the quality of daily life is a very important issue. Finding meaningful things to do and maintaining minimal social contacts are frequently problems. Aphasia clubs established throughout the country offer one possible solution. Here aphasic patients can meet and engage in appropriately designed activities.

SPEECH AND LANGUAGE CLINICIANS

Clinical linguists are neither acknowledged nor paid for by the National health system. Although they work with aphasic patients in only three or four institutions, their work has had an important impact on diagnostic approaches (e.g., spontaneous speech) and on the development of therapeutic techniques and materials. On the whole, however, speech therapists are responsible for conducting aphasia therapy. They collaborate closely with physiotherapists and occupational therapists, who have become increasingly interested in neuro-rehabilitation and aphasiology.

Education of speech therapists has changed considerably over the past 10 years. Formerly, a 2-year part-time training course, it has become a 4-year full-time education. Training is highly vocational and not strictly scientific in character. A part-time 2-year postgraduate course, specializing in aphasia therapy, is now offered at the "Hogeschool Rotterdam–Polytechnics." The Department of Neuropsychology (Erasmus University Rotterdam) and the Stichting Afasie Rotterdam (SAR, Rotterdam Aphasia Foundation) assist with this program.

Formerly, speech therapists were obliged to study Linguistics or Psychology to obtain an academic degree. A shorter course is now available in Groningen, and the University of Nijmegen offers an academic degree in speech-language pathology. Speech therapists now have a professional society, and they also participate in multidisciplinary societies.

Financial support for speech therapy is provided by health insurance companies and by health-related institutions. Some hospitals have departments of speech therapy. In others, speech therapists are housed in departments of Neurology, Otolaryngology, or Rehabilitation. Treatment must be prescribed by a physician. In most nursing homes, the rehabilitation team consists of speech therapists, physiotherapists, and occupational therapists. Generally speech therapists are employed only part-time and are rather isolated.

Although speech therapists have distinctive responsibilities in the health care system, they are frequently insufficiently trained in recognizing cognitive dysfunction, and often do not understand how to incorporate cognitive rehabilitation in their treatment. Limited status is given to clinical psychologists and neurolinguists, even within the university hospitals, with the result that these professions have little impact on the health care system and its facilities.

This situation has led to the formation of regional multidisciplinary aphasia diagnosis and treatment teams. Despite financial limitations there are a number of teams, which include speech therapists, linguists, neuropsychologists, and physicians who diagnose and plan treatment. The team decides which of two forms of treatment is appropriate (van Harskamp & Visch-Brink, 1989, 1991).

All aphasic patients and their families need care, in the sense of information, guidance, and support in coping with the communication disorder. Stimulation techniques and enhancement of communicative and social behavior play a central role in helping the patient cope with his disabilities and find meaning in life. A subgroup also needs activities aimed at improving communication. For this group Structural Therapy is used.

SELECTION OF PATIENTS FOR APHASIA THERAPY

No clear consensus exists among medical professionals concerning which aphasic patients are candidates for therapy. In most centers, the speech therapist neither selects patients, nor controls the selection process. Because effective treatment depends on many factors (some unrelated to aphasia), some good candidates for aphasia therapy are not treated. Others receive treatment from which little or no effect can be expected.

We believe it is important to "reapportion time for aphasia rehabilitation," but not as Marshall (1987) suggests. It is far too simple to say that mild aphasics should have intensive treatment and severe global aphasics should not be treated. Although contraindications for Structural Therapy exist, severe aphasia in itself cannot be considered one of them. However, severe aphasia limits both the goals and methods of Structural Therapy. Edelman (1984) asks, "which global aphasics should be treated, and which treatment methods are most likely to be effective?" In fact the same question should be answered for all types of aphasia.

THE SAR APPROACH

The Stichting Afasie Rotterdam (SAR, or Rotterdam Aphasia Foundation) diagnostic team consists of a neurologist, a neuropsychologist, a clinical linguist, and a speech therapist. Speech therapists in nursing homes provide information and therapy, and also refer patients to the diagnostic team. The team discusses the results of diagnostic tests and determines the goals and methods for therapy. The SAR uses "stepwise diagnosis," so that only patients who are suitable candidates for treatment receive an extensive diagnostic assessment.

After aphasia screening, biographical and family data are gathered. Mental status, somatic status, prognosis, and likelihood of complications are assessed. Communicative abilities are assessed, and neurolinguistic and neuropsychological investigations are conducted. An attempt is made to maximize learning conditions by trying to change factors that might interfere with progress. Exploratory therapy is conducted. Sometimes more than two decision levels are needed before Structural Therapy is begun; supplementary investigations help to define the precise goal of therapy. All of this information is structured along five axes analogous to the DSM III-R system (van Harskamp & Visch-Brink, 1991), as follows:

Axis I: Aphasia syndrome

Axis II: Somatic condition and neurological status

Axis III: Neurological and neuropsychological disturbances

Axis IV: Psychosocial stressors and personality

Axis V: Social circumstances

Relevant information is often gathered in parallel during pre-therapy assessment. Pre-therapy assessment includes: Disease-oriented diagnosis, therapy-oriented diagnosis, maximizing conditions, exploratory therapy, and structural therapy. Each is described below.

I. DISEASE-ORIENTED DIAGNOSIS

The neurologist is responsible for focusing on diagnosis and treatment of the disease. This usually begins while patients are still hospitalized, with the initial aphasia diagnosis being made as part of the mental status examination. This diagnosis is preliminary, because the clinical picture often changes rapidly during this time. At this time the severity of aphasia is more important than the exact type of aphasia.

Typically, hospital stay is short, and most of the time is spent on diagnostic procedures. Therapeutic efforts attempt to improve the patient's motor functioning and activities of daily living skills to maximize independence. Ameliorating verbal abilities is a secondary concern.

Speech therapists concentrate on enhancing the communicative interactions between patient, nursing staff, and family members, and on motivating the patient. Useful techniques include stimulation using various communicative channels simultaneously, and use of deblocking procedures. A communication notebook, in which family and professional visitors are asked to note some essential aspects of their visits, may also be important. Guidance, instruction, and support focusing on the patient's physical condition and expectations also play an important role.

Information gathered during this stage serves as background for an aphasia screening conducted at the beginning of the therapy-oriented diagnosis. The neurologist conducts a mental status and motor examination, and also considers the size and site of the lesion as well as looking for old infarcts and lacunae. Prognostic factors must be delineated at this time. Variables such as the level of activity at hospital discharge, age, sex, heart disease, hypertension, and vascular territory of infarction all influence mortality. Van Harskamp (1989) found a positive correlation between the complications occurring in hospital and those occurring later during therapy.

II. THERAPY-ORIENTED DIAGNOSIS

FORMAL LANGUAGE ASSESSMENT

The core of this assessment, usually carried out after discharge, is the identification of the specific disabilities related to the severity and type of aphasia, as well as concomitant disorders.

Classical aphasia batteries provide specific indications for therapy. They provide a systematic, practical examination of the patient's linguistic skills in several modalities. Until recently there was only one well-normed diagnostic test in the Dutch language, the Stichting Afasie Nederland-test (SAN) (Deelman, Liebrand, Koning-Haanstra, & Burg, 1981). The SAN investigates spontaneous speech, repetition, naming, sentence production, auditory word comprehension, and auditory morpho-syntactic comprehension. Some of the subtests show ceiling effects, and the SAN classifies the aphasic patient only as fluent or nonfluent. The test contains no reading or writing subtests. Because of these limitations, many therapists in the Netherlands use translated versions of the Boston Diagnostic Aphasia Exam (Goodglass & Kaplan, 1972) or the Western Aphasia Battery (Kertesz, 1982), but norms for a Dutch aphasic population are lacking. The Aachen Aphasia Test (Huber, Poeck, Weniger, & Willmes, 1983) has recently been translated and validated in Dutch. This test's psychometric characteristics are outlined in articles by Graetz, de Bleser, Willmes, and Heeschen (1991); Willmes, Graetz, de Bleser, Schulte, and Keyser (1991); and de Bleser, Willmes, Graetz, and Hagoort (1991).

We agree with Byng, Kay, Edmundson, and Scott (1990) that a number of patients should have a more detailed psycholinguistic investigation to specify the underlying deficit. Extensive case studies have shown that model-based and sufficiently detailed location of the deficit can be vital in planning successful therapy methods. If the level of the word-finding problem (Nettleton & Lesser, 1991) or the underlying problem in agrammatism (Black, Nickels, & Byng, 1991; Nickels, Byng, & Black, 1991) can be established, then explicit therapy methods can be applied.

In our setting, specific linguistic investigation is currently carried out for two types of disorders. For a patient with word-finding problems, semantic functioning is an important variable in planning therapy. The Pyramids and Palm Trees Test (Howard & Franklin, 1988) and similar measures are used to detect disorders in semantic processing and dissociations in input and output channels.

Aphasic patients with syntactic problems in spontaneous speech also can benefit from more detailed linguistic assessment. Therefore, patients with sentence production problems indicated on the AAT are further evaluated using a "syntactic battery," with subtests for verb naming, sentence production, production of prepositions, comprehension of reversible sentences, and syntactic judgment. Individual profiles indicate whether therapy for sentence production is likely to be effective.

Improved spontaneous speech is always an important therapy goal, but unfortunately, we have no system to measure such change. An extensive psycholinguistic group study was performed by Prins and coworkers (Prins, Snow, & Wagenaar, 1978; Wagenaar, Snow, & Prins, 1975). This study stressed the importance of the fluent-nonfluent dichotomy in analyzing aphasic speech. Vermeulen, Bastiaanse, and Wageningen (1989) conducted a similar investigation. However, these efforts have not yet resulted in a reliable instrument for evaluating changes in spontaneous speech. For Broca aphasic patients, a comprehensive system of analysis has been designed by Saffran, Berndt, and Schwartz (1989), with an elaboration by Byng and Black (1989).

ASSESSMENT OF FUNCTIONAL COMMUNICATION

We agree with many authors (Blomert, 1990; Herrmann, Koch, Johannsen-Horbach, & Wallesch, 1989; Holland, 1982; Lomas et al., 1989; Seron, 1979; Taylor-Sarno, 1969) that diagnosis should always include assessment of functional communication. For a full understanding of a patient's communicative abilities in daily life, one would like to follow the patient for a few hours, as Holland (1982) did. In clinical practice this is impractical and financially impossible. We have modified the Functional Communication Profile (FCP) (Taylor-Sarno, 1965) into the "Communicatie Profiel" (CP) (Wielaert & Visch-Brink, 1990) for use in assessing functional communication. Our measure differs from the original FCP primarily by including information provided by spouses and by using a standard observation. We agree with Lomas et al. (1989) that spouses' information is important and should not be ignored.

During the first 2 or 3 weeks after referral, the patient is observed in a variety of communicative situations. We try to incorporate the patient's pre-morbid communication level, as reported by family members, into our judgment about functioning after the onset of aphasia.

The first section of the CP assesses general communicative abilities independent of the output channel, such as showing initiative, use of yes and no, and participation in conversation. Section II concerns output channels and consists of tests of production and comprehension using oral language, gesturing, written language, and pictures. Section III focuses on production and comprehension of oral language. Section IV measures written language. Section V assesses practical abilities such as using the telephone, handling money, and shopping. This scale is also used to assess overall communicative performance, including gesturing, drawing, and pantomime.

Another measure for functional communication is the Amsterdam-Nijmegen Everyday Language Test (ANELT) by Blomert, Koster, and Kean (1991). The ANELT is a reliable tool for assessing functional oral language in a semi-structured setting. The test consists of a set of 10 scenarios to elicit oral verbal output.

NEUROPSYCHOLOGICAL ASSESSMENT

A neuropsychological evaluation assesses concomitant disorders that might restrict the effectiveness of therapy and helps to determine which patients are candidates for therapy. The aphasic patient, like other brain damaged people, may experience slowing of thought, emotional instability, reduced energy, and other disorders.

In some patients the language disorder is part of more diffuse cerebral disturbances. Aphasia may be embedded in a complex of cognitive disorders or be part of a picture of progressive disease such as a dementing illness. Differentiation of these syndromes is difficult (Au, Albert, & Obler, 1988); however, neuropsychological evaluation provides valuable additional information to help make such judgments. We believe that neuropsychological testing, including assessment of intelligence, concentration, memory and executive control should be part of the diagnostic process for aphasic patients.

In our experience many aphasic patients cannot choose the easiest, most effective response for a particular situation. Some may be "stuck" in a response set, such as gesturing. Such patients might not profit from therapy techniques such as PACE. Others may never use what they learn outside the therapist's room, a problem frequently seen in those using augmentative speech resources. When Structural Therapy is begun, problems emerge, such as an inability to explore a variety of options concerning a given task and the lack of flexibility in shifting from one response mode to another. Finding out about such characteristics before therapy is begun is desirable. Currently we are exploring how to modify other measures to observe concept-shifting, nonverbal abstraction, and planning.

One prerequisite for learning is intact memory. In aphasic patients information processing and transfer may be slow, with a buildup of information over many sessions. Previously learned information is assumed to be the basis upon which new material is learned. There is extensive literature on this topic (among others, Grober, 1984), but the number of tests available for the assessment of memory functions is small. The Rivermead Behavioural Memory Test (Wilson, Cockburn, & Baddeley, 1985) is one of the few tests with Dutch aphasia norms. Although it appears to be useful for assessing memory for everyday events, an assessment of memory should additionally test the specific skills needed in the therapeutic setting.

An aphasic patient's success in developing strategies and learning to make abstractions and generalizations in the newly acquired way of communicating depends partly on intelligence. The International Congress on Intelligence and Aphasia at Brussels (Lebrun & Hoops, 1974) concluded that no complete estimation of intelligence is applicable to aphasic individuals.

We have used the Raven Standard or Coloured Progressive Matrices (RSPM; RCPM) (Raven, 1958, 1962) to assess intelligence, but have found little relationship between Ravens scores and ability to make gains in treatment. In response to the need for an appropriate neuropsychological assessment, which is necessary for an accurate prognosis, the Global Aphasic Neuropsychological Battery (GANBA) was developed (van Mourik, Verschaeve, Boon, Paquier, & Harskamp, in press). The GANBA is especially designed for patients with a global aphasia. Besides general functions such as concentration, intelligence, and memory, it measures visual and auditory perception and language comprehension.

The GANBA profiles identify three treatment groups: The first is considered for Structural Therapy aiming at augmentative speech resources; the second group is considered for Structural Therapy, provided certain conditions are met; and the third is considered only for guidance.

We do not fully understand the mechanisms underlying aphasia and cognitive impairments in terms of coexistence, cause-consequence, and dissociability of functions. Nevertheless, it seems valuable to integrate cognitive rehabilitation into speech therapy, since the problems have much in common and require a unified approach.

III. MAXIMIZING CONDITIONS

We try to maximize conditions for the delivery of structural therapy. It may be necessary, for example, to introduce the patient to the conditions of Structural Therapy before it actually starts. Some problems which can accompany aphasia also need attention before structural therapy can be started. Vision and hearing should be corrected if possible. Factors such as a lack of motivation or serious depression will also impede structural therapy.

Difficulties with concentration, attention, and task dedication often occur. SAR developed the "Sorting Program for Global Aphasic Patients" to treat this kind of problem. It was designed to deal with functions such as attention, visual matching, persistence, and becoming accustomed to a therapeutic setting. The tasks involve matching and categorizing using real objects and photographs of fruit, drinks, animals, and money.

Goals differentiate maximizing conditions and exploratory therapy. When one is maximizing conditions, the goal is to arrange conditions under which optimal therapy can take place. In exploratory therapy, one is already working toward a communicative goal.

IV. EXPLORATORY THERAPY

Our first goal is to observe whether the patient is motivated and will respond to a specific therapeutic approach. The dynamics of the interaction between patient and therapist are important, and for maximum effectiveness, techniques, methods, and material used in therapy must be matched to the patient's specific problems and personality. Self-monitoring behavior, initiative and concept shifting, and some executive control functions are observed to provide information for planning therapy goals.

Although much information comes from direct assessment and from functional scales, trial and error in a therapeutic setting is still needed to develop a detailed therapy program. Basically, test batteries provide structured information about what is wrong. However, information about how a patient deals with his communication problems, what is still intact, and the right way to approach stimulation is also necessary. SAR has developed an instrument, the "Therapy-Oriented Assessment Set," a systematic approach that briefly tries out a variety of treatment methods, making it possible to judge the patient's abilities and the ways they can be used in a therapeutic setting. The therapist tries to determine the appropriate level of therapy, the applicable tasks, and the right material. Systematic observations in therapeutic situations reveal how a task is performed, what kind of cuing technique is useful, what material is appropriate, and which communication channel should be relied upon. The Therapy-Oriented Assessment Set has made us more aware of alternatives for therapy and their rationales. Tasks are grouped as follows: conversation, nonverbal techniques, semantics, syntax, phonology, and articulation. When administering this set the therapist is free to choose tasks based on earlier information. It is then possible to direct the tasks toward the kind of treatment that is most likely to succeed.

For example, Patient H was diagnosed as having severe Wernicke's aphasia with press of speech, phonemic jargon, and semantic neologisms. Comprehension was mostly poor but sometimes surprisingly adequate. The Therapy-Oriented Assessment Set demonstrated that phonemic cuing was of no use, that verbal input should be at word level, simultaneously visual and auditory, and that the patient could easily be stopped by a hand sign. This contrasts with patient B, who was also diagnosed as having severe Wernicke's aphasia with press of speech and poor comprehension. A hand sign was not helpful for him. A completely silent approach, where both patient and therapist use gestures, as in VAT (Groet, 1989), turned out to be very successful.

V. STRUCTURAL THERAPY

Structural therapy has three levels: Specification, integration, and generalization. The goal is to maximize linguistic abilities or to teach alternative means of communication that are complementary to speech. At a later stage, the patient must be assisted in using verbal and nonverbal strategies for information exchange. Unsuccessful strategies are corrected, and the patient is prepared to communicate with a naive partner.

Early assessment and prognosis can be carried out on the basis of what is known, and changes can be made as new information becomes available.

The reader might now have the impression that the process of diagnosis and planning a therapeutic approach takes months. It is true that in some cases determining the final therapeutic aim might take up to 3 months. On the other hand for some patients this process takes only a few days.

Of the 267 patients referred to us, structural therapy was recommended for 151 (57%). Guidance and support were recommended for the rest, a small proportion of whom later received therapy.

Ninety-four of those receiving treatment completed the therapy. Twelve patients continued to be seen as outpatients. Serious illness or death terminated therapy for 22 patients, and 33 dropped out because of diminished motivation or worsening of their physical condition. For 11 patients the speech therapist decided that further therapy would be of little use.

Only patients who perform at a given level on the Pre-therapeutic Assessment receive systematic aphasia therapy. The axis system provides information about general features which are important to the selection for Structural Therapy and the choice of a therapeutic approach.

Communicative goals must be specified before Structural Therapy is begun. The specification must be functional: "In all things related to rehabilitation, however, one must stay in touch with the pragmatics and constraints of the real world" (Howard & Patterson, 1989). An essential part of goal setting is a description of the patient as an interactive partner in language during daily situations. The patient's wishes (e.g., to shop on his own) and the therapist's expectations are both taken into account. Evaluation of functional communication is an important part of the therapy-oriented diagnosis.

GOALS IN STRUCTURAL THERAPY

Structural therapy pursues goals in the following areas: Basic skills, communicative strategies, conversational interaction with partner, and communication in daily life.

Basic Skills

Improvement of skills which may be relevant to the patient as a communicator in daily life is the main goal. The patient must become aware of his abilities at the level of the linguistic components of speech and/or at the level of augmentative speech resources. Therapy may be directed toward mastering or reinforcing basic communication skills. If the goal of therapy is to restore spontaneous speech, linguistic skills are emphasized. Augmentative speech resources are introduced only when speech as a channel of information transfer is expected to remain highly defective.

All augmentative speech resources impose restraints on the expression of individual needs and feelings. This is also true for more productive channels such as gestures, drawing, and writing. Moreover, concomitant disorders such as loss of motor skills, which are required for the use of augmentative speech resources, may impede adequate use. A communication board or Bliss symbols (Johannsen-Horbach, Cegla, Mager, Schempp, & Wallesch, 1985) may well be unfamiliar to a patient, because they are not part of a natural communicative situation.

Whether the objective is restoration of speech or development of augmentative speech resources, patients' learning patterns will differ, and this will influence the mode and the duration of therapy. A productive learner may invent new applications and require therapeutic assistance only in refining his technique. In such cases, the task of the therapist is essentially to make the patient aware of new modes of communication and ways to adapt his communicative behavior. Such is the case with ES, described below.

Patient ES

Description on the axes system, acute stage:

Axis I: Aphasia syndrome

Unclassifiable aphasia. Auditory and visual comprehension of sentences was moderately disturbed. At word level there was only a slight comprehension deficit. The patient was unsuccessful in initiating speech, but could repeat monosyllabic words. Articulation was inconsistent, and he could not write.

Axis II: Somatic condition and neurological status

TIAs resulting from right internal carotid stenosis. Infarction in the left middle cerebral artery with left internal carotid stenosis.

Axis III: Neurological and neuropsychological disturbances

Hemiparesis resolved largely within two weeks. Moderate buccofacial apraxia. Raven IQ 110.

Axis IV: Psychosocial stressors and personality

Poor relationship between patient and partner. One of his children lives in an institute for mentally retarded children.

Axis V: Social circumstances

52-year old male, right-handed, married, two sons. Profession: tram conductor. He had a poor social network. The most affectionate contact was with his sister. Hobbies: collector of stamps, history. Before his stroke he regularly visited the stamp market and exchanged stamps with a friend.

During exploratory therapy we unsuccessfully attempted to elicit spontaneous speech with MIT and deblocking techniques, suggested by Beyn and Shokhor-Trotskaya (1966) and Springer (1989). To offer the patient a way to express himself we used VAT. ES refused to use gestures, however, and made it clear that he wanted to speak. Exploratory therapy gave no cues for structural therapy except for auditory comprehension tasks, which were neither his most striking defect nor his desired goal. After some spontaneous speech appeared in conversation in the third month, structural therapy was begun.

We first used conversation only to gain insight into ES's attainable communicative level. Initially, he needed several minutes to prepare his utterances; his facial expression reflected his attempts. Mean length of utterances was 3–4 words. Content words were adequately used, although sometimes marred by slight phonemic paraphasias, and agrammatic features were prominent. When spontaneous speech became more Broca-like, we repeated MIT to facilitate ES's initiation and to make him aware of simple sentence structures.

To improve his word finding we used Intoned Sequence Units as proposed by Marshall and Holtzapple (1972–1976). ES completed the program in 6 weeks, having improved his spontaneous speech. The mean length of utterance increased to such a degree that we could apply the *Visuele Cue Program* (VCP) (van de Sandt-Koenderman, 1986). By the end of the program ES could produce most of the sentences alone, even constructions with three constituents. If the first word of the sentence was an article or preposition, however, he still had problems. During VCP-therapy he was noted to have a syntactic comprehension deficit, especially for verb tense, forms of plurality, and complex prepositions. We combined VCP and the Wilson Expanded Syntax Program (WESP) to improve his syntactic comprehension.

When his spontaneous speech and comprehension of sentences stabilized (after 2 months), we shifted to reading, since ES complained that he could no longer read history books. We combined silent reading with reading aloud; his problems in reading aloud were similar to his initial level of spontaneous speech. He could only read (with effort) the content words. Input material was a mystery thriller. When he completed one or two paragraphs, (first reading aloud, then reading silently), we questioned him about the contents, and he answered laboriously. Reading improved rapidly so that by 6 weeks he could read most function words. After 3 months, ES could retell, although effortfully, the essential part of what he had read without referring to the text.

We then changed to writing. Here too ES started laboriously. Rapid improvement occurred, with the necessary first steps directed toward eliciting written responses to written questions about his life or the news. He answered with single content words. After 3 months, he began to write his biography on the typewriter, and he continued this activity for a few months.

The primary goal of therapy for ES was improvement of verbal skills, especially syntax. The speech therapist merely guided ES, who successfully responded in all modalities. The tasks functioned as triggers for covert skills; ES seemed to learn immediately from his own responses. The main problem for him was that it seemed unlikely that he could practice his verbal abilities sufficiently in daily life. However, we successfully stimulated ES to resume collecting stamps, forcing him into verbal interaction with colleagues.

Patient AD

Structural Therapy started 1½ years post-onset. AD was not a candidate for therapy initially because of his problems in accepting his handicap.

He was aggressive and manifested behavioral changes that were probably consequences of the stroke. Prior to therapy AD was observed every 3 months by an interdisciplinary team. The neurologist tried to control his epilepsy, and the neuropsychologist and the speech therapist gave guidance, especially to the partner, and were waiting for a positive change in the patient's behavior. Pre-therapeutic assessment started as soon as AD called for the interview and tried to follow the events in his environment instead of walking away, jumping up and desperately pointing to himself with aggressive exclamations, or trying to slap his communicative partner's face.

Description on the axes system, 1 year and 3 months post-onset:

Axis I: Aphasia syndrome

Global aphasia with fluent CVCV recurring utterances.

Axis II: Somatic condition and neurological status

Infarction in the area of the left middle cerebral artery, infarction in the right occipital lobe.

Axis III: Neurological and neuropsychological disturbances

Right-sided hemiplegia, hemianopsia, severe ideomotor and constructional apraxia. Ambulatory after three months.

Axis IV: Psychosocial stressors and personality

After stroke aggressive behavior, outbursts of temper, domineering.

Axis V: Social circumstances

54-year old man, married, one daughter, living at home. Profession: head crane-driver. Hobbies: fishing.

Initially on the BDAE, AD scored 0 on all subtests. His spontaneous functional communication was ineffective. Spoken speech consisted exclusively of CVCV random utterances and cursing, and he made no attempt to use gestures communicatively. AD's head movements for yes/no were inadequate. The therapy-oriented diagnosis provided no direction for a therapeutic approach. During exploratory therapy Melodic Intonation Therapy seemed to have a strong positive influence on various aspects of the patient's behavior. He could almost immediately repeat the intoned sequences, in strong contrast to his reaction to words or spoken sentences. Furthermore, the method seemed to improve his attending and turn taking. Finally, due to his success, AD became strongly motivated for therapy.

Consequently, MIT was administered as a tool to maximize conditions. However, the outlook for the recovery of speech seemed poor. After 3 weeks, AD began to answer questions about the earlier trained sentences. All sentences were constructed in consultation with his partner so that AD could use the content words or the whole sentences spontaneously at home. Sentences were written during therapy so that he could point to the words during the auditory presentation. However, immediately after the MIT procedure, spontaneous speech occurred only during therapy. After 3 months AD made no progress beyond the level he had reached after 3 weeks. However, AD's attitude during therapy and in daily life was positively changed. In therapy he was more seriously involved, and his error-awareness was heightened, as was his attention to spoken speech. At home he started to repeat or to complete parts of his wife's utterances. According to his wife, AD's auditory comprehension was better in daily life.

Because the patient accepted only tasks in which he was to speak, we changed to the "Visual Cue Program," a method requiring only verbal repetition of utterances. After 2 months he could produce 50% of the SVO-sentences with a small cue: The first function word, the first phoneme, or even an initial mouth movement. He was able to produce spontaneously some content words associated with pictures. We then tried to improve his naming performance, using Sarno's Aphasia Therapy Kit with 100 pictures of common objects. After a few months of therapy AD could spontaneously name 70% of the pictures, but only when cued with the preceding article, a mouth movement, or the first phoneme of the noun. When a sentence was made with two pictures, he could name only the second noun. At home his functioning was stable.

AD's speech did not change in therapy. Consequently, we directed attention to comprehension. We used auditory word-picture matching at the single word level, with big pictures from different semantic fields. For sentence level comprehension, we administered the Wilson Expanded Syntax Program (WESP).

After 6 months of comprehension therapy we resumed work on language production, with the help of a communication aid, the "Language Pocket Book" ("Taalzakboek"). This book provided AD with a practical pointing mechanism for functional communication. Because choosing a word from the book required selecting a semantic category and then its exemplar, he depended on his partner's guidance to manage.

Summary

The therapy, initially aimed at improving AD's oral speech, influenced speech comprehension in daily life and thus his attitude in communicative situations, according to his wife and his therapist. However, this change was not reflected in test results.

We question whether any structural therapy is useful in a patient with fluent CVCV random utterances. Would the same effect not be observed after a period of adequate guidance? In this case guidance would have been psychosocial, medical, and communicative. Structural therapy may create false expectations, as was true in this case when the patient made substantial progress in a short period of time within a specific therapeutic approach aimed at oral production. However, imitation of words proved to be an insurmountable obstacle for AD. Perhaps an elaborate investigation of his executive functions prior to therapy-planning would have predicted his lack of success. An extra complication was that the patient would only participate in therapy directed toward eliciting utterances other than his CVCV concatenations.

The therapist must make educated decisions about when to move to a different level. Most therapy focuses on different skills consecutively, beginning with the most severely impaired. When the therapy focuses on linguistic skills, assessment directed toward uncovering the underlying deficit is often required (Howard & Patterson, 1989). An additional complicating factor is that some disorders are difficult to influence directly. Therapeutic intervention in phonology, especially in the phonemic planning of words, is problematic. Error awareness may be perfect, as is recognition of distorted spoken or written words. We have obtained relatively good results when patients were asked to read written words or sentences with graphically indicated stress patterns and syllabification. The effect of psychomotor therapy on neologisms is described by Hadar (1989) who also suggests using semantic therapy to reduce neologisms. For patients with conduction aphasia, Cubelli, Foresti, and Consolini (1988) proposed therapy directed toward the analysis of the phonological form. In the Netherlands, most therapeutic intervention for Broca's aphasia focuses more on syntax than on semantics. Despite the fact that treating semantics has been shown to be effective (Patterson, Purell, & Morton, 1983), careful descriptions of therapeutic methods are lacking.

We have designed two therapeutic programs for patients with Broca's aphasia; the "Visual Cue Program" (Visuele Cue Programma, VCP) (van de Sandt-Koenderman, 1986, 1987; van de Sandt-Koenderman & van Harskamp, 1987), and a Dutch version of "Melodic Intonation Therapy" (van der Lugt-van Wiechen & Verschoor, 1987).

VCP aims to improve the syntactic quality of utterances in spontaneous speech by teaching sentence production through the use of visual symbols. The idea stems from the Romanian neurologist Voinescu, who based his idea on Luria and Tsvetkova. They presented patients pictures of a situation, together with a linear array consisting of one card for each word of the target sentence. These blank cards form an external scheme by which agrammatic patients can be cued to produce a complete sentence. VCP also uses a sentence scheme, but different symbols are used for nouns, verbs, prepositions, and determiners. The program provides exercises for several sentence types, progressing from simple to more complex forms. The central role of the verb in the process of sentence construction (Black et al., 1991) is stressed throughout the program.

Once the patient is able to produce a given construction, the visual cue is removed. Tasks can focus on manipulation of surface structures (e.g., changing a positive sentence into a negative, changing a declarative sentence into a question, changing nouns into personal pronouns) or manipulating the underlying argument structure and the role of the verb (e.g., making different sentences with one verb, making several sentences by changing the verb).

Kolk and van Grunsven's adaptation hypothesis (1985) suggests that agrammatic constructions should not be discouraged, because they represent a strategy to avoid slow and effortful production of complete sentences. Nevertheless, we have had rather good results with VCP. Although spontaneous speech is rarely as good as performance on sentence production tasks, our experience indicates that syntactic therapy positively influences speech tempo and the use of verbs. Without this therapy, the patients' speech often remains hesitant and effortful, at the expense of the transfer of information.

Patient TL

Patient TL was referred to the SAR by the speech therapy department of a general hospital, where she had received aphasia therapy from 2 to 24 months post-onset. At 3 weeks post-onset she was diagnosed as having Broca's aphasia, with good auditory comprehension. TL began to speak in one-word utterances at about 6 weeks post-onset. She received individual therapy during the first year, which consisted of "Language Pocket Book" training, PACE (drawing, writing), and exercises for word finding, naming, and syntax. AT 13 months post-onset individual therapy was discontinued, and TL began to participate in group therapy.

The question was whether her spontaneous sentence production could be still influenced by using VCP. To decide whether or not to use

VCP, TL was examined by a neurologist and a neurolinguist. In this case linguistic assessment included our syntactic battery.

At 2 years post-onset, the information on the five axes was as follows:

Axis I: Aphasia syndrome

Broca's aphasia, alert and communicative. Spontaneous speech nonfluent and agrammatic, predominantly single NP's occasionally simple sentences. Hardly any verbs, but when using verbs, production of the inflected form. Comprehension of reversible sentences 65%, naming verbs 40% (lower level than naming nouns), production of simple sentences possible, production of prepositions relatively good.

Axis II: Somatic condition and neurological status

Infarction in the territory of the left middle cerebral artery.

Axis III: Neurological and neuropsychological disturbances

Right hemiplegia, right hemianopsia, mild buccofacial apraxia, no ideomotor apraxia, no signs of speech apraxia. Mental status examination: no indication for formal neuropsycholgical assessment.

Axis IV: Psychosocial stressors and personality

No stressors besides aphasia. Good motivation.

Axis V: Social circumstances

56-year old woman, right-handed, assistant on the nursing staff of a nursing home. Married, supportive husband, retired from his job as a hospital administrative clerk. Three children who all live in the same town as TL.

It was concluded that TL's problems producing verbs in sentences and, to a lesser degree, in naming tasks could be treated using VCP. This decision was based on her good motivation and her excellent psychosocial situation. It was expected that the whole family would support TL during treatment. To control the effect of VCP treatment, two 3-month therapeutic periods were planned, preceded by a baseline period.

Following therapy, most of the AAT and syntactic scores remained the same. The sentence production score did not change but the test took much less time, indicating that TL's sentence construction had become less effortful. In addition, naming of actions (verbs) improved while naming of objects (nouns) remained stable.

Analysis of spontaneous speech, based on Saffran et al., (1989) and Byng and Black (1989) yielded the following results: There was a clear improvement in the production of verbs versus the production of nouns (noun-verb ratio). As in naming tasks, TL used many more verbs in her spontaneous speech after each therapy period. The argument structure of the utterances also improved.

Our observations of TL were reinforced by reports from the patient, her family, and even people who did not know that she had received individual therapy that, suddenly, she talked much better.

Melodic Intonation Therapy (MIT) is appropriate for several groups of patients: Patients with severe chronic Broca's aphasia; patients with Broca's aphasia with apraxia of speech; and patients with global aphasia and nonfluent recurring utterances, consisting of words or CVCV concatenations. As mentioned by Springer (1989), MIT may be applied in the acute stage to trigger oral speech in mute patients with a mild to moderate comprehension disorder. In our experience the process of deblocking speech may take just a few days. The patients to whom we administered MIT during the acute stage were evolving into non-agrammatic Broca's aphasics, which may be an intriguing observation in view of the hypothesis of Beyn and Shokor-Trotskaya (1966) that it is possible to prevent agrammatism. In one case we administered MIT to a patient with Broca's aphasia and nonfluent CVCV recurring utterances at 10 months post-onset. Our hypothesis was that the patient was confined in an overt articulatory loop by his apraxia of speech (Blanken, Wallesch, & Papagnos, 1990; Poeck, de Bleser, & Graf van Keyserlingh, 1984). After 6 weeks of therapy the recurring utterances had been replaced by one- to three-word sentences with phonemic paraphasias (Visch-Brink & Wielaert, in preparation).

The use of MIT with globally aphasic patients is described by van der Lugt-van Wiechen and Visch-Brink (1989). Nine patients with stroke-induced global aphasia, right-sided hemiplegia, and buccofacial apraxia were studied. Five patients made nonfluent recurring utterances in spontaneous speech, and one patient was a fluent CVCV global aphasic. All patients received at least 6 weeks of MIT. The recurring utterances of the nonfluent global aphasics disappeared, as described by van Eeckhout, Meillet-Haberen, and Pillon (1981). This effect was independent of the time post-onset. Two patients with initially nonfluent recurring utterances developed spontaneous speech, mostly isolated content words. The method failed to work in the patient with fluent CVCV recurring utterances. One of the three other patients without recurring utterances also developed spontaneous speech.

Motivated by the literature on the effectiveness of semantic therapy (among others Howard, Patterson, Franklin, Orchard-Lisle, & Morton, 1985), a Semantic Therapy Program was recently developed for patients with mild to moderate semantic impairment. The program consists of three parts: Word, sentence, and text level. Each part has three degrees of difficulty. To give the therapist the opportunity to switch levels, from word to sentence level and back, which may have a facilitating effect, the same words are incorporated at both levels. Patients are asked to perform tasks such as classification, matching, judgments of correctness, answering questions, and detecting material that is out of context. The more complex tasks occur at the level of text. Another semantic therapy program, which is part of the "Auditory Language Comprehension Program" ("Auditief Taalbegripsprogramma") developed by Bastiaanse, van Groningen-Derksen, Nijboer, and Taconis (1986), requires the patient to match a word with a picture. The difficulty of the task is manipulated by varying the degrees of semantic relatedness between the target and the distractors.

Since the early 1980s, when microcomputers became available, computer-assisted programs for aphasia therapy have been developed (Robertson, 1990; Stachowiak & Willeke, 1987). Such programs have become increasingly sophisticated, and it is generally agreed that the computer can be useful for a number of tasks. The advantages have often been stressed. The patient can work independently, supervised by the therapist. Consequently therapy sessions can emphasize other tasks, such as generalization of learned skills. Working independently is often very satisfactory for the patient, because the computer reacts to his activities, but does not judge the way a therapist does. In addition the computer allows unlimited response time.

Considering these advantages, it is surprising how long it has taken to incorporate microcomputers into aphasia therapy. In the Netherlands only a few centers use microcomputers, partly because of the shortage of adequate software. Many patients can spend a great deal of time at the computer and thus need a range of programs. The first program for aphasia, the "System for Therapy for Aphasic Patients" (STAP), was developed in 1980 through the cooperation of the Rehabilitation Center "de Hoogstraat" and the Technical University Delft (Janssen et al., 1986; de Vries, 1984, 1987). After an 8-year experimental period the program became commercially available. It contains a treatment system for therapists, and a training system for patients. In the treatment system, the therapist chooses the exercise and, for each patient, adjusts the type of words or sentences, the kind of feedback, and the help to be provided. The program includes exercises at the word and sentence level.

In addition, a set of diskettes containing exercises and games of various types, "Compro," was published by the AVN, the Dutch Aphasia Association (Köbben & Nibbering, 1992). These are not presented as aphasia therapy, but as recreation. As mentioned, a specific problem of Dutch aphasiologists is that the potential market is rather small. Therefore, in this area as in others, international cooperation is essential.

A German program, "Lingware/Stach," developed by Stachowiak, and colleagues, has been translated into English, Italian, and Dutch as a result of European Community concerted action. This program provides many different types of exercises and uses spoken language in addition to pictures and written text. The system also provides an authoring system that enables the therapist to create new exercises.

We have developed a program specifically for word finding, called "Multicue" (van Mourik & van de Sandt-Koenderman, 1992). This program demonstrates that the computer can also be used for learning strategies. The basic principle is to let the patient experience the effect of several cues on his word-finding problems, and to learn to choose among these different possibilities. The long-term effect of the program is that the patient internalizes the various possibilities presented in the program and learns to choose among them in everyday situations. Each cue provides different kinds of information. For example, if a patient cannot name the picture of a bicycle, he can choose from a variety of categories of cues to help him. One cue, for example, provides associations such as "traffic" and "flat tire." Another suggests that the patient imagine aspects of the target such as use, movement, how it feels, and so forth. Another presents specific semantic features such as "vehicle," "two wheels," and so forth. Two cues provide extensive semantic information about the target. The patient's choices during therapy sessions are registered.

COMMUNICATIVE STRATEGIES

The patient must integrate his basic communicative skills to produce an information-carrying message. The speech therapist arranges various situations that permit patients to develop strategies for facilitating information transfer. Patients must become aware of their abilities through experience. Therapy leads to optimizing verbal strategies or alternative systems in the context of a structured communicative situation, as advocated in PACE therapy (Davis & Wilcox, 1981). The main objective is to increase success in exchanging information. Functioning at discrete linguistic or nonlinguistic levels is of value only in relation to the information value of the utterance. A syntactically ill-formed utterance with adequate semantic structure will be successful in a functional context; numerous syntactic self-corrections may decrease the listener's attention. Unsuccessful strategies can be modified by using more facilitative strategies (Golper & Rau, 1983).

The role of the speech therapist is to arrange communicative situations to optimize patients' use of their abilities, to observe patients' communicative behavior, and to model effective communication strategies. There are some pitfalls. Patients often simulate modeling the speech therapist without really choosing that kind of behavior, with the result that they use this behavior even in situations in which another strategy would be better. The therapist must help them to develop flexibility in selecting communicative strategies appropriate to the particular situation. The time required for information transfer and the clarity of the message are measures of the success of therapy.

The following illustrates how AG, a 66-year-old male with chronic moderate amnesic aphasia, learned to modify his message through PACE therapy.

AG participated in PACE for 2 hours weekly over 2 months. His AAT scores did not change over time. AG was asked to read and retell short journal reports. The therapist modeled differentiation between main points and side issues. The following journal entries compare pre- and post-therapy.

Pre-therapy: duration 2 minutes, 40 seconds.

AG: There is the environment of Woensdrecht (place name) there has of Woensdrecht there they took a new com com commander. That that that is the 48 year old sergeant, I don't know exactly, of the base. That man is there took for the head, appointed to be a head. Yes, that's it, I believe. The old Emmerich (person's name), that man became (neol.) [neol.], no, that of the of the year before, before, yes no, the new Emmerich the the Emmerich we don't take, no. Yes, that is easy now. He found the present commander Emmerich oh, oh, now that on that new commander that is the 48 year of that. I don't know, to the base Woensdrecht, takes eh Oendrecht the.

TH: So in Woensdrecht there is a new 48-year-old commander. You do not know his name. But you said Emmerich.

AG: Yes, that man they picked up. Yes, he goes in, he leaves.

TH: Oh, that man is succeeded by someone.

AG: Yes, yes, then he is on.

Post-therapy: duration 30 seconds.

AG: There is a commander of to Woensdrecht, there is there is [neol.] nominated mayor no the commander Schut (person's name) to eh Woensdrecht. She is nominated there by 28 February. The man who the [neol.] who leaves is the commander Emmerich.

Successful therapy essentially means that a patient knows his communicative limits and tries to find the best strategies to convey his message and to receive messages from his conversational partner.

Training conversation is not always a necessary component of aphasia therapy. For example, patients with mild to moderate phonological deficits may not need such therapy. Most such patients are very aware of errors and will spontaneously integrate into conversation what they have learned in therapy.

CONVERSATIONAL INTERACTION WITH PARTNER

As the patient and his conversational partner adjust to the linguistic handicap, they learn how to resolve blockages during conversation. Therapy leads to mastery of verbal strategies or alternative systems in the context of a structured communicative situation. The partner may actually be more involved in the therapy than the patient. Better communication in daily life often has its roots in the changed behavior of the partner. Therapy may increase the understanding of family members and friends of the nature of the patient's problems. Perceptions of spouses' problems were more concordant in a treated than in an untreated group (Shewan & Cameron, 1984). The treated group also appeared to have learned more ways to communicate with aphasic patients, such as rewording sentences and assisting with word retrieval problems, than the untreated group. In our experience, guidance and counseling is not enough to facilitate the communicative interaction between the partner and the patient. Many observations of patient and spouse in a verbal communicative interaction are necessary to assess the problems which may arise and to determine the limits and the terms of adequate assistance, as exemplified by patient DL and patient JT below.

Patient DL

Axis I: Aphasia syndrome

Transcortical sensory aphasia, no dysarthria. In the acute stage there was no speech production. Comprehension was severely disturbed.

Axis II: Somatic condition and neurological status

Infarction in the posterior left temporal lobe. Medical history: atrial fibrillation with cardioversion and hypertension.

Axis III: Neurological and neuropsychological disturbances

Severe acalculia, lack of initiative, slight disorder in visual perception.

Axis IV: Psychosocial stressors and personality

No stressors.

Axis V: Social circumstances

70-year-old retired physician, three children, many social contacts.

Structural Therapy: For the first 6 months we used semantic therapy with visual verbal material, his best input channel. Much time was spent grouping words from the same semantic category, labeling semantic categories, making yes/no judgments about a picture/word presentation, semantic feature recognition and other semantic tasks. When DL's naming performance improved, we shifted to PACE therapy to try to increase his initiative, with little progress.

A positive side effect of PACE therapy was that DL became accustomed to auditory input. We returned to semantic therapy which combined auditory and visual presentation of verbal material. To improve his verbal comprehension, we presented spoken texts on tape, and DL was asked to detect utterances or combinations of words which did not fit into the text. When necessary, we showed him the written text to detect the errors. After 6 months of therapy, the patient could understand tape recorded books for the blind.

The patient's wife had great difficulty accepting the severity of the disorder. It took a year-and-a-half for her to interpret his behavior more realistically. She attended almost every therapeutic session and repeatedly told the therapist that DL could have done much better: she said that his shyness caused his lack of initiative and erroneous responses.

To improve their communicative interaction we began conducting therapy at their home. At first the therapist observed DL and his wife during a conversation about shared experiences. The therapist noted the types and frequency of the spouse's intervention, and tape recorded the conversation for future analysis. This revealed that the partner used many unfinished sentences in rapid succession to try to elicit information. Further, she frequently asked for names and dates which the patient could not produce, causing unnecessary blocks. When miscommunications occurred she forced the patient to use gestures, most of which were unsuccessful. DL appeared to function rather well in conversation when his partner gave semantically associated words or descriptions. She led him to the topic of interest or to an answer through a semantic context.

We began to use family and magazine photographs. The wife was taught to comprehend DL's semantic paraphasias by presenting related words and asking him to say whether they were the word he was seeking.

After 3 months, DL's wife had become more attentive to her husband's utterances. She stopped using the rapid unfinished sentences that confused him and helped him to structure his message by guiding him semantically to the answer. To resolve the blocks caused by DL's difficulties producing names, we gave him a "Language Pocket Book" with written names of shops, friends, and family, as suggested by his wife.

Patient JT

Axis I: Aphasia syndrome

Mild to moderate Wernicke's aphasia, most problems in spontaneous speech, including word finding difficulties, semantic paraphasias and empty speech. He had slight logorrhea but succeeded in conveying his message. He was sometimes aware of his problems. On the Token Test he scored in the normal range but he clearly had comprehension difficulty with spoken language. He denied this almost completely and usually blamed his wife for not being precise.

Axis II: Somatic condition and neurological status

A long-standing hearing loss, unchanged after the cerebral hemorrhage, which he suffered while staying in his summer house in southern France. After unsuccessful embolization, he was taken to the Rotterdam Academic Hospital. Physically he recovered quite quickly and his aphasia improved quickly as well.

Axis III: Neurological and neuropsychological disturbances

No problems.

Axis IV: Psychosocial stressors and personality

Not willing to accept his language problem in addition to his hearing loss. Blamed the latter for all of his problems.

Axis V: Social circumstances

Right-handed, 73-year-old male retired financial manager of a medium-sized company. Intelligent and a strong personality.

Despite denial of some of his problems, JT agreed to a weekly visit with his wife to our outpatient clinic for therapy and guidance. It was often very hard to determine whether he could not hear speech or could not understand language, but it was clear that his comprehension was poorer after the hemorrhage, although his audiogram remained the same. His wife discovered that he understood written better than spoken language. They came to the clinic for 4 months.

The goals for structural therapy for JT were: Convey on-topic information, listen to wife's questions, let her know when not quite understanding, and ask for written information. Goals for Mrs. T were: Help him to stick to the subject, tell him when not understanding, and continue to use written information, especially when changing the subject.

The tasks included giving JT a short newspaper story both auditorily and visually, and then having him answer direct questions. He was allowed to make comments only after the tasks were completed. JT and his wife participated in PACE therapy. They described newspaper photographs to one another. The therapist supplied the material and discussed the process afterwards.

During this period, JT began to recognize the difference between not hearing speech and not understanding language. He admitted that he sometimes used wrong words or even strange words and that he did not always understand what his wife meant. He also admitted that he was afraid of becoming demented and of having another hemorrhage. He had great difficulty accepting what had really happened to him.

His wife learned a great deal from participation in the therapeutic sessions. Mr. and Mrs. T were informed about the Dutch Aphasia Association, a society for aphasic patients and their families, and some recent literature was recommended. Both welcomed the books, but preferred further backup from their own children and a few friends.

COMMUNICATION IN DAILY LIFE

In daily life situations, speech therapists may guide patients in situations such as shopping, using the telephone, and writing or reading a letter or a postcard. Therapists also can help people to use communication aids creatively in everyday life.

Clinical experience has suggested that there is a great discrepancy between the use of augmentative speech resources in therapeutic settings and in natural environments. Patients sometimes do not recognize the communicative value of a communication aid, and further, lack flexibility, not necessarily a consequence of the aphasic disorder, but possibly a consequence of brain damage.

For severely impaired patients, this stage of therapy often focuses on the use of the "Language Pocket Book" ("Taalzakboek") (van Haaften-van Bekkum, Vries, Stumpel, & van Loon-Vervoorn, 1981; de Vries, 1989). This book provides word lists and pictures organized by categories or situations, as an aid to communication. To find words, the patient must select the appropriate semantic categories. To do this, the patient must be able to categorize words and concepts. Therefore, with severe patients much attention is focused on learning to use the book.

A new communication book has recently been developed by Verschaeve (in press; Verschaeve & van Mourik, in press). This "Conversation Book" (*Gespreksboek*) provides written words and pictures organized in a unique way. To classify the words and concepts, five main categories corresponding to semantic characteristics are used: Who and what, doing and happening, where, when, and how.

The aphasic person's conversational partner must play an active role, asking the same questions about each semantic characteristic each time. These questions are provided in a communication scheme: The patient can point to the correct answer, and the answers refer to "chapters" in the book. For example, at first the patient has to indicate about "whom or what" he wants to tell something, and the first question is whether it is about a human being, an animal, or a thing. The partner has to check regularly whether he has understood everything correctly. It is recommended that the patient's choices be written down so that the course of the conversation is evident.

COMMENTS

When a patient achieves less in therapy than had been expected, the therapist should try to figure out why, beginning with a re-evaluation of the choice of therapy. The failure of model-inappropriate therapy has been demonstrated by Nettleton and Lesser (1991), who provide a strong argument for a detailed model-based language assessment as a prerequisite for planning therapy.

However, an analysis of the language deficit alone is not necessarily sufficient. Extralinguistic factors also influence the effectiveness of Structural Therapy. Thus, multi-axial evaluation is necessary, both to reconsider any disturbing circumstances and to refocus the patient's clinical picture. Such a review should be conducted at each turning point during the course of Structural Therapy to prevent at the end of therapy a bewildering gap between expectations and the actual level of progress.

As important as specifying the skills that respond to treatment is the enumeration of unreachable speech levels. Patients must be guided in both directions: Their awareness of optimum communicative skills and acceptance of the fact that some situations will be too difficult to manage without help (e.g., the wish to read the newspaper or a book is unrealistic for most patients, even those who are labeled as nonaphasic by a diagnostic test battery). After some aphasic individuals succeed in reading a favorite book, they may complain that they do not know why they admired it before. Their sensitivity to linguistic aspects other than literal meaning seems to have disappeared.

EPILOGUE

We have presented our approach to aphasia rehabilitation, resulting from many years of clinical experience. Our multidisciplinary team meets weekly to discuss treatment for patients with neurological speech and language disorders who have been referred to the diagnostic team of the Stichting Afasie Rotterdam.

The SAR was designed to simplify diagnostic procedures and to stimulate the development of new therapeutic techniques. With the extension of diagnostic tools in the domain of neuropsychology and aphasia, influenced in part by linguists' growing interest in aphasia, test results began to influence therapeutic decisions. Newly developed therapeutic approaches required specific selection criteria, which were then reflected in assessment. Our enthusiasm for Structural Therapy based on formal analysis of the language disorder initially diverted our attention from patients' psychosocial and medical realities. However, in clinical practice the impact of psychosocial factors on the success of therapeutic methods was so great that we were required to affirm the importance of checking these essential features.

The axes system provides a starting point for the selection of aphasic patients for Structural Therapy. The complex of features described on the various axes predicts the effect of remediation on the patient's communicative level in daily life.

The assessment of the aphasia syndrome (axis I) has been well developed since the founding of SAR, because standardized test batteries and tests for subcomponents of the aphasic disorder have become available. Detailed assessment in terms of cognitive neuropsychology often leads to a hypothesis about the effect of model-based therapy.

Clearly somatic condition and neurological status (axis II) influence the course and duration of therapy. Well-described systematic speech therapy directed at improving the patient's communicative level succeeds only if therapy is not frequently interrupted by illness.

Knowledge about which neurological and neuropsychological disturbances (axis III) are relevant for aphasia therapy is limited. We lack clear insight into the impact of neuropsychological disorders on speech therapy. As a first step, the SAR has directed attention to patients with global aphasia, to determine the weight of neuropsychological factors for several types of treatment.

One of the most difficult factors to assess accurately is the extent to which psychosocial stressors, personality, and social circumstances (axes IV and V) affect selection of patients for Structural Therapy and development of appropriate approaches to therapy. We recognize that it is hard to make generalizations. It is not always easy to detect relevant features such as depression, which may greatly influence both the patient's motivation for therapy and his functioning on cognitive tasks, including language.

Despite its uncertainty the axis system appears to be clinically useful. Using this method of describing patients, we are in a better position to identify favorable conditions for Structural Therapy. Previously, the decision-making process was opaque for people who did not know the patient personally. It became clearer when pre-therapeutic assessment was divided into well-described subcomponents and subgoals of therapy were recognized. For insiders, the system gives structure to the stream of information and provides an opportunity to note the patient's life situation. For outsiders, the system clarifies the arguments that supported the decision for a specific therapeutic approach.

New developments in pre-therapeutic assessment will be reflected in the system; executive control functions (Glosser & Goodglass, 1990) may be an indispensable issue in relation to the success of Structural Therapy. Refinements in the selection criteria for specific therapeutic approaches will also be incorporated in the axes system for individual patients. For example, the intactness of phonemic discrimination may be a prerequisite for the rehabilitation of writing in brain-damaged patients (Carlomagno & Parlato, 1989).

The axes system requires interdisciplinary cooperation. Such cooperation is necessary not only during pre-therapeutic assessment, but also during Structural Therapy. As patients' nonlinguistic features change, the therapeutic program also will change. It is possible that a communicative impairment is the consequence of a primary nonverbal deficit (Davis, 1989), which may require a nonlinguistic therapy.

The main goal of evaluation and of aphasia therapy is to establish adequate communicative abilities in daily life. However, our knowledge about the essential aspects of communication is limited. Since the development of the Rating Scale of Speech Characteristics (Goodglass & Kaplan, 1972), much progress has been made in the ways spontaneous speech can be analyzed (e.g., Saffran et al., 1989). Still lacking, however, is a clinically applicable design for analyzing communicative acts. We believe that "Still there are very few tools to measure the ability to communicate" (Frattali, 1992). The available scales for measuring functional communication are designed primarily to describe the communicative channels that the aphasic patient uses. They do not provide an in-depth analysis of important communicative features. The most devastating aspect of aphasia is its resultant difficulties with the transactional and interactional functions of language (i.e., the content-bearing aspect and the social aspect, respectively; see Brown & Yule, 1983). A realistic therapy program must take those functions into account. To that end, aphasic patients must be observed in different communicative situations. Patients with residual aphasia, however minimal, continue to complain about their inadequate functioning in conversation. Knowledge of why they fail might help us to elaborate on a workable definition of functional communication. At the same time we must realize that, especially in the field of communication, remediation has its limits. "The linguistic meaning of an uttered sentence falls short of encoding what the speaker means" (Sperber & Wilson, 1986).

REFERENCES

Alderse Baes, I., Leipoldt, T., Dharmaperwira-Prins, R., & Verschaeve, M. (1991). Een model voor het beschrijven van afasie-onderzoek en afasiebehandeling. *Logopedie en Foniatrie, 63,* 10–13.

Au, R., Albert, M. L., & Obler, L. K. (1988). The relation of aphasia to dementia. *Aphasiology, 2,* 161–173.

Bachy-Langedock, N., & de Partz, M. P. (1989). Coordination of two reorganization therapies in a deep dyslexic patient with oral naming disorders. In X. Seron & G. Deloche (Eds.), *Cognitive approaches in neuropsychological rehabilitation* (pp. 211–248). London and Hillsdale, NJ: Lawrence Erlbaum.

Basso, A., Capitani, E., & Vignolo, L. A. (1979). Influence of rehabilitation on language skills in aphasic patients: A controlled study. *Archives of Neurology, 36,* 190–196.

Bastiaanse, R., Groningen-Derksen, M. J. I. J. van, Nijboer, S. F., & Taconis, M. P. (1986). *Het Auditief Taalbegripsprogramma; een taalbegripsprogramma op woordniveau.* Enschede: het Roessingh.

Beyn, E. S., & Shokhor-Trotskaya, M. K. (1966)'. The preventive method of speech rehabilitation in aphasia. *Cortex, 2,* 96–108.

Black, M., Nickels, L. A., & Byng, S. (1991). Patterns of sentence processing deficit: Processing simple sentences can be a complex matter. *Journal of Neurolinguistics, 6,* 79–102.

Blanken, G., Wallesch, C. W., & Papagnos, C. (1990). Dissociations of language functions in aphasics with speech automatisms (recurring utterances). *Cortex, 26,* 41–63.

Bleser, R. de, Willmes, K., Graetz, P., & Hagoort, P. (1991). De Akense Afasie Test. *Logopedie en Foniatrie, 63,* 207–217.

Blomert, L. (1990). What functional assessment can contribute to setting goals for aphasia therapy. *Aphasiology, 4,* 307–320.

Blomert, L., Koster, Ch., & Kean, M. L. (1991). Amsterdam-Nijmegen Test voor Alledaagse Taalvaardigheid. *Logopedie en Foniatrie, 63,* 368–374.

Brown, G., & Yule, G. (1983). *Discourse analysis.* Cambridge and Sydney: University Press.

Byng, S., & Black, M. (1989). Some aspects of sentence production in aphasia. *Aphasiology, 3,* 241–263.

Byng, S., Kay, J., Edmundson, A., & Scott, Ch. (1990). Aphasia tests reconsidered. *Aphasiology, 4,* 67–91.

Carlomagno, S., & Parlato, V. (1989). Writing rehabilitation in brain-damaged adult patients: A cognitive approach. In X. Seron & G. Deloche (Eds.), *Cognitive approaches in neuropsychological rehabilitation* (pp. 175–211). London and Hillsdale, NJ: Lawrence Erlbaum.

Crevel, H. van (1991). Consensus cerebrovasculair accident. *Nederlands Tijdschrift voor Geneeskunde, 48,* 2280–2288.

Cubelli, R., Foresti, A., & Consolini, T. (1988). Reeducation strategies in conduction aphasia. *Journal of Communication Disorders, 21,* 239–249.

Davis, G. A. (1989). Pragmatics and cognition in treatment of language disorders. In X. Seron & G. Deloche (Eds.), *Cognitive approaches in neuropsychological rehabilitation* (pp. 317–355). London and Hillsdale, NJ: Lawrence Erlbaum.

Davis, G. A., & Wilcox, M. J. (1981). Incorporation parameters of natural conversation in aphasia treatment. In R. Chapey (Ed.), *Language intervention strategies in adult aphasia* (pp. 169–193). Baltimore, MD: Williams & Williams.

Deelman, B. G., Liebrand, W. B. G., Koning-Haanstra, M., & Burg, W. van de. (1981). *SAN-test: Een afasietest voor auditief begrip en mondeling taalgebruik.* Lisse: Swets & Zeitlinger.

Edelman, G. M. (1984). Assessment of understanding in global aphasia. In F. C. Rose (Ed.), *Advances in neurology, progress in aphasia* (pp. 277–289). New York: Raven Press.

Eeckhout, P. van, Meillet-Haberen, C., & Pillon, B. (1981). Utilisation de la mélodie et du rythme dans les mutismes et les stéréotypies. *Rééducation Orthophonique, 19,* 109–124.

Frattali, C. M. (1992). Beyond barriers: A reply to Chapey, Sacchett and Marshall, Scherzer and Worral. *Aphasiology, 6,* 111–117.

Glosser, G., & Goodglass, H. (1990). Disorders in executive control functions among aphasics and other brain-damaged patients. *Journal of Clinical and Experimental Neuropsychology, 12*(4), 485–501.

Golper, L., & Rau, M. (1983). Systematic analysis of cueing strategies in aphasia: Taking your cue from the patient. In R. H. Brookshire (Ed.), *Clinical aphasiology conference proceedings* (pp. 52–62). Minneapolis: BRK Publishers.

Goodglass, H., & Kaplan, E. (1972). *The assessment of aphasia and related disorders.* Philadelphia: Lea & Febiger.

Graetz, P., Bleser, R. de, Willmes, C., & Heeschen, C. (1991). De akense afasie test. *Logopedie en Foniatrie, 63,* 58–68.

Grober, E. (1984). Nonlinguistic memory in aphasia. *Cortex, 20,* 67–73.

Groet, E. (1989). Een patient met een Wernicke afasie. In E. G. Visch-Brink, F. van Harskamp, & D. de Boer (Eds.), *Afasietherapie* (pp. 259–262). Lisse: Swets & Zeitlinger.

Haaften-van Bekkum, I. J. van, Vries, L. A. de, Stumpel, H. J. E. J., & Loon-Vervoorn, W. A. van (1981). *Handleiding taalzakboek en language master programma.* Arnhem: Boek- en Leermiddelencentrale.

Hadar, U. (1989). Sensory-motor factors in the control of jargon in conduction aphasia. *Aphasiology, 3,* 593–610.

Harskamp, F. van (1989). Behandeling van afatische patiënten in het verpleeghuis; een verkennend onderzoek. In J. J. F. Schroots, A. Bouma, G. P. A. Braam, A. Groeneveld, D. J. B. Ringoir, & C. J. J. Tempelman (Eds.), *Gezond zijn is ouder worden* (pp. 155–162). Assen, Maastricht: van Gorcum.

Harskamp, F. van, & Visch-Brink, E. G. (1989). Inleiding tot de afasietherapie. In E. G. Visch-Brink, F. van Harskamp, & D. de Boer (Eds.), *Afasietherapie* (pp. 11–27). Amsterdam: Swets & Zeitlinger.

Harskamp, F. van, & Visch-Brink, E. G. (1991). Goal recognition in aphasia therapy. *Aphasiology, 5,* 529–539.

Herrmann, M., Koch, U., Johannsen-Horbach, H., & Wallesch, C. W. (1989). Communicative skills in chronic and severe nonfluent aphasia. *Brain and Language, 37,* 339–354.

Holland, A. L. (1982). Observing functional communication of aphasic adults. *Journal of Speech and Hearing Disorders, 47,* 50–56.

Howard, D., & Franklin, S. (1988). *Missing the meaning? A cognitive neuropsychological study of the processing of words by an aphasic patient.* Cambridge, MA and London: MIT Press.

Howard, D., & Hatfield, F. M. (1987). *Aphasia therapy. Historical and contemporary issues.* London and Hillsdale, NJ: Lawrence Erlbaum.

Howard, D., & Patterson, K. (1989). Models for therapy. In X. Seron & G. Deloche (Eds.), *Cognitive approaches in neuropsychological rehabilitation* (pp. 39–64). London and Hillsdale, NJ: Lawrence Erlbaum.

Howard, D., Patterson, K., Franklin, S., Orchard-Lisle, V., & Morton, J. (1985). Treatment of word retrieval deficits in aphasia. *Brain, 108,* 817–829.

Huber, W., Poeck, K., Weniger, D., & Willmes, K. (1983). *Der Aachener Aphasietest.* Göttingen: Verlag fr psychologie Dr. J. C. Hogrefe.

Janssen, R. J., Messing-Peterson, J. J. M., Stumpel, H. J. E. J., Vries, L. de, Wenneker, B. J. M., & Graaf, A. de. (1986). *Het verslag van een onderzoek naar het gebruik van het STAP in de thuissituatie* (Report No. N-268). Delft: TH-Lab.

Johannsen-Horbach, H., Cegla, B., Mager, U., Schempp, B., & Wallesch, C. W. (1985). Treatment of chronic global aphasia with a nonverbal communication system. *Brain and Language, 24,* 27–43.

Kertesz, A. (1982). *Western aphasia battery.* New York and London: Grune & Stratton.

Köbben, A. H., & Nibbering, B. (1992). Compro. *Logopedie en Foniatrie, 64*(5), 154–156.

Kolk, H. H. J., & Grunsven, M. J. F. van (1985). Agrammatism as a variable phenomenon. *Cognitive Neuropsychology, 2,* 347–384.

Lebrun, Y., & Hoops, R. (1974). *Intelligence in aphasia. Neurolinguistics, 2.* Amsterdam: Swets & Zeitlinger.

Lincoln, L. B., Mully, G. P., Jones, A. C., McGurk, E., Lendrem, W., & Mitchell, J. R. A. (1984). Effectiveness of speech therapy for aphasic stroke patients. *Lancet, 1,* 1197–1200.

Lomas, J., Pickard, L., Bester, S., Elbard, H., Finlayson, A., & Zoghiab, C. (1989). The communicative effectiveness index: Development and psychometric evaluation of a functional communication measure for adult aphasia. *Journal of Speech and Hearing Disorders, 54,* 113–124.

Lugt-van Wiechen, K. van der, & Verschoor, J. (1987). Een voor het Nederlands taalgebied uitgewerkt programma voor afasietherapie, gebaseerd op de Melodic Intonation Therapy. Stichting Afasie Rotterdam.

Lugt-van Wiechen, K. van der, & Visch-Brink, E. G. (1989). Die Melodic Intonation Therapy bei Patienten mit einer globalen Aphasie; das Hemmen von Recurring Utterances. *Sprache-Stimme-Gehör, 13,* 142–145.

Marshall, N., & Holtzapple, P. (1972–1976). Melodic intonation therapy: Variations on a theme. In R. H. Brookshire (Ed.), *Clinical aphasiology, collected proceedings* (pp. 285–309). Minneapolis, MN: BRK Publishers.

Marshall, R. C. (1987). Reapportioning time for aphasia rehabilitation: A point of view. *Aphasiology, 1,* 59–73.

Mourik, M. van, & Sandt-Koenderman, W. M. E. van de. (1992). Multicue. *Aphasiology, 6,* 179–184.

Mourik, M. van, Verschaeve, M. A. W., Boon, P., Paquier, P., & Harskamp, F. van (1992). Cognition in global aphasia: Indicators for therapy. *Aphasiology, 6*(5), 491–499.

Nettleton, J., & Lesser, R. (1991). Therapy for naming difficulties in aphasia: Application of a cognitive neuropsychological model. *Journal of Neurolinguistics, 6* (2), 139–157.

Nickels, L., Byng, S., & Black, M. (1991). Sentence processing deficits: A replication of therapy. *British Journal of Disorders of Communication, 26,* 175–199.

Patterson, K., Purell, C., & Morton, J. (1983). Facilitation of word retrieval in aphasia. *Cognitive Neuropsychology, 3,* 149–177.

Poeck, K., Bleser, R. de, & Graf van Keyserlingh, D. (1984). Neurolinguistic status and localization of lesion in aphasic patients with exclusively consonant-vowel recurring utterances. *Brain, 107,* 199–217.

Prins, R. S. (1987). *Afasie: Classificatie, behandeling en herstelverloop.* Dissertatie, Universiteit van Amsterdam.

Prins, R. S., Snow, C. E., & Wagenaar, E. (1978). Recovery from aphasia: Spontaneous speech versus language comprehension. *Brain and Language, 6,* 192–211.

Raven, J. C. (1958). *Coloured progressive matrices.* London: H. K. Lewis.

Raven, J. C. (1962). *Standard progressive matrices.* London: H. K. Lewis.

Robertson, I. (1990). Does computerized cognitive rehabilitation work? A review. *Apahasiology, 4,* 381–405.

Saffran, E. M., Berndt, R. S., & Schwartz, M. (1989). Quantative analysis of agrammatic production: Procedure and data. *Brain and Language, 37,* 440–479.

Sandt-Koenderman, W. M. E. van de (1986). *Het visuele cue programma.* Stichting Afasie Rotterdam: Stichting Afasie Nederland.

Sandt-Koenderman, W. M. E. van de (1987). Afasiebehandeling met het visuele cue programma. *Logopedie en Foniatrie, 59,* 39–43.

Sandt-Koenderman, W. M. E. van de, & Harskamp, F. van. (1987). The effect of aphasia therapy on linguistic functioning in elderly aphasic patients. In E. Scherzer, R. Simon, & J. Stark (Eds.), *First European conference on aphasiology* (pp. 146–149). Vienna: Conference Proceedings.

Seron, X. (1979). *Aphasie et neuropsychologie.* Brussels: Pierre Mardaga.

Shewan, C. M., & Cameron, H. (1984). Communication and related problems as perceived by aphasic individuals and their spouses. *Journal of Communication Disorders, 17,* 175–187.

Sperber, D., & Wilson, D. (1986). *Relevance: Communication and cognition.* Oxford: Basil Blackwell.

Springer, L. (1989). Fasen in de afasietherapie. In E. G. Visch-Brink, F. van Harskamp, & D. de Boer (Eds.), *Afasietherapie* (pp. 63–76). Amsterdam: Swets & Zeitlinger.

Stachowiak, F. J., & Willeke, A. (1987). Computer als werkzeug der sprachtherapie. *Neurolinguistik, 1,* 57–94.

Taylor-Sarno, M. (1965). A measurement of functional communication in aphasia. *Archives of Physical Medicine and Rehabilitation, 46,* 101–107.

Taylor-Sarno, M. (1969). Observing functional communication of aphasic adults. *Journal of Speech and Hearing Disorders, 47,* 50–56.

Vermeulen, J., Bastiaanse, R., & Wageningen, B. van. (1989). Spontaneous speech in aphasia: A correlational study. *Brain and Language, 36,* 252–274.

Verschaeve, M. A. W. (1992). *Het gespreksboek: een communicatiemiddei voor afasie patiënten.* Therapy program published by Stichting Afasie Nederland.

Verschaeve, M. A. W., & Mourik, M. van. (1992). Communicatietherapie bij een globale afasie. *Logopedie en Foniatrie, 64*(7/8), 222–229.

Visch-Brink, E. G., & Wielaert, S. (in preparation). The influence of melodic intonation therapy on recurring utterances.

Vries, L. A. de (1984). Computergestuurd oefenprogramma voor de behandeling van afasie. *Logopedie en Foniatrie, 56,* 9–10.

Vries, L. A. de (1987). Computergestuurd oefenprogramma's in de afasietherapie. *Tijdschrift voor Gerontologie en Geriatrie, 18,* 77–78.

Vries, L. A. de (1989). Totale communicatie therapie. In E. G. Visch-Brink, F. van Harskamp, & D. de Boer (Eds.), *Afasietherapie* (pp. 156–165). Amsterdam: Swets & Zeitlinger.

Wagenaar, E., Snow, C. E., & Prins, R. S. (1975). Spontaneous speech of aphasic patients: A psycholinguistic analysis. *Brain and Language, 2,* 218–303.

Wertz, R. T., Collins, M. J., Weiss, D., Kurtzke, J. F., Friden, T., Brookshire, R. H., Pierce, J., Holtzapple, P., Hubbard, D. J., Porch, B. E., West, J. A., Davis, L., Matovitch, V., Morley, G. K., & Resurreccion, E. (1981). Veterans Administration cooperative study on aphasia: A comparison of individual and group treatment. *Journal of Speech and Hearing Research, 24,* 580–594.

Wertz, R. T., Weiss, D. G., Aten, J. L., Brookshire, R. H., Garcia-Buñuel, L., Holland, A. L., Kurtzke, J. F., LaPointe, L. L., Milianti, F. J., Brannegan, R., Greenbaum, H., Marshall, R. C., Vogel, D., Carter, J., Barnes, N. S., & Goodman, R. (1986). Comparison of clinic, home, and deferred language treatment for aphasia. *Archives of Neurology, 43,* 653–658.

Wielaert, S., & Visch-Brink, E. G. (1990). *Communicatie Profiel: Een Nederlandse uitgave van het functional communnication profile.* Rotterdam: Stichting Afasie Rotterdam, Erasmus University.

Willmes, K., Graetz, P., Bleser, R. de, Schulte, B., & Keyser, A. (1991). De akense afasie test. *Logopedie en Foniatrie, 63,* 375–386.

Wilson, B., Cockburn, J., & Baddeley, A. (1985). *The Rivermead Behavioral Memory Test (RBMT).* Reading: Thames Valley Test Company.

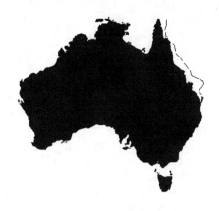

CHAPTER 11

Aphasia Rehabilitation: A Sociolinguistic Perspective

ELIZABETH M. ARMSTRONG

School of English and Linguistics
Macquarie University
Sydney, Australia

The clinical approach taken to the rehabilitation of aphasic speakers depends very heavily on the perspective from which the clinician views communication and, in particular, language. Although many such perspectives exist in the field of clinical aphasiology, which indeed are not necessarily mutually exclusive, they appear to fall basically into two main categories. The first includes those who view the language system as a set of rule-governed principles, driven by internal processes, existing within an individual (the intrapsychological perspective). The second includes those who view language as a social process in itself, the means by which meanings are created and negotiated between individuals (the interpsychological perspective). Having worked with aphasic adults for over 15 years in the acute stage and in the longer term, I have utilized aspects of both of these approaches at one time or another, often taking what I think is a typical eclectic approach to treatment. However, in recent times, my approach has reflected the latter perspective, the interpsychological one, in which language as a social process is central to my treatment strategies. In this chapter I attempt to outline why I am pursuing this approach, and how I am implementing it clinically. Finally, I offer some ideas that may stimulate further discussion of such approaches.

When I started working in the area of aphasia rehabilitation in the 1970s, resources for investigating intrapsychological language processes were relatively highly developed and indeed constituted the main focus of assessment and treatment. Aphasia tests such as the Minnesota Test for the Differential Diagnosis of Aphasia (MTDDA) (Schuell, 1965), the Boston Diagnostic Aphasia Examination (BDAE) (Goodglass & Kaplan, 1972), the Porch Index of Communicative Ability (PICA) (Porch, 1967, 1981), and later the Western Aphasia Battery (WAB) (Kertesz, 1982) all examined a range of psycholinguistic abilities. They were utilized clinically for diagnosis, planning of treatment, and monitoring of progress.

Although treatment strategies varied, the nature of language treatment usually followed a basic principle of grammatical constituency, working from the lowest level to the highest. In aphasia treatment, this usually meant working from the word level to the phrase to the sentence and more recently to the discourse level. Inherent in aphasia treatment was the principle that the lowest level of constituency was necessarily the easiest and therefore should be the starting point of therapy. As the sentence was usually seen as the upper limit of manipulable language units, conversation or discourse was considered a "carryover" level. That is, one would work on a particular syntactic structure or skill, such as naming ability, and then examine samples of spontaneous speech to see if they were used in this context.

Research into intrapsychological processes has continued to provide significant insights into the aphasic deficit and directions for intervention, particularly with the advent of cognitive neuropsychology (Behrmann & Lieberthalm, 1989; Byng, 1988; Byng & Coltheart, 1986; Caramazza, 1984, 1986; Coltheart, 1980, 1985; Coltheart, Sartori, & Job, 1987; Ellis & Young, 1988; Jones, 1986; Schwartz, Linebarger, Saffran, & Pate, 1987) and recent applications of Chomsky's (1981) Government and Binding Theory (Grodzinsky, 1986; Shapiro & Levine, 1989; Shapiro & Thompson, 1992; Thompson & Shapiro, 1992). However, equally illuminating insights into aphasia have been provided in more recent years by researchers concerned with the social/functional aspects of the disorder. These insights formed the basis of my initial excursions into interpsychological functioning and have become my primary focus of interest.

During the late 1970s and 1980s, Holland (1975, 1980, 1982) Davis and Wilcox (1985), and others began looking at aphasia from a social/functional perspective, shedding light on the ways in which aphasic individuals communicated in everyday contexts. Of course, the seed had been sown in 1969, with the publication of Sarno's Functional Communication Profile, but I think it would be fair to say that the functional perspective as a significant movement in aphasiology was not adopted with any great enthusiasm until the late 1970s. Whereas the standardized aphasia tests (BDAE, PICA, WAB) concentrated on psycholinguistic skills involving component parts of the language system, these "functional" analyses probed more general communicative skills of speakers during conversation. They examined the performance of speakers in everyday situations (Communicative Abilities in Daily Living-CADL) (Holland, 1980), their ability to convey new information (Promoting Aphasics' Communicative Effectiveness, the PACE technique) (Davis & Wilcox, 1985), and their ability to perform such conversational skills as turn-taking, maintaining eye contact, maintaining topic, and asking relevant questions (Damico, 1985; Prutting & Kirchner, 1983). The era of pragmatics was thus ushered into Speech Pathology, offering speech pathologists new ideas on how aphasic speakers communicated and challenging clinicians with decisions as to what components of communication required remediation.

One of the main challenges inherent in this way of looking at aphasia was that it required clinicians to focus not only on what aphasic clients could not do, but what they could do. As Holland (1991) noted, a pragmatic-centered approach to aphasia treatment is a "strength-centered" approach, rather than a "deficit-centered" one, which had previously been the prevailing perspective.

However, whereas pragmatic analyses tended to describe the status of general speech functions such as questions, denials, assertions, and so on, they said little about how these functions were realized linguistically by a speaker. The different ways in which a speaker could produce such speech acts was scarcely discussed in any aphasiology literature. Most of the clinical discussion to date has focused on the speech act as a single entity without specific reference to the potential for variation in its realization for different purposes. For example, a denial can be achieved through a number of syntactic structures, numerous choices of lexical items involving varying levels of conviction, and with a number of different intonation patterns, all with specific semantic intent. Similarly, functional analyses which looked at performance during everyday activities, such as those sampled in the CADL, did not provide information on how the speakers achieved adequate responses.

Concurrent with the interest in pragmatic skills during discourse was the introduction of a number of spontaneous speech analyses which were concerned with the incidence of certain types of linguistic behaviors during connected speech (Berko-Gleason, Goodglass, Obler, Green, Hyde, & Weintraub, 1980; Shewan, 1988; Wagenaar, Snow, & Prins, 1975;

Yorkston & Beukelman, 1980). These analyses encouraged clinicians to look at the frequency of verbal behaviors such as verbal paraphasias, neologisms, and word-order mistakes as well as the so-called "efficiency" of communication, that is, the amount of content conveyed within a certain time frame (Yorkston & Beukelman, 1980). Such analyses have been used mainly for monitoring change over time and for examining certain aspects of carryover from psycholinguistically based treatments.

Clinically, such analyses enabled me to look at the connected discourse of my clients in a systematic fashion, but these measures only vaguely directed me into therapy involving spontaneous speech. This, of course, was not surprising, because they were not based on theories of discourse, but were merely aimed at the monitoring of single word and sentence skills at the discourse level.

In the early 1980s I became aware of discourse analysis as it had developed in the field(s) of linguistics/sociolinguistics. As a clinician, I was becoming increasingly convinced that analysis of language performance during conversation and in other meaningful contexts could shed significant new light on the aphasic deficit. The pragmatic and other "functional" analyses were already beginning to yield such new insights (Aten, Caligiuri, & Holland, 1982; Gurland, Chwat, & Wollner, 1982; Holland, 1980, 1982; Lubinski, Duchan, & Weitzner-Lin, 1980; Wilcox & Davis, 1977). I became convinced that a more comprehensive knowledge of linguistic theory, and discourse grammar in particular, could provide further insights into the ways in which aphasic speakers communicated. Although functional analyses offered significant new perspectives, it also seemed important to call upon linguistic theory in an effort to document the linguistic realizations of the speech functions under focus. Linguistic accuracy was not the issue, as Holland (1975) discussed, but the aphasic speaker's utilization of linguistic resources needed to be addressed. With text linguistics and discourse analysis developing at an amazingly rapid rate, it appeared that a linguistic theory, based on the notion of discourse and language use, would have much to offer the description of the aphasic deficit. Indeed, the work of Ulatowska and her colleagues (Ulatowska, North, & Macaluso-Haynes, 1980, 1981; Ulatowska, Weiss-Doyell, Freedman-Stern, & Macaluso-Haynes, 1983) was beginning to demonstrate the usefulness of applying notions of text grammar to aphasia, by drawing on the work of linguists such as Van Dijk (1977), Kintsch and Van Dijk (1978), and Longacre (1976) in the analysis of the narrative and procedural discourse of aphasic speakers.

I was fortunate enough to have the opportunity to study with professor Ruqaiya Hasan, an accomplished sociolinguist, who had written extensively in the field of text/linguistics, that is, discourse analysis. This experience changed my perspective on language and the role of language in social organization, providing me with the framework for subsequent research in aphasic discourse, on which I have based my clinical diagnostic and treatment procedures. This framework was based on the work of Michael Halliday (1985a) and his version of a systemic-functional grammar.

SYSTEMIC-FUNCTIONAL GRAMMAR

Systemic-functional grammar provides a way of looking at language as a set of meaning resources rather than a set of rules. For the last 50 years, linguistics has emphasized structural or formal grammar, such as Chomsky's transformational grammar, which focuses predominantly on syntactic rules, separating form from meaning. A functional grammar, on the other hand, focuses on meaning and the ways in which the lexis (wording) and syntax realize meanings. It is of interest to note Halliday's (1985a) explanation of the three main ways in which a functional grammar operates, differentiating it from a formal one. First, a functional grammar is "designed to account for how the language is used" (p. 13), and is explained in terms of the context in which it is functioning. Halliday stresses the fact that language is not an arbitrary system — it is organized relative to its ability to express human needs — hence, it is functional in nature.

Second, the fundamental components of the grammar are related to meaning. Halliday distinguishes two main types of meaning: interpersonal and ideational. Hence, language has two purposes: (a) to help individuals to understand the environment (ideational) and (b) to permit them to act on others (interpersonal). The content of discourse assists in the realization of the former two components. Finally, each part of the grammar is seen in the context of the whole. As Halliday explains, "each element in a language is explained by reference to its function in the total linguistic system" (p. 13). All levels (e.g., phrases, clauses) are described in terms of their ability to perform a particular function; thus, one can see that the focus of a functional grammar is to relate form to function.

The "systemic" part of systemic-functional grammar involves the notion of choice within the linguistic system and provides a way of focusing on paradigmatic relations rather than the syntagmatic ones that have been the focus of syntactically oriented formal grammars. The paradigmatic axis of language is the axis from which selections are made by the speaker from within certain linguistic categories such as speech function (e.g., request, denial) or lexical class (e.g., noun). The syntagmatic axis of language is the axis on which the language linearly unfolds in time and syntactic ordering of the above choices is achieved, with one lexical class combining with another to create meaning, as for example the noun + verb formation.

One example of using a system of choices is selecting a semantic function for regulating a situation (see Figure 11–1, based on an example given by Halliday, 1973). The speech function choices available to a speaker in this situation are hypothesized as (a) threat, (b) warning, and (c) rule. These are realized grammatically in certain ways according to the mood system of the language. If the option taken is a "threat" or "warning," the grammatical feature "declarative" is selected. On the other hand, if "rule" is chosen, the grammatical realization will involve an imperative clause.

This is a simple example of use of *system networks*, as these choice systems are called. These networks are exhaustive, encompassing all aspects of the linguistic system. They range from simple mood system choices such as declarative/interrogative and their grammatical realizations, to systems for pronoun choices, lexical choices serving numerous semantic functions, and choices involving logical relations between clauses. Although there is insufficient space to pursue the notion of systemics in this chapter (the reader is referred to Fawcett & Young, 1988; Martin & Halliday, 1981; and Matthiesson & Halliday, in press, for exten-

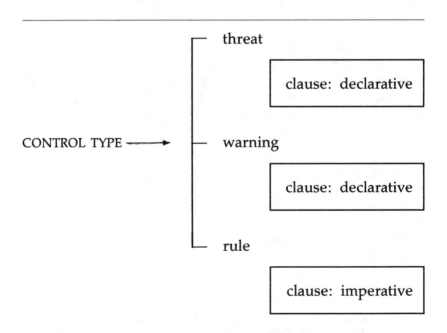

Figure 11–1. Small section of a regulatory semantic network, based on Halliday (1973).

sive descriptions), it will suffice to say that systemic-functional grammar is concerned with the different types of meanings that speakers wish to convey and how they create these meanings through a grammatical system.

Such a grammar appeared to offer great potential to the analysis of aphasic language as it enabled one to examine what meanings are and are not available to the aphasic speaker and what grammatical resources are and are not being utilized. Rather than emphasizing linguistic accuracy, the focus can be the meanings conveyed and how the speaker achieves them successfully, as well as how the remaining linguistic resources could be best put to use.

Because it emphasizes the social nature of language, this type of grammar most comfortably sits under a sociolinguistic umbrella. Although such categories occasionally can foster unnecessarily dichotomous thinking, the term will be used here to highlight new insights that the approach has to offer, which differ theoretically from previous perspectives on aphasia.

DISCOURSE: LANGUAGE IN USE

One of the basic differences between sociolinguistic and psycholinguistic approaches, that is, between inter- and intrapsychological ones, is that the former regard the text (or discourse) as the basic unit of language whereas the latter regard the word as the basic unit. From a psycholinguistic point of view, one needs words and indeed sentences before one can construct a discourse. Hence, the distinction relates to length and complexity rather than to meaning. Sociolinguists such as Halliday and Hasan (1976), however, view text as a semantic unit, not a grammatical one. Its length is irrelevant — a text may be a sign consisting of a single word such as "STOP," a single sentence, or a complete novel. It is "any message, spoken or written of whatever length, that does form a unified whole" (Halliday & Hasan, 1976). Unity is a basic characteristic as is functionality. Therefore, text is not defined in terms of its size; it does not form the next level above the sentence in a constituency model. It is a semantic unit in the sense that it is a unit of meaning that functions as a unity within itself and with its environment. de Beaugrande (1980) reinforces Halliday and Hasan's concept of a text by contrasting it with the syntactic basis of a sentence:

> A text cannot be fully treated as a configuration of morphemes or symbols. It is the manifestation of a human ACTION in which a person intends to create a text and INSTRUCTS the text receiver to build relationships of various kinds . . . Texts also serve to MONITOR, MANAGE, and CHANGE a situation. (p. 13)

Text, then, is language in use.

Hence, a basic principle of treatment performed in a sociolinguistic framework is that any remediation of language must involve a meaningful context of situation in which language plays a central and constitutive role. Using this philosophy, one cannot simply be satisfied with using what would be considered "meaningful" materials in treatment. The whole context in which language plays a role must be considered. The notion of "context of situation" has been elaborated on by numerous theorists (Firth, 1959; Halliday, 1973, 1974, 1977, 1985b; Hymes, 1967), and if we are to use constructs such as "context" in treatment, we might as well utilize the rich theoretical notions behind them. These notions provide a framework for treatment as well as assessment of functional language.

WHAT IS CONTEXT?

Halliday has proposed a model in which there is direct interaction between the context of situation and the language itself. The way the context of situation motivates the choice of expressed meanings forms the basis of Halliday's model. Halliday postulates three aspects of the context of situation: field, tenor, and mode. *Field* refers to what is actually taking place, that is, what the participants are actually doing, for example, a buying/selling encounter in a store. The *tenor* of discourse refers to who is taking part and what agency they carry (e.g., customer, salesperson) as well as the status they possess in relation to each other (e.g., authority, familiarity, social distance) (Hasan, 1973). The *mode* refers to the part language plays in the interaction, both in terms of genre and of the channel through which the language is being transmitted (e.g., writing, spoken language).

Given a certain configuration of situational features, one will find a corresponding set of linguistic features; these constitute a register. These linguistic features correspond to Halliday's three metafunctions of language: ideational, interpersonal, and textual metafunctions. The *ideational* metafunction is concerned with meanings representing events, actions, states, or other aspects of the real world. The ideational includes the grammatical system of transitivity, which delineates numerous verbal processes described below. Other elements, including agent, recipient, phenomenon, and circumstance, also exist within the clause. Finally, the ideational metafunction encompasses vocabulary and the logico-semantic relations existing between clauses. The *interpersonal* metafunction covers the role relationship related to the situation (e.g., questioner-respondent). At the clause level, the output of this metafunction is the grammar of mood and modality. The *textual* metafunction includes the expression of theme/rhyme and cohesive relations which enable the text to function as a coherent whole. For further description of these three metafunctions, the reader is referred to Halliday (1985a).

The clinically useful idea is that, in the case of verbal interaction, the situation and the language used within it are interdependent. Given a certain field, for example, one can anticipate what sorts of meanings will be conveyed. In terms of the ideational metafunction, one can then plan for the range of vocabulary being used and the possible transitivity patterns. Consider the following example.

In a buying and selling encounter, one might create the following situation: A person is entering a large department store to buy some new furniture. The sort of vocabulary that could be used in this situation might include the following: outdoor, indoor, cedar, mahogany, desk, table, chair, design, material, expensive, inexpensive, practical, and decorative. Verbal processes might include both material ones (e.g., sit, work, paint, assemble) relating to what the buyer might like to do with the furniture itself, and mental ones (e.g., think, like, prefer) relating to the buyer expressing interest in the furniture available.

From the tenor perspective, a certain amount of politeness may be expected from the salesperson, with some authority being vested in the buyer as the prospective client. In such a situation, the interpersonal metafunction would realize this in the seller's use of words of politeness such as *"sir"* and *"madam"* or in the use of modalization in the grammar, such as *"would you like . . . ?" "can I help . . . ?" "if you think you prefer that one, I could . . ."*. If the buyer were very forthright, assertive, or even aggressive, his or her language might entail the use of many imperatives and declaratives, leaving little room for negotiation. If, on the other hand, the buyer really wanted to enter into a negotiating situation or genuinely wanted information and advice from the salesperson, the buyer might utilize more tag questions and modality, such as *"I'd be better off with this one, wouldn't I?" ". . don't you think?"*

The mode of this situation is oral, not written, discourse. Hence, language consistent with oral language (Halliday, 1985c) and language operating as part of a dialogue will be used. This would include certain patterns of adjacency pairs (Sacks, Schegloff, & Jefferson, 1974). Because both participants are in the same physical situation and can see what is being discussed (as opposed to a situation in which a buyer is purchasing by telephone), references can be made to items in an inexplicit manner, such as "this," "that," or "it".

This example provides some idea of the way in which the lexico-grammar realizes the situational meanings. Considerations such as these should be taken into account in planning treatment. One can manipulate the context of situation to direct the sorts of meanings which are to be "practiced" or encouraged. For example, if the aphasic speaker needs to be able to make requests more often due to physical incapacitation and consequent dependence on others to fulfill everyday physical needs, the general context of situation can be set and then varied according to the sorts of goods and services required, the people from whom they are required (e.g., familiar vs. unfamiliar), and the way in which they can be requested (e.g., over the phone, face to face, one room to another). The word and syntactic choices can be varied appropriately according to each of these factors. The situations can be role-played or acted out in the actual home or environment in which the aphasic speaker must function, with words, sentences, and turn-taking cues supplied as needed to facilitate the completion of the interaction. Thus the clinician has a logical and theoretically motivated way to conduct functional activities, and the aphasic client receives concrete help in regaining functional status.

THE IMPORTANCE OF FUNCTION: FUNCTION AS FOCUS

The importance of the function of a particular word or clause is central to an interpsychological perspective in which function and form are not divorced from each other. Function is the driving force and the focus of attention. Thus, treatment tasks are necessarily communicatively motivated and have to have a functional point. To this end, therapy should provide aphasic speakers with a variety of conversational partners, social contexts, and topics. Conversation/dialogue, as well as monologic discourse, must be part of treatment.

Whether the aphasic patient is globally involved or only mildly impaired is irrelevant to the principle that language remediation must occur in a meaningful context. In the case of global or severely impaired Broca's type patients, it may be realistic to expect only single word utterances. However, these single words must have a significant function — not merely meaning in a referential sense, such as the name of an object, but in an interpersonal sense as well. The clinician can ask, "What is the function of that word in an interaction situation? What is it conveying to a listener?" For example, rather than focusing predominantly on nouns only as names of objects, one can focus on a variety of lexical items, including the verb, recently promoted by practitioners of treatment conducted in the cognitive psychological framework (Jones, 1986; Shapiro & Levine, 1989). In focusing on function rather than form, a grammar such as Halliday's systemic-functional grammar provides a variety of contextual foci for lexical items.

The noun provides a good example of the ways in which lexical items perform a variety of functions in discourse. This fact can be overlooked if one views the isolated word as representing solely a particular concept in the lexicon. The name of an object in its referential sense is only one small part of the way nouns are used. Identifying an object by name when the object is in front of the speaker serves very few interpersonal functions. We are rarely required to name objects in our everyday lives.

However, nouns are used for a variety of functions, such as to call for someone's attention, to request particular goods at a store, to inform a listener of a particular person who was involved in events under discussion, or to direct a person to give something to someone. Within a clause, a noun can be an actor, a recipient, or an object. It can be the theme of the clause (used in Halliday's sense to mean the starting point of the clause) which can emphasize a particular perspective on a story. A noun can be maintained through the text to create continuity in topic, and it can participate in lexical cohesion relations to unite complete discourse. Thus, when looking at the variety of functions a noun can perform, one opens a gamut of possibilities for treatment, rather than limiting treatment of lexical retrieval to the very restricted area of naming.

In therapy, it is possible to emphasize the noun's role as an element at the clause level by employing strategies similar to those outlined by Jones (1986), that is, by having the client respond to questions regarding the noun's role in the clause. For example, given the clause *the boy was playing with the ball*, the clinician asks the client "Who was playing with the ball?" or "What was the boy playing with?" Probably the main difference between this type of activity as performed by Jones, and the way I might use it is that I always use clauses that make up part of a story or discourse. Unrelated sentences are never presented successively to the client as stimuli. Usually, the clauses are taken from the context of a video just watched, a topic that has just been informally discussed, or an activity that has just been performed. In this way, the language has a functional meaning and it is hypothesized that the client is more likely to attach meaningful associations to the tasks and hence achieve better retrieval and carryover.

The role of the noun as a theme in certain clauses also can be explored. Halliday defines "theme" as the starting point of a message. For example, in the clause *the girl walked along the road, the girl* constitutes the theme and is the initial point of departure of the message. However, rather than always being an actor, as in many therapy tasks, the theme may also be the goal of the action, as in the passive *the ball was given to the boy*. Rather than teaching the passive construction, however, the clinician may encourage the client to produce utterances (possibly incomplete) in which he or she thematizes aspects of clauses which may not be actors. In the above situation in which a ball was given to a boy, the speaker may perceive the act of giving as the important aspect of the situation. The speaker may try to convey this by commencing the utterance with the word "give." Rather than correcting, and then encouraging the traditional noun-verb-noun construction, the clinician should encourage such thematization, if it appears to be a meaning resource for the client. Thematization also can be generalized to a number of different situations. The client is freed from having to produce strictly accurate noun-verb-object constructions and is allowed to focus on conveying the meanings which are personally important. For example, if a client trying to relate an event, he or she is encouraged to describe many different aspects of it, rather than simply the main actions. If a story involves going to the store, the clinician may ask not only what the client did at the store or what was bought, but who else was there, what the store was like, and so on.

Similarly, the clinician may emphasize elaboration of the nominal group/noun phrase so that the client feels free to focus on any aspect of the situation being considered, rather than simply producing a correct grammatical structure focusing on actions. A client describing a picture or sequence of pictures could be encouraged to thematize any part of the story, rather than only the central action. For example, in a sequence of pictures depicting a man losing his hat on a windy day and trying unsuccessfully to retrieve it from a tree, a client could give any number of responses, focusing on the man, the hat, the wind, or the tree, in any sequence. Any of these responses as the initiating utterance would be encouraged and facilitated when necessary. Such an approach provides much leeway for the patient. It allows for divergent rather than convergent use of language (Chapey, 1981) and gives the client many choices of meaning, rather than designating one particular grammatical structure, such as an agent-action-object utterance, as the predetermined "correct" response.

One can also view verbs in a number of ways, depending on function. A verb (or process, according to Halliday) can be of several types: material (walk, catch, break), relational (is, represent, seem), mental (like, please, realize, know), verbal (sit, tell, ask), or behavioral (laugh, watch, listen). The verb process can be modulated according to interpersonal meaning. For example, the modals (can, will, and should) are used to signal degrees of certainty and possibility of duress. Tense variations denote the event in time. Voice variations, such as passive versus active, create particular meanings by the thematization of certain aspects of the clause. The verb can be thematic in a clause such as "Walk along the road," usually present in the imperative, or it can participate in an interrogative such as "Can you walk along the road?" Its form changes according to its function. The meaning of the utterance is central to the form the verb will take. Hence, to teach only the unmarked or the present progressive verb form, as is often done in treatment, limits the function of the verb and thus limits the chances for aphasic speakers to trigger connections with premorbid functional language.

Verbs, like nouns, participate in the lexical collocation or cohesion patterns forming a text. Hence, one should attempt to incorporate the verbs taught into a meaningful context, in which lexically and situationally related associations are also available to the speaker, to facilitate word retrieval.

REMEMBERING THE IMPORTANCE OF FORM

In treatment from a sociolinguistic perspective the function of the utterance, rather than the form, motivates the treatment goals. One might work on a particular speech function such as making requests rather than a psycholinguistically based goal such as naming. However, one cannot work on making requests without considering how they are realized in their lexicogrammatical forms — the syntactic patterns and word choices. This appears to be a weakness of many current pragmatic approaches to treatment, in which the grammatical form is relegated to secondary status. Such an approach is understandable, because aphasic speakers often perform functions of language, such as requesting, without using the correct form of the interrogative. Indeed, emphasis on correct grammatical form should not take precedence over the ability to get meaning across. However, we must not overlook form altogether, because form constitutes an important and central meaning resource.

Only by seeing *how* aphasic speakers actually convey meaning through language will the clinician be able to determine how to encourage them or to build on particular abilities. How does a clinician provide therapy at a speech act level without referring at some point to the way in which speakers might achieve such an act verbally? One might simply try to reinforce requests using a behavior modification approach, but such a perspective is quite limited. The treatment might be much more effective if it also provided speakers with the verbal means for making requests in a variety of situations to a variety of people.

Clients can be re-taught several different forms of questions, each of which is used in particular sorts of situations and for different purposes. Attention also can be given to intonation and stress patterns to alter meaning. For example, questions can be either Wh-questions ("Who took the last cake?"), yes/no questions ("Did you take the last cake?"), or tagged questions ("You took the last cake, didn't you?"). Altering stress or intonation on any of these questions, further alters the meaning. Practicing such utterances in different functional situations can provide rich linguistic experiences as well as fun, as speakers begin to manipulate their language.

The level of linguistic accuracy is not the focus of the exercise. Rather, the central point is the function of the forms. This central point can be achieved at different levels of linguistic accuracy depending on the severity of the client's aphasia. An approach taken by Doyle, Goldstein, Bourgeois, and Nakles (1989) to train requesting behavior in aphasic speakers of the Broca's type is an interesting example of how such treatment could be undertaken. Doyle et al. used a behavior modification technique to encourage the use of requesting behaviors during conversation over a variety of topics and conversational partners. I believe the variety of functional categories associated with requesting behavior as provided in a functional grammar could further enrich the technique. Based on a systematic framework for the speech function of requests, modeling could be more focused.

Underlying Halliday's systemic-functional theory is the notion that meaning is realized throughout the linguistic system. Semantics is realized throughout the lexicogrammar which in turn is realized through the phonological system. Because each aspect of language contributes to the other, the realization arrow is bi-directional. This means that lexicogrammatical form can contribute to meaning and that phonology can modulate the meaning produced in the lexicogrammar. Halliday's model sees the three levels of language as absolutely interrelated. Hence, one cannot discuss meaning without discussing lexicogrammar and one cannot discuss lexicogrammar without including phonology. One needs to draw on all speaker resources to present such options to a client.

SPECIFIC TECHNIQUES

In discussing her Conversational Coaching technique, Holland (1991) offers direct intervention at a conversational level using such resources. She incorporates the use of simple scripts and involves both aphasic speakers and their families in everyday situations and verbal interactions. In a similar approach, I focus a session on a series of texts, providing specific lexicogrammatical patterns, including individual lexical items, intra-clausal syntactic patterns, and inter-clausal structuring (via text elements — ways to join clauses using different types of semantic relationships as well as by using conjunctions). The amount of cuing (or coaching, as Holland would describe it) a client requires depends on the severity of the aphasia. The more severe client may simply be required to repeat different utterances at appropriate times, may be asked to read complete texts, or be provided with key words and be required to fill in the rest, or may be provided with facilitatory pictures, with cues being faded as appropriate. The texts are always meaningful to the client and usually involve family. Obviously, one needs to focus on one particular aspect of text construction at a time, but the speaker as a creator of meaning remains the central issue.

An example of the way in which particular lexicogrammatical items can be patterned for discourse purposes is given below, focusing on cohesion, an aspect of text construction that has been repeatedly demonstrated to be problematic for aphasic speakers (Armstrong, 1987; Bottenberg, Lemme, & Hedberg, 1985; Lemme, Hedberg, & Bottenberg, 1984; Ulatowska et al., 1980, 1981, 1983). A more detailed discussion of cohesion is available in Halliday and Hasan (1976), whereas Armstrong (1991) discusses potential treatment techniques.

COHESION TREATMENT

Because narrative frequently provides the most structure for facilitated production of discourse, the narrative genre is probably most often chosen. The client is asked to choose a story of particular personal significance, whether it be happy, sad, or frightening. If the client is unable to generate a story, pictures may be presented so that the client can choose a sequence to make up a story (recommended by Ulatowska & Bond-Chapman, 1989). Once the topic/story is chosen, the essential text structure is outlined: Introduction of participants and setting, complicating action(s), and resolution. Discussion of structure depends on the level of the client. Vocabulary which is likely to occur in such a text is then selected. A variety of categories of lexical items including nouns, verbs, and adjectives are elicited, with synonyms, antonyms, and other lexically related items. Cuing is used as required by the client's ability. The words can then be represented visually, with participant names linked together to form one chain, action words related to each other forming another chain, and other chains composed of adjectives which may be linked semantically. An example is given in Figure 11–2, with lexical items related to a car accident described by an aphasic speaker.

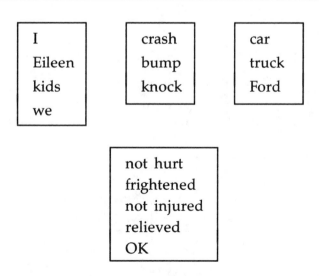

Figure 11–2. Chains formed as basis of text construction for aphasic speaker during treatment.

These chains can be referred to as cues throughout the story attempt, with the clinician guiding the aphasic speaker in the order for introducing each item, stressing each word's relation to the others, and encouraging continuity of meaning. If the client is capable of more than single word utterances, the interrelationships among the noun, verb and adjective chains can be made more explicit (see Figure 11–3).

These text plans can be utilized in a number of different ways, depending on the client's type of aphasia. Given the framework, a fluent aphasic speaker could use the key words and fill in the rest to construct largely grammatical sentences whereas a nonfluent speaker may benefit simply from reading or imitating the key words, with no emphasis on achieving morphological accuracy. The visual plans can be faded gradually, with the aphasic speaker taking increasing responsibility for reproducing the chains/text without the visual cues. Then the client can begin to create more original chains or complete chain interactions. Work such as this can be achieved through activities such as traditional sentence completion tasks, in which one interacting chain is taken out of the picture and the speaker has to supply the missing word to complete the meaning (e.g., "I crash . . ."). The crucial difference between sentence completion work in the traditional aphasia handbook sense and this kind of task, however, is that the speaker is working within a text framework

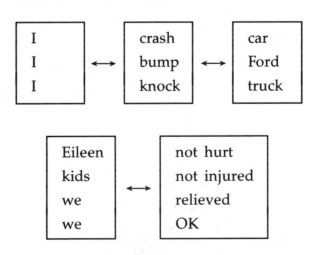

Figure 11–3. Chain interaction visually displayed for aphasic speaker during recount of a car accident.

and knows that each sentence must follow from the previous one and that each fulfills a certain meaning function, rather than being divorced from reality.

Text plans can range from the extremely simple ones just described to complex ones involving a variety of participants, actions, and events.

STRENGTHS RATHER THAN DEFICITS

Another important aspect of a sociolinguistic framework is the focus it places on the retained skills rather than deficits. Working in the systemic-functional framework, the clinician can map out the aphasic speaker's system for conveying meanings. Initially, the focus is the function of the speaker's communication rather than its form. What the speaker is capable of communicating and what language patterns are used for these purposes are examined in detail. For example, when looking at the aphasic speaker's ability to ask questions, it is often noted that an utterance can perform the function of asking a question without being in typical question form. As Doyle et al. (1989) noted, aphasic speakers "characteristically present with propositional aspects of language disproportionately impaired relative to language pragmatics" (p. 169). A systemic-functional description of such a speaker's language would include a description of the resources available to that speaker when asking questions. These might include a variety of intonation patterns overlaid on simple two-word utterances consistently taking the form of either *Subject + Predicator* (e.g., "you walk?" meaning "are you going to walk to the store?") or *Subject + Adjunct* (e.g., "you home?" meaning "are you going home?"). One could compare these structures with a non-brain-damaged speaker's productions and then try to teach the omitted structures to the aphasic speaker. However, the systemic-functional approach suggests another avenue as well. The clinician can examine in detail the resources the speaker is using (utilizing the functional concepts associated with phonological, syntactic, and semantic aspects of discourse in the systemic-functional model) and then capitalize on them. For example, the aphasic speaker may be able to use simple question forms but rarely does so and only with a very limited variety of lexical items. One might stay with the question form used intitially, but incorporate it into a wider variety of situations, with a more varied use of lexical items and intonation patterns, modulating the meaning in more subtle ways.

Recent preliminary work by Armstrong (1992) and Ferguson (1992a) in the systemic-functional framework has suggested that, in many cases, mildly to moderately impaired aphasic adults have a normal range of meaning resources available to them, but simply use these resources with different frequency from normal speakers. Ferguson demonstrated a wide range of speech functions available to aphasic speakers in conversation, although they were used only in limited circumstances. Armstrong documented the use of the complete range of logico-semantic relations between clauses (Halliday, 1985a) in the extended texts of a moderately aphasic speaker, but found a different frequency of use by aphasic relative to normal speakers.

When focusing on strengths rather than deficits, one must ask why speakers are using retained resources in certain ways. What might they be achieving through using certain patterns of language? Rather than seeing their new pattern of discourse only in terms of what is missing or abnormal, this approach looks at how they are using their resources to communicate, given their restrictions. While one might still work on increasing a skill that is used rarely if at all (such as qualifying a description of an event with enhancing circumstances — time, place, manner, causal connections), one could also work on increasing use of the skills the speaker is already using. For example, the use of elaboration may be reinforced by having the speaker rephrase, clarify through restatement, or emphasize a point through repetition. Such elaboration appears circumlocutory from a deficit perspective, but indeed may fulfill a useful function for the speaker with limited resources (as suggested by Penn, 1988).

OTHER MODALITIES

So far, I have concentrated on verbal expression. However, the sociolinguistic framework has equal ramifications for treatment in the areas of auditory and visual comprehension and writing. Although these will not be explored in detail here, it should be said that language in context forms the basis for my treatment of aphasic individuals in these modalities as well. Rather than working purely from a bottom-up processing approach to comprehension, in which the smallest constituent parts of the language (the phoneme or the word) are the usual initial focus of comprehension tasks, I work in a top-down manner, using everyday texts and encouraging the aphasic client to use world knowledge, script knowledge, and text schemata to facilitate comprehension. The work of Kintsch (1974), Kintsch and Van Dijk (1978), Rumelhart (1980), and the research findings of clinical aphasiologists such as Brookshire and Nicholas (1984) can be drawn upon in this area. Brookshire (1987) provides a clear overview of relevant work.

In terms of writing, meaningful language use is also an integral part of treatment. As with verbal expression, the client may have one of several types of writing difficulty. Severe spelling impairment may be one client's major difficulty and specific treatment procedures can be planned following evaluation with the Psycholinguistic Assessments of Language Processing in Aphasia test (PALPA) (Kay, Lesser, & Coltheart, 1991). Other clients may have difficulties with lexicogrammar or with planning overall text structure in written discourse. The latter examples lend themselves more easily to discourse-level treatment, but even spelling work can be undertaken in a meaningful discourse context. For example, a client may write a narrative in the form of a letter to a friend, an entry in an ongoing diary (a clinical task successfully used by Ulatowska & Bond-Chapman, 1989), or a procedural discourse in the form of a recipe for a friend. The level of cuing needed to create such texts requires the speech pathologist to adapt the procedure to clients of varying severity and type of aphasia. Although the emphasis of intervention differs according to type of aphasia or type and severity of processing disorder, the background against which intervention occurs is again that of language in context.

THE APHASIC SPEAKER'S ROLE IN TREATMENT

Another important aspect of the sociolinguistic framework is the notion that all communicators are active participants in constructing meanings — whether one is asking or replying, demanding or complying, narrating or comprehending. Aphasic communicators are at a distinct disadvantage since they no longer have the same access to all their previous linguistic resources. Because they are restricted in this way, they are perceived as being passive recipients of other people's communication rather than as active participants in interactions. Several studies have demonstrated that stereotyped and limited patterns of speech acts predominate between aphasic and normal speakers in a variety of situations (Armstrong, 1989; Gurland et al., 1982; Ripich, Hambrecht, & Panagos, 1985; Wilcox & Davis, 1977). In a representative study, Kimbarow (1982) reported a predominant question/answer paradigm in clinical settings, with the clinician asking the questions and the client answering.

As speech pathologists, it is important to ask ourselves whether we actually perpetuate and in some instances encourage the perception of aphasic speakers as passive recipients in conversation through our treatment paradigms. Certainly behavior modification paradigms view the client as someone to be acted upon rather than as an active participant in the treatment program. The client's responses are reinforced or punished as the paradigm sees appropriate, with external goals established which clients must aim to reach. Language is seen as a behavior that clients perform either correctly or incorrectly. Clients are given little opportunity to manipulate the paradigm. Although not usually contained within strict behavior modification regimes, much aphasia treatment is carried out with the client acting as the recipient of stimulation, and treatment tending to be "clinician-directed" rather than "client-directed." Many tasks are pre-arranged by the clinician; with target utterances already predetermined (e.g., naming tasks and materials supplied by the

clinician). Even many seemingly spontaneous clinical conversational interactions are relatively predetermined and leave little room for the creation of new meanings by the aphasic speaker. How many of us are guilty
of asking our clients questions to which we already know the answers?

In an effort to facilitate aphasic speakers' active roles in treatment and
indeed in their communication environments, I employ a number of
techniques which have been traditionally used in therapy, such as group
treatment and use of therapy materials that are relevant and meaningful
to the client's everyday life. However, when participating in treatment
within a discourse framework, aphasic speakers constantly communicate in everyday conversational genres rather than participating in artificial language games or stimulus-response situations. In both group
and individual work, aphasic speakers are encouraged to choose topics
for discussion that are relevant to their own life styles and interests, to
plan the sessions with the clinician as much as possible, to include or not
to include relatives, and generally to become active partners in treatment.
The severity of aphasia will strongly influence the degree to which an aphasic person will be able to participate in these aspects of treatment. Nevertheless, it is important for people to feel empowered rather than disem-
powered by their treatment. Even those with severely restricted auditory
comprehension usually can respond to some visual tasks or cues, so their
ability to make choices within each session is encouraged. An innovative clinician can design most topics of conversation and activities as
choice situations for even the most impaired clients, so that they can
have some control over what is happening.

Clients' rights to independence within a traditionally "sick" role and
within a traditional medical institutional setting in the community are
difficult concepts to convey. The medical system is very much geared to
the patient/health worker paradigm, in which patients are passive recipients of treatment. Hence, initial work often focuses on conveying to clients that their aphasia may be a handicap, but will not be "treated" as
their other medical conditions are probably being treated, with the patients fulfilling a compliant role. Treatment of the communication disorder will actually focus on speakers' roles as active participants in their
own life situations. This begins with encouraging clients to see themselves as having some control over language treatment. Initially, this might
be deciding frequency and length of sessions, location of sessions (e.g.,
on the ward, in the clinic, at home, if possible, or in the nursing home),
and the duration of treatment. Clients can also decide who should be included in the session in terms of family members or friends.

With the medical system and speech pathology treatment still operating in a traditional professional-dominated paradigm, the goal of em-
powering clients is difficult to achieve. However, I believe it is important because it corresponds to a functional orientation to language. If one

is to assist aphasic clients in regaining some degree of communication empowerment, the language system cannot be seen solely in terms of rules. From the sociolinguistic perspective, language is the vehicle for empowerment. Using this vehicle, and the aphasic speaker's attitude about it, are the real goals in rehabilitation of functional communication skills.

THE FAMILY'S ROLE IN TREATMENT

Much has been written about the importance of counseling and education of families of aphasic clients (Buck, 1968; Derman & Manaster, 1967; Linebaugh & Young-Charles, 1978; Pannbacker, 1972; Rice, Paull, & Muller, 1987; Sarno, 1980) and of their involvement in treatment regimes (Goodkin, Diller, & Shah, 1973; Lesser, Bryan, Anderson, & Hilton, 1986). Although the value of emotional counseling seems to be unchallenged, the optimum way of involving families in language treatment remains controversial. Approaches vary, and can include supplying families a list of ways to facilitate interactions (Green, 1982; Collins, 1986), having them sit in on treatment sessions which they can then replicate at home, or providing behavior modification programs for relatives to train specific interactive behaviors (Goodkin et al., 1973) or to extinguish family verbal behaviors not considered conducive to conversational interaction, such as interruptions and convergent questions (Simmons, Kearns, & Potechin, 1987).

More recent approaches (Lubinski et al., 1980; Milroy & Perkins, 1992) have attempted to look at the conversational dynamics between aphasic speakers and their partners. Applying the ethnomethodological principles used in Conversational Analysis (Ferguson, 1992b; Schegloff, Jefferson, & Sacks, 1977) goes beyond the notion that there are optimal ways to interact with aphasic speakers in general and suggests that intervention should be based on individual patterns of interaction between the aphasic clients and their families. Consideration is given to such aspects of communication as the effectiveness of interactions and the use of successful repair strategies when a breakdown in the conversation occurs. This approach acknowledges the cognitive deficit underlying the aphasia, but places it in the context of aphasic individuals' communication skills, as well as the communicative performance of partners. A breakdown in conversation is seen as a joint problem, not just the aphasic speaker's problem. The verbal behaviors of aphasic persons and the communication partners are analyzed throughout the conversation, and the moments when either partner experiences difficulty in communication are noted. The way the difficulty is identified and managed by the participants is analyzed (Ferguson, 1993). For example, the partner's response to aphasic word-finding difficulty is examined. Does the partner supply what is thought to be the sought-after word or expression? Does the nonaphasic partner offer alternatives to the aphasic speaker? What method facilitates successful continuation of the interaction for this couple? No generic rules exist for facilitation of communication for relatives of aphasic speakers. Each dyad's negotiation of meaning during conversation is investigated. Discussion with the aphasic speaker and family member follows, with the aim of mutually exploring the many possible ways to facilitate their interaction.

My own perspective on family involvement in treatment is largely congruent with this latter view. Consistent with the view of the individual as a social being, rather than a cognitive entity, I see involvement of relatives and friends of aphasic speakers as essential at some level in the treatment process. As mentioned earlier, it is the client's choice whether or not the family is always involved in treatment sessions. However, if communication is conveyed as a social interaction from the beginning of contact, aphasic clients rarely object to family involvement. Hence, there must always be someone with whom clients can interact during a treatment session, and I encourage a variety of people to participate, particularly those with whom clients will interact the most frequently.

I encourage the family to participate in therapy sessions, rather than merely to observe them. They assist in the selection of topics and materials and do much of the facilitation of the aphasic speaker.

To date, most of my treatments have focused on aphasic speakers in largely monologic discourses. Hence, the relative is often facilitating the production of a recounting or expository discourse. However, the ultimate goal is for family members to converse with aphasic relatives in a true dialogue, with the clinician acting as facilitator only when necessary. Because dialogue involves many complex parameters, it is much more difficult to control. This complexity (and until recently, lack of theoretical frameworks within which to handle it) has certainly inhibited much research into assessment and treatment of this vital aspect of communication, but Ferguson's work and further investigations using Conversational Analysis (Lesser & Milroy, 1992) and Exchange Structure (Ventola, 1988; Fawcett, van der Mije, & van Wissen, 1988; Martin, 1992) should shed productive insights into ways in which clinicians can incorporate more dialogue into treatment of aphasic individuals.

CONCLUSION

In approaching aphasia rehabilitation from a sociolinguistic perspective, the clinician can focus on communicative function in everyday situations, taking linguistic resources into account to show how these functions are achieved. Rather than separating language structure from pragmatic function, Halliday's systemic-functional grammar has provided a framework in which the two are intimately interrelated. Using such a framework, the clinician is able to analyze the ways in which aphasic speakers convey meaning via their phonological, syntactic, and lexical choices and utilize these analyses to direct treatment strategies designed to maximize or expand the aphasic speaker's remaining resources. The main focus of a sociolinguistic approach is language in use. Therefore, treatment involves the text/discourse as the basic unit of meaning and the focus of treatment in all modalities. The approach also recognizes involvement of relatives and significant others as crucial to efficacious treatment, as is the notion that the aphasic speaker is an active participant in the treatment procedure. Because the concept of language as a social process is inherent in this approach, language remediation aims at re-empowerment of aphasic individuals in society by facilitating the use of their still-available language resources.

ACKNOWLEDGMENT

The author gratefully acknowledges the useful comments of Alison Ferguson on previous drafts of this chapter.

REFERENCES

Armstrong, E. M. (1987). Cohesive harmony in aphasic discourse and its significance in listener perception of coherence. In R. H. Brookshire (Ed.), *Clinical aphasiology: Conference proceedings.* Minneapolis, MN: BRK Publishers.

Armstrong, E. M. (1989, November). *Conversational interaction between clinician and aphasic client during treatment sessions.* Paper presented at the American Speech-Language-Hearing Association annual conference, St. Louis, MO.

Armstrong, E. M. (1991). The potential of cohesion analysis in the analysis and treatment of aphasic discourse. *Clinical Linguistics and Phonetics, 5*(1), 39–51.

Armstrong, E. M. (1992). *The logical metafunction in aphasic discourse: A case study.* Paper presented at the 19th International Systemic Functional Congress, Sydney, Australia.

Aten, J. L., Caliguiri, M. P., & Holland, A. L. (1982). The efficacy of functional communication therapy for chronic aphasic patients. *Journal of Speech and Hearing Disorders, 47,* 93–96.

Behrmann, M., & Lieberthal, T. (1989). Category-specific treatment of a lexical-semantic deficit: A single case study of global aphasia. *British Journal of Disorders of Communication, 24,* 281–299.

Berko-Gleason, J., Goodglass, H., Obler, L., Green, E., Hyde, M. R., & Weintraub, S. (1980). Narrative strategies of aphasic and normal-speaking subjects. *Journal of Speech and Hearing Research, 23,* 370–382.

Bottenberg, D., Lemme, M., & Hedberg, N. (1985). Analysis of oral narratives of normal and aphasic adults. In R. H. Brookshire (Ed.), *Clinical aphasiology: Conference proceedings.* Minneapolis, MN: BRK Publishers.

Brookshire, R. H. (1987). Auditory language comprehension disorders in aphasia. *Topics in Language Disorders, 8*(1), 11–23.

Brookshire, R. H., & Nicholas, L. E. (1984). Comprehension of directly and indirectly stated main ideas and details in discourse by brain-damaged and non-brain-damaged listeners. *Brain and Language, 21,* 21–26.

Buck, M. (1968). *Dysphagia: Professional guidance for family and patient.* Engelwood Cliffs, NJ: Prentice-Hall.

Byng, S. (1988). Sentence processing deficits: Theory and therapy. *Cognitive Neuropsychology, 5,* 629–676.

Byng, S., & Coltheart, M. (1986). Aphasia research: Methodological requirements and illustration results. In E. Hjelmquist & L. B. Nilsson (Eds.), *Communication and handicap.* Amsterdam: North-Holland, Elsevier.

Caramazza, A. (1984). The logic of neuropsychological research and the problem of patient classification in aphasia. *Brain and Language, 21,* 9–20.

Caramazza, A. (1986). On drawing inferences about the structure of normal cognitive systems from the analysis of patterns of impaired performance: The case for single-patient studies. *Brain and Cognition, 5,* 41–66.

Chapey, R. (1981). Divergent semantic intervention. In R. Chapey (Ed.), *Language intervention strategies in adult aphasia.* Baltimore, MD: Williams & Wilkins.

Chomsky, N. (1981). *Lectures on government and binding.* Dordrecht, Holland: Foris.

Collins, M. (1986). *Diagnosis and treatment of global aphasia.* London: Taylor & Francis.

Coltheart, M. (1980). Deep dyslexia: A review of the syndrome. In M. Coltheart, K. E. Patterson, & J. C. Marshall (Eds.), *Deep dyslexia.* London: Routledge & Kegan Paul.

Coltheart, M. (1985). Cognitive neuropsychology and the study of reading. In M. I. Posner & G. S. M. Marin (Eds.), *Attention and performance XI.* Hillsdale, NJ: Lawrence Erlbaum.

Coltheart, M., Sartori, G., & Job, R. (Eds.) (1987). *The cognitive neuropsychology of language.* Hillsdale, NJ: Lawrence Erlbaum.

Damico, J. (1985). Clinical discourse analysis: A functional approach to language assessment. In C. S. Simon (Ed.), *Communication skills and classroom success: Assessment of language-learning disabled students.* San Diego, CA: College-Hill Press.

Davis, G. A., & Wilcox, M. J. (1985). *Adult aphasia rehabilitation: Applied pragmatics.* San Diego, CA: College-Hill Press.

de Beaugrande, R. (1980). *Text, discourse and process: Toward a multi-disciplinary science of texts.* Norwood, NJ: Longman.

Derman, S., & Manaster, A. (1967). Family counseling with relatives of aphasic patients at Schwab rehabilitation hospital. *Asha, 9,* 175–177.

Doyle, P. J., Goldstein, H., Bourgeois, M. S., & Nakles, K. (1989). Facilitating generalized requesting behavior in Broca's aphasia: An experimental analysis of a generalization training procedure. *Journal of Applied Behavior Analysis, 22*(2), 157–170.

Ellis, A. W., & Young, A. W. (1988). *Human cognitive neuropsychology*. East Sussex, England: Lawrence Erlbaum.

Fawcett, R. P., van der Mije, A., & van Wissen, C. (1988). Towards a systemic flowchart model for discourse structure. In R. P. Fawcett & D. J. Young (Eds.), *New developments in systemic linguistics. Vol. 2: Theory and application*. London: Printer Publishers.

Fawcett, R. P., & Young, D. J. (Eds.) (1988). *New developments in systemic linguistics. Vol. 2: Theory and application*. London: Printer Publishers.

Ferguson, A. J. (1992a). *Interpersonal aspects of aphasic conversation*. Paper presented at the 19th International Systemic Functional Congress, Sydney, Australia.

Ferguson, A. J. (1992b). *Conversational repair in aphasic and normal interaction*. Unpublished dissertation, Macquarie University, Sydney, Australia.

Ferguson, A. J. (1993). Conversational repair of word-finding difficulty. In M. Lemme (Ed.), *Clinical aphasiology: Conference proceedings* (Vol. 21, pp. 299–307), Austin TX: Pro-Ed.

Firth, J. R. (1959). Personality and language in society. In J. R. Firth, (Ed.), *Papers in linguistics 1934-1951*, London: Oxford University Press. (Original work published in 1950.)

Goodglass, H., & Kaplan, E. (1972). *The assessment of aphasia and related disorders*. Philadelphia: Lea & Febiger.

Goodkin, R., Diller, L., & Shah, N. (1973). Training spouses to improve the functional speech of aphasic patients. In B. Lahey (Ed.), *The modification of language behavior* (pp. 218–269). Springfield, IL: Charles C. Thomas.

Green, G. (1982). Assessment and treatment of the adult with severe aphasia: Aiming for functional generalization. *Australian Journal of Human Communication Disorders, 10*(1), 11–23.

Grodzinsky, Y. (1986). Cognitive deficits: Their proper description and its theoretical relevance. *Brain and Language, 27*, 178-191.

Gurland, G., Chwat, S., & Wollner, S. (1982). Establishing a communication profile in adult aphasia: Analysis of communicative acts and conversational sequences. In R. Brookshire (Ed.), *Clinical aphasiology: Conference proceedings*. Minneapolis, MN: BRK Publishers.

Halliday, M. A. K. (1973). *Explorations in the function of language*. London: Edward Arnold.

Halliday, M. A. K. (1974). *Language and social man*. London: Longman for the Schools Council.

Halliday, M. A. K. (1977). Text as semantic choice in social contexts. In T. A. Van Dijk & J. S. Petofi (Eds.), *Grammars and descriptions* (pp. 176–225). Berlin: de Gruyter.

Halliday, M. A. K. (1985a). *An introduction to functional grammar*. London: Edward Arnold.

Halliday, M. A. K. (1985b). Context of situation. In M. A. K. Halliday & R. Hasan (Eds.), *Language, context and text: Aspects of language in a social-semiotic perspective* (pp. 3–48). Geelong, Australia: Deakin University Press.

Halliday, M. A. K. (1985c). *Spoken and written language*. Geelong, Australia: Deakin University Press.

Halliday, M. A. K., & Hasan, R. (1976). *Cohesion in English*. London: Longmans.

Hasan, R. (1973). Code, register and social dialect. In B. Bernstein (Ed.), *Class, codes and control. Vol. 2: Applied studies towards a sociology of languages* (pp. 252–292). London: Tourledge & Kegan Paul.

Holland, A. L. (1975, November). *Aphasics as communicators: A model and its implications.* Paper presented to the American Speech-Language-Hearing Association, Washington, DC.

Holland, A. L. (1980). *Communicative abilities in daily living.* Baltimore, MD: University Park Press.

Holland, A. L. (1982). Observing functional communication of aphasic adults. *Journal of Speech and Hearing Disorders, 47,* 50–56.

Holland, A. (1991). Pragmatic aspects of intervention in aphasia. *Journal of Neurolinguistics, 6*(2), 197–211.

Hymes, D. H. (1967). Models of the interaction of language and social setting. *Journal of Social Issues, 23,* 8–28.

Jones, E. V. (1986). Building the foundations for sentence production on a non-fluent aphasic. *British Journal of Disorders of Communication, 21,* 63–82.

Kay, J., Lesser, R., & Coltheart, M. (1991). *Psycholinguistic assessment of language processing in aphasia.* Hillsdale, NJ: Lawrence Erlbaum.

Kertesz, A. (1982). *Western aphasia battery.* New York: Grune & Stratton.

Kimbarow, M. (1982, November). *Discourse analysis: A look at clinicians' conversational strategies in treatment.* Paper presented at the Annual Meeting of the American Speech-Language-Hearing Association, Toronto.

Kintsch, W. (1974). *The representation of meaning in memory.* Hillsdale, NJ: Lawrence Erlbaum.

Kintsch, W., & Van Dijk, T. E. (1978). Toward a model of text comprehension and production. *Psychological Review, 85,* 363–394.

Lemme, M. L., Hedberg, N. L., & Bottenberg, D. F. (1984). Cohesion in narratives of aphasic adults. In R. H. Brookshire (Ed.), *Clinical aphasiology: Conference proceedings* (pp. 215–222). Minneapolis, MN: BRK Publishers.

Lesser, R., Bryan, K., Anderson, J., & Hilton, R. (1986). Involving relatives in aphasia therapy: An application of language enrichment therapy. *International Journal of Rehabilitation Research, 9,* 259–267.

Linebaugh, C. W., & Young-Charles, H. Y. (1978). The counseling needs of the families of aphasic patients. In R. H. Brookshire (Ed.), *Clinical aphasiology: Conference proceedings.* Minneapolis, MN: BRK Publishers.

Longacre, R. (1976). *An anatomy of speech notions.* Lisse: The Peter de Ridder Press.

Lubinski, R., Duchan, J., & Weitzner-Lin, B. (1980). Analysis of breakdowns and repairs in aphasic adult communication. In R. H. Brookshire (Ed.), *Clinical aphasiology: Conference proceedings* (pp. 111–116). Minneapolis, MN: BRK Publishers.

Martin, J. (1992). *English text: System and structure.* Amsterdam: John Benjamins.

Martin, J., & Halliday, M. A. K. (Eds.). (1981). *Readings in systemic linguistics.* London: Batsford Academic and Educational Ltd.

Matthiesson, C., & Halliday, M. A. K. (in press). Systemic functional grammar. In F. Peng & J. Ney (Eds.), *Current approaches to syntax.* Amsterdam and London: Benjamins & Whurr.

Milroy, L., & Perkins, L. (1992). Repair strategies in aphasic discourse: Towards a collaborative model. *Clinical Linguistics and Phonetics, 6,* 27–40.

Pannbacker, M. (1972) Publications for families of adult aphasics. *Rehabilitation Literature, 33*(3), 72–78.

Penn, C. (1988). The profiling of syntax and pragmatics in aphasia. *Clinical Linguistics and Phonetics, 2,* 179–207.

Porch, B. E. (1967). *Porch index of communicative ability.* Palo Alto, CA: Consulting Psychologists Press.

Porch, B. E. (1981). *Porch index of communicative ability* (3rd ed.). Palo Alto, CA: Consulting Psychologists Press.

Prutting, C. A., & Kirchner, D. M. (1983). Applied pragmatics. In T. M. Gallagher & C. A. Prutting (Eds.), *Pragmatic assessment and intervention issues in language.* San Diego, CA: College-Hill Press.

Rice, B., Paull, A., & Muller, D. J. (1987). An evaluation of a social support group for spouses of aphasic partners. *Aphasiology, 1*(3), 247–256.

Ripich, D., Hambrecht, G., & Panagos, J. (1985). Discourse analysis of aphasia therapy. *Aphasia-Apraxia-Agnosia, 3*(4), 1–10.

Rumelhart, D. E. (1980). Schemata: The building blocks of cognition. In B. Spiro, B. Bruce, & W. Brower (Eds.), *Theoretical issues in reading comprehension.* Hillsdale, NJ: Lawrence Erlbaum.

Sacks, H., Schegloff, E., & Jefferson, G. (1974). A simplistic systematics for the organization of turn taking for conversation. *Language, 50,* 696–735.

Sarno, M. T. (1980). Review of research in aphasia: Recovery and rehabilitation. In M. T. Sarno & O. Hook (Eds.), *Aphasia: Assessment and treatment* (pp. 485–529). New York: Masson.

Schegloff, E. A., Jefferson, G., & Sacks, H. (1977). The preference for self-correction in the organization of repair in conversation. *Language, 53,* 361–382.

Schuell, H. (1965). *The Minnesota test for differential diagnosis of aphasia.* Minneapolis: University of Minnesota Press.

Schwartz, M., Linebarger, M. C., Saffran, E. M., & Pate, D. S. (1987). Syntactic transparency and sentence interpretation in aphasia. *Language and Cognitive Processes, 2,* 85–113.

Shapiro, L. P., & B. A. Levine (1989). Real-time sentence processing in aphasia. In T. E. Prescott (Ed.), *Clinical aphasiology* (Vol. 18, pp. 281–296). Boston, MA: College-Hill Press.

Shapiro, L. P., & Thompson, C. K. (1992). *The use of linguistic theory as a framework for treatment studies in aphasia.* Paper presented at the Clinical Aphasiology Conference, Durango, CO.

Shewan, C. M. (1988). The Shewan spontaneous language analysis (SSLA) system for aphasic adults: Description, reliability and validity. *Journal of Communication Disorders, 21,* 103–138.

Simmons, N. N., Kearns, K. P., & Potechin, G. (1987). Treatment of aphasia through family member training. In R. H. Brookshire (Ed.), *Clinical aphasiology: Conference proceedings.* Minneapolis, MN: BRK Publishers.

Thompson, C. K., & Shapiro, L. P. (1992). *A linguistic-specific approach to treatment of sentence production deficits in aphasia.* Paper presented at the Clinical Aphasiology Conference, Durango, CO

Ulatowska, H. K., & Bond-Chapman, S. (1989). Discourse considerations for aphasia management. *Seminars in Speech and Language, 10*(4), 298–314.

Ulatowska, H. K., North, A., & Macaluso-Haynes, S. (1980). Production of discourse and communicative competence in aphasia. In R. H. Brookshire (Ed.), *Clinical aphasiology: Conference proceedings.* Minneapolis, MN: BRK Publishers.

Ulatowska, H. K., North, A. J., & Maculuso-Haynes, S. (1981). Production of narrative and procedural discourse in aphasia. *Brain and Language, 13*, 345–371.

Ulatowska, H. K., Weiss-Doyell, A., Freedman-Stern, R., & Macaluso-Haynes, S. (1983). Production of narrative discourse in aphasia. *Brain and Language, 19*, 317–334.

Van Dijk, T. E. (1977). *Text and context: Explorations in the semantics and pragmatics of discourse*. New York: Longmans.

Ventola, E. (1988). Text analysis in operation: A multilevel approach. In R. P. Fawcett & D. J. Young (Eds.), *New developments in systemic linguistics. Vol. 2: Theory and application* (pp.52–75). London: Pinter Publishers.

Wagenaar, E., Snow, C., & Prins, R. (1975). Spontaneous speech of aphasic patients: A psycholinguistic analysis. *Brain and Language, 2*, 281–303.

Wilcox, M. J., & Davis, G. A. (1977). Speech act analysis of aphasic communication in individual and group settings. In R. H. Brookshire (Ed.), *Clinical aphasiology: Conference proceedings* (pp. 166–174). Minneapolis, MN: BRK Publishers.

Yorkston, K., & Beukelman, D. (1980). An analysis of connected speech samples of aphasic and normal speakers. *Journal of Speech and Hearing Disorders, 45*, 27–36.

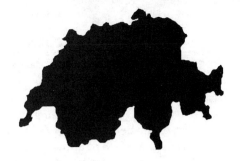

CHAPTER 12

Which Route to Aphasia Therapy?

DOROTHEA WENIGER
BRIGITTE BERTONI
Department of Neurology
University of Zurich
Zurich, Switzerland

Most people concerned with aphasia therapy would agree that without some knowledge about the pattern of retained and lost language skills a reasonable treatment program cannot be designed. However, more than an inventory of diagnostic test scores is needed to determine the goals of treatment. A description of surface symptoms fails to capture the functional deficits underlying the linguistic disorders assessed in formal diagnostic testing. The information processing models developed during recent years have purported to provide a framework for identifying the different processes and representations of knowledge which could be impaired in aphasia and thus could be responsible for disruptions in language processing. These models have served as the basis for the formulation of a number of hypotheses about the processing of spoken and written words. Of particular relevance for decisions concerning the focus of treatment, they allow determination of whether the patient's deficits reflect problems in availability or in accessibility. But, as has been

discussed by Seidenberg (1988), these models of the functional architecture of the language processing system amount to a "kind of descriptive, first-order decomposition" of the tasks involved in formal diagnostic testing. In cases of impaired accessibility, more information about
the affected linguistic units and their rule-governed behavior needs to be
known if effective deficit-oriented therapy materials and procedures are
to be constructed. It is only when a patient's performance is analyzed
in terms of the structural features which characterize the different units
of the language system that deficit-oriented treatment programs can
be designed.

Our chapter is organized as follows. The first section discusses the contribution of processing models to designing treatment procedures. In
particular, it will be argued that materials should highlight the linguistic
structure of the impaired language component. The second section focuses on the need to consider issues of brain plasticity. Depending on
site and size of lesion, different repair processes become operative after
brain damage. Many patients interested in improving their language
skills unfortunately lack the required processing capacities to do so. In
the third section, some nonlinguistic impairments that frequently accompany aphasic language disturbances are pointed out, and their implications for treatment procedures discussed.

PROCESSING MODELS IN LANGUAGE THERAPY: WORD-FINDING DEFICITS

Word-finding difficulties are a ubiquitous aphasic symptom. As a number of recent case studies (Caramazza & Hillis, 1990; Hillis & Caramazza, 1991; Hillis, Rapp, Romani, & Caramazza, 1990; Howard & Orchard-
Lisle, 1984; Kay & Ellis, 1987) have demonstrated, they can result from
problems at different stages in the process of retrieving and articulating
words. The models currently popular in cognitive psychology share the
assumption that there are modality-specific input and output components which are interconnected by a semantic component. The different
components can be impaired selectively, resulting in predictable patterns of impaired performance. With damage to the semantic component, deficient performance should be found in all lexical tasks. If damage is restricted to the phonological output lexicon, selective deficits
should be found only in tasks requiring spoken word production. A
model-based distinction between word-finding difficulties arising at the
semantic level and at the phonological level can thus be made. (For a discussion of semantic errors resulting from damage to the phonological
output lexicon, see Caramazza & Hillis, 1990.)

Patients displaying the same pattern of deficient performance in naming tasks and in tasks of auditory word comprehension are likely to have problems in processing semantic information. The semantic information available to these patients may be insufficient to specify the exact target name. When these patients are cued in a picture-naming task with the initial phoneme of a word semantically related to the target name, semantic paraphasias are more likely to occur than when the cue is the initial phoneme of the target name. Other patients with naming problems will reject quite reliably the initial phoneme of semantically related words which are offered as cues to object names that cannot be retrieved. In contrast to patients whose word-finding difficulties reflect semantic impairments, these patients often are able to generate phonological approximations. They appear to have some rough idea of the phonological form of the correct name. The problem seems to be one of reduced activation: Not all phonemes that make up a word's spoken form and are activated by the word's (intact) semantic representation receive sufficient activation to boost their resting levels high enough for articulation. These patients might be expected to have comparable difficulties in oral reading of irregular words, as exemplified by the patient EST, described by Kay and Patterson (1985).

The best illustration of an attempt to derive treatment procedures from a model-based analysis of the patient's word processing problems has been presented by de Partz (1986). The patient in this study (SP) was found to have deep dyslexia; SP was unable to read nonwords aloud, had difficulties with abstract words and function words, and made semantic errors when reading real words. The nonlexical route to reading appeared to be inoperative, and the lexical one was hampered by an inability to monitor the transcoded written words. If the patient could be trained to relate spelling to sound, the lexical routes to reading might be expected to benefit from the acquired transcoding skills. The patient was taught to transcode graphemes into phonemes by means of a lexical relay code. The code consisted of associating written letters with the initial sound of familiar words. The patient learned to sound out letters with the aid of visuo-lexical associations. After 9 months of treatment the patient displayed remarkable improvement in his oral reading of both words and nonwords. However, difficulties persisted when letter pronunciation was context-dependent or when the sound corresponded to a complex grapheme configuration. This aspect of the training program will be discussed further in the next section.

According to the functional architecture of word processing models, reading is tied to two distinct translation mechanisms. On the one hand, the phonological representation of a printed word is taken as a stored entity which corresponds to the whole string of letters making up a word. On the other hand, it is taken as a code which must be cobbled together from orthographic subcomponents of the printed letter string. The former procedure is known as addressed phonology, whereas the latter is known as assembled phonology (see Patterson & Coltheart, 1987). Roughly speaking, addressed phonology may be associated with a lexical route to reading, assembled with a nonlexical route. The training program for SP exploited the mechanistic feature of assembled phonology, namely the one-to-one correspondence between a particular letter and its sound. The success of de Partz's treatment approach resides in the patient's retained ability to attend to a one-to-one mapping strategy that can be performed (with a considerable degree of reliability) on the basis of a limited set of fixed identity relations. Had the patient's reading problems been a matter of impaired comprehension rather than impaired oral production of written words (commonly associated with surface dyslexia), a different treatment approach would have been required. Word meanings cannot be related to word forms in the same manner as letters to sounds. What kind of approach is to be followed in patients with marked difficulties in accessing the meaning of words?

In recent times, case studies of patients displaying selective impairment in specific classes of words have pervaded discussions of semantic impairments (for a review of the various cases that have been reported, see Shallice, 1988). The implication of these studies is that knowledge is organized categorically according to the relative prominence of the sensory associations which enter its neuronal representation. Damasio (1990) has summarized the state of affairs succinctly:

The fact that lesions in some neural systems disturb processing relative to some knowledge domains more than others suggests that such systems are dedicated to the processing of some prevailing characteristics of entities and events in these domains. It does not indicate dedication to the representation of a conceptual category. (p. 98)

By and large, impairments in semantic processing are characterized by difficulties in differentiating among related word meanings. Although patients frequently retain the ability to assign words to a broad semantic field, they fail when required to attend to the defining features of a word's meaning (Grober, Perecman, Kellar, & Brown, 1980; Zurif, Caramazza, Myerson, & Galvin, 1974). It has been a matter of some debate whether such difficulties are to be interpreted as problems of access or problems of store (Blumstein, Milberg, & Shrier, 1982; Milberg & Blumstein, 1981; Shallice, 1987). Within the framework of cognitive processing models the two interpretations entail different treatment procedures. Training the patient to generate semantic cues has been found to facilitate word retrieval. With problems of storage such reactivational strategies offer little promise of help. The degradation of semantic store calls for techniques designed to help the patient compensate for lost information. However, if a distributed memory system is adopted to account for impairments associated with the semantic component of the language system (Allport, 1985), "store" and "access" cease to be of any theoretical relevance. In these models the meaning of a word is not taken as a network of concept nodes with labeled and directed links but is viewed as a code which is manifested in a specific pattern of activity; accessing a word's meaning amounts to "turning on" the activity pattern the system has "learned" for that word. In somewhat more technical terms: The recoverability of an activity pattern is a joint function of the strength with which the elements of a pattern are inter-associated and the strength of association between the retrieval cue and the to-be-recovered pattern (Allport, 1985). Consistency of performance does not reflect a loss of stored information but the strength of particular (retained) associations and the capacity of the system to suppress competing patterns of activity.

Such a distributed model of processing calls for remediation procedures aimed at activating the patient's awareness of word meanings as a specific configuration of lexical-semantic features. Improvement in the semantic availability of words should be achieved by training patients to attend to the lexical-semantic structure of semantically related words.

We examined the effects of such a therapeutic rationale by requiring patients to observe semantic selection restrictions in sentences which had to be constructed from their constituent parts. Five patients with moderate to severe word-finding difficulties and fairly good auditory word comprehension skills participated. Patients ranged in age from 31 to 53 years old, with an average age of 36 years; duration of illness ranged from 9 to 32 months, with a mean of 16 months. Forty bisyllabic nouns denoting common everyday objects were used as subjects in simple declarative sentences in which the predicate consisted of a finite auxiliary verb with a noun or adjective as the complement. For each target word three such sentences were constructed. The predicate complement in these sentences always specified a particular property of the target word serving as subject of the sentence (e.g., the window is narrow). Three cards were made for each of these 120 sentences. On each card was written the subject, auxiliary verb, or noun/adjective complement of a given sentence. The three cards making up a sentence were presented in a random array together with two distractor cards for the predicate complement. For half of the target words, the distractor cards contained a semantically related word in the same syntactic category as the predicate complement (e.g., the window / is / narrow / thin / slender). For the other half of the target words, the distractor cards contained words merely belonging to the same syntactic category as the predicate complement (e.g., the carpet / is / soft / full / weak). The selection of the distractors for complement nouns was guided by morphological considerations; the patients were discouraged from relying on formal rather than semantic features of the individual constituents (in German the article of noun phrases is case-marked). Once they had assembled and read the target sentence aloud the patients were asked to copy the sentence and then say it. These practice steps were the same for both types of sentences. Patients were given this treatment program in three hour-long sessions a week for 8 weeks.

To determine whether the necessity to differentiate among semantically related words had a stimulating effect, patients were asked to produce as many associations as possible for the 40 target words. This task was administered just before the treatment period, immediately after the treatment period, and 4 weeks after the end of the treatment period; during the latter period patients received no treatment. As can be seen in Figure 12–1, the average number of associations elicited for the two sets of words was about the same before treatment; the two sets of words were thus of comparable associative power. Treatment proved to have a stimulating effect on both lists of words. The average number of associations was not affected by whether more precise semantic differentiations had been required in assembling the sentence constituents. Four weeks post-treatment, a further increase in the average number of associations was found. However, the words used in the target sentences with semantically related distractors appeared to have been more specifically activated. With these words the variability in response was largely due to a steady increase in the number of associations produced; with the words that did not occur in sentences with semantically related distractors no such trend was served.

The differential increase in the average number of associations elicited for the two sets of words may be attributed to a greater semantic stimulation effect generated by therapy materials designed to activate specific features of word meanings. Such an interpretation of the patients' performance fits well with the results obtained by Cohen, Engel, Kelter, and List (1979) in a picture naming study. These authors compared the effects of two types of prompts in facilitating aphasic patients' naming abilities. Whenever the name of a depicted object could not be produced, an overlearned sequence or an open-ended sentence was given to the patient for completion. Overlearned sequences proved to be more effective prompts than open-ended sentences; however, one day later, picture names that had been cued by open-ended sentences were more likely to be available than picture names cued by overlearned sequences. The authors argue that the open-ended sentence prompts called for a

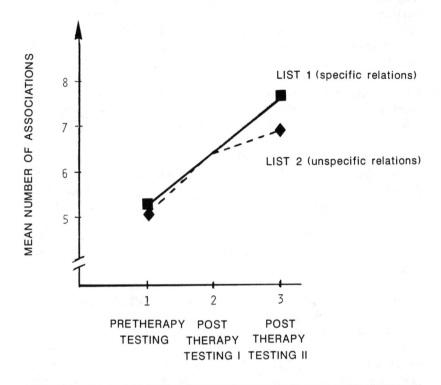

Figure 12-1. Mean number of associations elicited before treatment, immediately after treatment, and 1 month later, after a period of no treatment.

search in semantic memory, which resulted in a longer lasting stimulation effect than did the completion of an automatized sequence of words.

The treatment of BRB's word-finding difficulties, described by Byng (1988), also provides supportive evidence for the greater activation effects of remediation approaches that require the patient to attend to specific features of word meanings. To achieve an improvement in BRB's comprehension skills, Byng had the patient match written words with their pictorial representations in a set of four pictures consisting of the correct response and three distractors, one of which had a semantic relationship to the target picture. The only aid given to the patient was a list of the correct picture numbers against which he could check his responses. Treatment effects were assessed with two types of comprehension tasks: a picture-word matching task and a synonym judgment task. For the latter task, treated words were paired with appropriate as well as incorrect synonyms. The patient was asked to sort the pairs of words. In the picture-word matching task, item-specific treatment effects were found. These effects proved to be task-specific, as no improvement of the synonym judgment performance was obtained. The treatment procedure taught the patient to match a word with a particular instance of its meaning; in performing these matching tasks the patient did not have to perceive the full meaning of the individual words, as is required in a synonym judgment task. It seems reasonable to assume that the stimulating effect of a treatment procedure is dependent on the depth of processing required.

This assumption finds confirmation in the experimental findings of studies using different cuing techniques to elicit picture names. Phonemic cues have been found to be effective prompts in word retrieval (Kohn & Goodglass, 1985; Pease & Goodglass, 1978), but as Patterson, Purell, and Morton (1983) have demonstrated, such phonological information about the form of a word does not result in long-term facilitation; benefits from phonemic cuing dissipated after half an hour. Comparable results were obtained by Bruce and Howard (1987) who studied the feasibility of teaching patients to generate their own phonemic cues with a microcomputer. The words under study were words for which subjects could specify the initial letter, but not the whole word. The five patients in this study achieved significantly better naming performances when they were allowed to use the computer as an aid than when they received no help. The effects generalized to untreated items, but there was a trend for greater effects with the treated items. However, the overall difference in performance between the treated and the untreated items was fairly small; one is again led to conclude that phonemic cuing only has short-term effects.

The effects of different semantic facilitation techniques were explored by Howard, Patterson, Franklin, Orchard-Lisle, and Morton (1985). An improvement in naming performance was found after auditory as well as written word-to-picture matching. But when patients were given the naming task again 2 weeks later, their performance dropped to the level of the control condition. Pointing to a different object from the same semantic category as the target picture that could not be named was a less effective technique than having to judge whether a particular property applied to the target name. The results of these studies seem to indicate that only short-term improvements are achieved in naming tasks if the treatment procedure does not involve intentional processing of semantic information.

PROCESSING MODELS IN LANGUAGE THERAPY: SYNTACTIC AND MORPHOLOGICAL DEFICITS

The language system also has a syntactic component which specifies the constituent structure of connected speech and the syntactic relationships that enter the grammatical encoding of lexical items in the form of bound and free closed class vocabulary. A comprehensive representation of words must include information about the syntactic frames into which they may be inserted, the morphosyntactic markings which they take on, and the semantic selection restrictions which the retrieved lexical items must meet.

Until recently, impairments in sentence production have been examined largely within the confines of the classical clinical syndromes of agrammatism and paragrammatism. In the days when the focus of interest was classification, checklist approaches dominated: The symptoms characterizing disorders in sentence production were analyzed to provide a more detailed definition of these clinical syndromes (see Gleason, Goodglass, Green, Ackerman, & Hyde, 1975; Goodglass, Gleason, Bernholtz, & Hyde, 1972; Tissot, Mounin, & Lhermitte, 1973; von Stockert & Bader, 1976; Zurif, Caramazza, & Myerson, 1972). But because the combination of symptoms displayed by patients with impaired grammar is rather heterogeneous (for examples, see Miceli, Silveri, Romani, & Caramazza, 1989), checklist approaches were found to have little promise of leading to significant generalizations regarding the underlying deficit (for a discussion of the theoretical issues, see Badecker & Caramazza, 1985). A more thorough explanation can be gained by using an approach that allows inferences to be made about the nature of the sentence processing deficit.

In a number of proposed accounts of processing, the symptoms observed are analyzed in terms of a functional deficit associated with a particular component of the language system. The assumption underlying these approaches is that aphasic language disorders reflect failures in the central representation of some component of the language system. Supportive evidence for such an assumption comes from empirical observations and experimental findings showing that defects manifested in one modality are paralleled in other modalities. Focusing her attention on the deficient processing of grammatical morphemes, Kean (1977, 1979) found agrammatism to be a phonologically based disorder in which the syntactic representation of a sentence is reduced to those morphemes that contribute to its stress pattern. On the basis of their findings in lexical decision tasks, Bradley, Garrett, and Zurif (1980) interpreted the deficient processing of grammatical morphemes as a problem involving the lexical component. Studying the ability of agrammatic patients to distinguish between subject and object in word order tasks led Saffran, Schwartz, and Marin (1980) to conclude that the locus of the functional deficit is at the level of the syntactic component. Caramazza and Berndt (1985) have challenged such efforts to relate the symptoms of impaired grammar to disruptions in the processing mechanisms of a single component of the language system. They have suggested that dif-

ferent patterns of sentence production impairments reflect different dys-
functions of the individual components of the sentence production system. But without a sufficiently articulated model of the sentence production process, it is hard to formulate a theoretically coherent functional
account of sentence production impairments. The model developed by
Garrett (1976, 1982) has been adopted as a possible framework for interpreting the various constellations of co-occurring and dissociating symptoms found in disorders of sentence processing (Caramazza & Hillis, 1989;
Saffran, 1982).

In this production model, different levels of representation are distinguished, each associated with specific processing operations (only
broadly sketched in Garrett's presentation of the model). The linguistic
encoding of an intended message (a conceptual construct referred to as
the message level representation of a surface sentence) begins with the
lexical identification of semantic information and the computation of
functional structure roles that specify the relations among the selected
lexical formatives. The sentence frames thus generated can also be described as a set of argument functions, assigned to nouns in accordance
with the predicate structure of the verb. On the basis of such functional
level representations, the phrasal geometry of a sentence is determined,
closed class vocabulary items are selected, and the word forms of the
identified lexical items are retrieved. The ensuing positional level representation consists of a string of phonologically specified units to which
procedures for constructing a phonetic level representation are applied.
The theoretically relevant feature of this model is that syntax and morphology, the two formal aspects of grammar, are interpreted in terms
of processing procedures yoked to the selection of open and closed
class vocabulary items. The syntactic constituents making up sentence
frames are semantically motivated (i.e., they are generated by the semantic structure of the lexical items designated to fill the slots of the sentence pattern). The subsequent morphological structuring of the generated sentence frames then entails the incorporation of the various
types of closed class items (articles, pronouns, prepositions, auxiliaries, inflections).

Such a computational account of the syntactic and morphological
aspects of grammar offers a framework for identifying the presumed
locus of the functional deficits in the sentence production process. It also
encompasses theoretical constructs that could be exploited in designing
deficit-oriented therapy materials. Related to the concept of a functional
level representation are other linguistic notions, such as thematic structure of a sentence (Fillmore, 1971; Gruber, 1965; Jackendoff, 1972,
1983). Words, more specifically verbs, can be described as predicates
taking a certain number of conceptually required "arguments." Depend-

ing on the conceptual structure of the predicate, these arguments are ascribed particular thematic roles. For example, the verbs *lend* and *borrow* are three-argument predicates, the arguments representing the one who receives some object for temporary use, the one who is eligible to grant permission for use, and the object that is transferred for temporary use. A distinction is made between the number of conceptually required arguments and the number of arguments that must be explicitly identified in a grammatically well-formed sentence. With *lend*, the argument identifying the recipient of the object transferred for temporary use can be omitted; whereas with *borrow*, it must be specified because it has the syntactic function of being the subject of the sentence. The thematic roles played by the different arguments of a predicate generally can be matched on a one-to-one basis with the constituent syntactic frames that are associated with the predicate. Which arguments can be left out of the surface structure of a sentence is a matter of case hierarchy and not of particular relevance here.

Patients with difficulties in sentence processing have been found to have problems in mapping thematic roles onto syntactic structures (Linebarger, Schwartz, & Saffran, 1983). But few attempts have been made to improve sentence processing abilities in these patients by training them to identify the different thematic roles associated with particular predicates and then to map these roles onto the corresponding syntactic structures. Jones (1986) and Byng (1988) have reported the results of teaching patients to perform such mapping routines in comprehension tasks. The treatment program followed by Jones consisted of giving the patient BB sentences of increasing syntactic complexity, beginning with intransitive sentences, proceeding to transitive SVO sentences with reversible as well as nonreversible noun phrases, and then going on to sentences with prepositional and adverbial phrases. The patient was required to identify the constituents which "responded" to such questions as "who," "what," "when," "where," and "how."

Working with the patient BRB, Byng concentrated on sentences with a locational preposition. This patient's task was also one of identification; he had to choose the picture that went with a written stimulus sentence. The target picture was paired with a distractor picture representing the opposite role from the target picture. To aid the patient in perceiving the expressed relationship, the stimulus materials were color coded. The two noun phrases in the sentence were written in the colors corresponding to the colors in which the two objects in the pictures were drawn. For the sentence "The pan is in the jug," the correct picture had a red pan in a blue jug whereas the distractor picture had a red jug in a blue pan. Four prepositions were selected for treatment, with each preposition being used in five sentences. After working with these materials at home for a week, BRB correctly matched 17 of the 20 practice sentences — using colorless sentences and pictures. The patient also scored better on a test which comprised untreated items. The improvement in performance therefore cannot be attributed to rote learning of the practice sentences.

Structural changes were noted in the sentences that BRB produced in retelling a story; more two-argument structures occurred. However, the proportion of open and closed class items remained unbalanced. Closed class items are intricately tied to the shades of meaning that a verb may have. As has been pointed out by Fillmore (1971), the two sentences, "He smeared mud on the fender," and, "He smeared the fender with mud," are not quite paraphrases of each other. An appropriate paraphrase of the second sentence would be, "He covered the fender with mud." In the second sentence "the fender" functions syntactically as direct object. However, its thematic role is the same as in the first sentence where it is not the direct object of the verb and its thematic role is signaled by a preposition. Such interrelationships between the conceptual argument structure of a verb and the (syntactic) surface realization of these arguments call for more complex mapping capacities than is entailed by the tasks generally designed for treatment.

REPAIR PROCESSES AND LANGUAGE THERAPY

As maintained in the previous section, treatment programs aimed at remediating disruptions in language processing cannot be designed without some hypothesis about the functional locus of the deficit. Information processing models provide a theoretical framework for setting up such hypotheses. But this is just one side of the coin. To benefit from a treatment program the patient must have the necessary processing capacities. The proponents of a model-based approach to therapy tend to evoke the impression that all patients with aphasic language impairments have retained the cognitive abilities to improve their residual language skills, given a proper analysis of the patient's language problems and the implementation of the appropriate approach to treatment.

Howard and Patterson (1989) distinguish between treatment approaches directed toward restoration of function, reconstitution of function, and facilitation of function. Neurologically, *functional restitution* is understood to be a restoration of the original function and is evidenced with functions that are widely distributed and organized with some redundancy (Singer, 1982). From this point of view, functional restitution in aphasia is limited to instances in which the patient has regained the ability to perform linguistic tasks according to the rules of the language system. Improved performance on a particular linguistic task cannot be taken as evidence that the respective rules of the language system are again available to the patient. Patient SP's improvement in reading aloud, resulting from his learning to sound out letters of written words, did not amount to a restoration of his premorbid reading ability. The patient continued to have difficulties when the letter pronunciation was context-dependent or when the sound corresponded to a complex grapheme-phoneme configuration. Only certain aspects of the functional deficit were "made up for"; a behavioral difference in performance may be discerned when comparisons are made with the pre-lesion state. The same arguments must be put forward in appraising the improvements achieved by the two patients BB and BRB who were treated for their sentence processing problems.

These three cases have been discussed by Howard and Patterson (1989) as examples of restitution of function brought about by the "patients' ability to relearn procedures that normally underlie the performance in question." Such an interpretation can be challenged. The observed improvements might well be the result of a response strategy developed by patients to solve the tasks with their residual processing abilities. We prefer to interpret the improvement of the three patients as the result of their ability to adapt to their processing impairments. Such adaptation can take various forms, depending on the nature of the deficit. With some deficits, functional improvement can be obtained by applying a one-to-one matching technique. When such a procedure is possible, there is little need to consider the rules of context-sensitivity, because the technique turns out to be rather effective. This was demonstrated by the patient SP in reading aloud and the patients BB and BRB in comprehending syntactically more structured sentences. However, not all deficits permit a context-free matching procedure. As soon as it becomes necessary to observe contextual selection restrictions, the technique becomes too taxing for many patients.

The term *reconstitution of function* refers to the ability of the patient to achieve some functional success with his or her remaining processing abilities by reorganizing function. Functional reorganization is conceptualized two ways: Preserved elements are either internally re-structured or lost cerebral links are replaced by the integration of intact functions that were not previously part of the damaged functional system. In either case, the "re-developed" functions (Luria, 1963) are only substitutes, which usually differ markedly from the original functions. The crucial question with regard to efforts at remediation is whether, in cases of language disruption, there are inherent limitations on the kind of functional substitution that is possible. Another way of putting the question is to ask whether some of the cognitive operations involved in natural language may persist in the presence of a severe aphasia.

To shed some light on the this conceptual issue Gardner, Zurif, Berry, and Baker (1976) explored the capacities of severely aphasic patients to circumvent their oral-aural communication deficits by acquiring a visual symbol system, known as VIC (Visual Communication). This symbol system consists of simple geometric forms with arbitrary meanings and simple line drawings of objects with representational meanings. Both types of symbols are drawn on individual cards. Basic semantic relations between the various symbols can be expressed by a linear arrangement of the cards. The authors distinguished two levels of use: At level 1, patients were taught how to carry out commands, answer questions, and describe events; and at level 2, patients were required to employ this alternative mode of communication more spontaneously to convey immediate needs and to express feelings. The patients selected for VIC training had little or no usable speech but demonstrated comprehension skills equivalent to the demands of level 1 and were able to match objects with ideographic drawings of the objects. The latter two screening conditions led to the elimination of seven of the 22 patients initially selected for treatment. Only five patients succeeded in mastering the basic properties of VIC, and only two of them satisfied the criteria for level 2 training.

The vexing question is whether the patients learned to use VIC only as a sort of language game rather than as a vehicle of communication. Both games and communication systems call for rule-governed behavior. When manipulating their component elements the subject must attend to specific conditions of use. A prerequisite for the successful use of a communicative system is the ability to code intended messages according to the rules of the system. It is this ability which appears to be lacking in aphasia — commensurate with the overall severity of the language disorder. Interestingly enough, of the two patients who attained level 2 performance with VIC, one had a lesion resulting from trauma and the other, who was left-handed, had a large left hemisphere lesion affecting predominantly prerolandic areas.

An earlier attempt (Glass, Gazzaniga, & Premack, 1973) to teach severely aphasic patients an alternative symbol system produced similar results. The symbols utilized by these authors were borrowed from studies of communication in chimpanzees. They consisted of geometric forms cut from paper and varying in size and color. Subjects received training aimed to teach them to use the symbols communicatively and to perform logical operations with them. Of the seven globally aphasic patients in the study, two progressed sufficiently to express and comprehend simple declarative statements. Certain cognitive abilities may be preserved in the face of severe language dysfunction. But can the cognitive operations underlying these abilities subserve the processing of a symbol system such as language?

More recent studies with a visual symbol system called Blissymbolics (Funnell & Allport, 1989; Johannsen-Horbach, Cegla, Mager, & Schempp, 1985; Sawyer-Woods, 1987) have supplied further evidence of the limited capacities of aphasic patients to acquire an alternative visual symbol system. As Funnell and Allport were able to demonstrate, whenever a patient succeeds in learning and using a particular visual symbol, the equivalent written word sharing the same conceptual base as the learned symbol is also available.

Aphasic patients' difficulties in acquiring an alternative symbol system are not restricted to the visual modality. Coelho and Duffy (1987, 1990) found a significant relationship between severity of aphasia and success in the acquisition of manual signs. The varying degrees of success with which manual signs are learned suggests that alternative nonverbal symbol systems tap the same cognitive abilities that are required for natural language processing. Aphasic patients are not only impaired in their use of language; they also display difficulties in nonverbal category decision tasks (e.g., categorization of pictured objects; see Cohen, Kelter, & Woll, 1980). It is when isolated features must be detected and integrated into larger contextual settings that processing problems arise. What appears to be impaired in aphasia is the capacity to process compound featural information. The alternative symbol systems that have been introduced as aids in circumventing expressive communication problems require the patient to assign some functional value to an arbitrary symbol and then to relate this functional value to a certain situational setting. If less arbitrary symbols were adopted perhaps greater communicative effectiveness could be achieved with a nonverbal symbol system. Pictographs appear to be less demanding symbols. They are simplified pictorial representations of objects occurring in common everyday situations and activities. We have set up a training program that exploits the iconicity of pictographs and is aimed at making patients aware of the functional relevance of the discriminating pictorial features of object drawings (Bertoni, Stoffel, & Weniger, 1991). The program proceeds from the receptive and expressive use of pictographs encountered in everyday life to the spontaneous production of line drawings in response to questions. The results of a pilot study have shown that pictographs are a promising aid in augmenting the communicative capacities of patients with little or no usable speech. Despite intensive treatment over a period of 18 months, a global aphasic patient, PC's spontaneous speech continued to be limited to the automatism *"ja."* When PC was first introduced to the pictograph training program he was hardly able to produce an intelligible drawing of a presented pictograph. In time, his drawings became more structured, and PC began modifying trained pictographs to convey messages of his own. To indicate that he was feeling better after having been ill for 5 days, he drew a row of five stick figures in horizontal position, separated by a vertical line from a stick figure in upright position (see Figure 12–2).

A notion which is associated with repair processes but not tied explicitly to any reorganizational mechanism is that of adaptation. It has its roots in Jackson's (1878–79) interpretation of a symptom. We are prone to analyze a patient's performance in terms of its deficiency, taking the impaired behavior as the more or less direct expression of the underlying deficit. But some symptoms that look like behavioral abnormalities are manifestations of the organism's struggle to cope with the deficit by resorting to an evolutionarily more primitive but intact processing mechanism. Jackson contrasts such symptoms which occur in a positive condition with the symptoms occurring in a negative condition (i.e., the damaged system) and "representing" the deficit. Heeschen (1985) has applied this concept of a symptom to the phenomenon of agrammatism (see also Kolk & Heeschen, 1990). The omission of grammatical morphology which characterizes agrammatic speech can be shown to reflect the adoption of elliptical speech, which is also used by nonaphasic speakers in certain contexts. To avoid sentence structures that exceed their available processing abilities, agrammatic patients frequently resort to formulations "within their reach." It is of particular significance that, when they phrase their utterances elliptically, they observe the rules of elliptical speech, differing from normal speakers only in the frequency with which they use this style of speech. Not all patients with sentence production problems change their style of speech to circumvent their processing difficulties. For example, patients with paragrammatic speech produce the same type of sentence constructions as before the onset of the illness due to a reduced ability to control for their erroneous speech production.

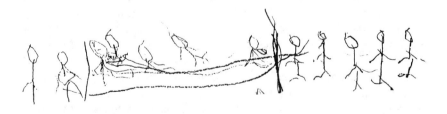

Figure 12–2. Drawing of the patient PC indicating that he was ill for 5 days.

The mechanized elements of speech that frequently occur in states of word-finding difficulties (the negative condition) are another example of the two-sidedness of a symptom. Unless words are chosen with some referential specificity, the hearer fails to capture the message the speaker is trying to convey. Not having words with the necessary referential specificity available, aphasic speakers tend to rely on the ability of the non-aphasic hearer to "catch on" to the intended message with the clues they are capable of offering. Interjections and deictic phrases are a common feature of the empty speech that characterizes the discourse of many fluent aphasic patients. Although such forms of expression lack referential specificity, they can help the listener identify the particular objects, properties, places, and events that the patient is trying to signal, provided the participants share sufficient background information.

Improvements in performance due to mechanisms of functional reorganization are to be distinguished from the effects of facilitating interventions. As the examples given illustrate, the retrieval of target words can be triggered by giving the patient an appropriate semantic or phonemic cue. Following Weigl's (1961) argument, the success of such cues rests on their potential to elicit a verbal response by "clearing" a functionally blocked pathway. The effect of deblocking techniques such as cuing is temporary. It disappears after some minutes but has been shown to persist for longer periods of time (hours, days) with appropriate stimulation. The phenomenon of deblocking is a physiological process and consists of breaking through the patient's raised threshold levels. The extent to which repeated activation of a given type of information can result in a longer lasting breakthrough is an unresolved issue. The differential effect of semantic and phonemic cues was pointed out in the previous section. The persistent treatment effects reported in the study with therapy materials that were aimed at inducing the patient to attend to certain structural features of the language system could result from specific arousal of threshold levels in a modular subsystem (see also Weniger, Springer, & Poeck, 1987).

NONLINGUISTIC IMPAIRMENTS AND LANGUAGE THERAPY

In setting goals for treatment, different types of information need to be considered. A model-based deficit analysis is certainly important in deciding which language problem is to be the focus of treatment. However, the assessed language disorders are often accompanied by additional impairments such as motor speech difficulties, short-term verbal retention disturbances, and reductions in cognitive flexibility. Such impairments, which are not intricately tied to the language system proper, can be masked by the more dominant disruptions of the language system that have been chosen for treatment; and they can affect the outcome of the linguistically motivated treatment approach.

Two examples of non-linguistic impairments that can influence performance on tests designed to assess language skills are presented in this section. The first example touches on the ability to set up a "plan" of the verbal utterance to be generated and is associated with what Luria (1970) has termed "dynamic aphasia."

In a recent study, de Lacy-Costello and Warrington (1989) examined the expressive language difficulties of the patient ROH. ROH could produce the names of depicted objects and actions, achieved satisfactory scores on tests of auditory as well as written word comprehension, and could repeat polysyllabic words, sentences, and cliches accurately and with normal articulation. His literacy skills were dull average with his reading somewhat better than his spelling. However, the patient's spontaneous speech was characterized by enormous problems in initiating speech and generating sentences; responses to questions were extremely sparse and very slow. In contrast to his relatively short onset latencies when naming objects from pictorial stimuli, ROH displayed slow response latencies in sentence and phrase completion tasks. When asked to produce a sentence containing a given word, the patient managed to generate grammatically complete sentences for only 13 of the 23 stimulus words. Comparable results were obtained when a sentence context was given and a second sentence had to be generated around the theme of this stimulus sentence; either a grammatically correct sentence followed the presentation of the stimulus sentence or there was a total absence of a response. But when presented with a pictorial context from which to generate a sentence, the patient succeeded in producing a sentence for 17 of the 18 pictures.

Pictorial prompts appear to have been more effective than verbal prompts in eliciting propositional speech. The authors attributed this finding to the fact that the pictorial stimuli provided the patient with a framework for organizing verbal output. The functional locus of this patient's difficulties in producing sentences lies in his impaired ability to generate a verbal plan on the basis of which a sentence can then be constructed. It is not knowledge about syntactic structuring and morphological processing that is deficient in patients like ROH. Therapeutic procedures must therefore be aimed at training such patients how to "find" a verbal plan. As has been suggested by Luria, Naydin, Tsvetkova, and Vinarskaya (1969), these patients need to be given some external aid to support them in their search for a sentence scheme. For example, to initiate the generation of a sentence scheme, patients are confronted with the

picture of a familiar everyday activity or event. Their first task is to identify the elements that constitute the central activity; then they are asked
to sequence the identified elements in such a way that the linear arrangement of the elements reflects the message conveyed by the picture.
Training consists of getting patients to look for an external pivot from
which a sentence scheme can be developed.

Let us now turn to the second example pertaining to impairments of
auditory-verbal short-term memory that have been associated with deficits of phonological encoding in aphasia (e.g., Allport, 1984; Friedrich,
Glenn, & Marin, 1984; Shallice & Warrington, 1977). It has been argued
(e.g., Howard & Franklin, 1990; Martin & Saffran, 1990) that the ability
to hold linguistic information briefly in store is a property of the processing mechanisms involved in language production and comprehension. It
might therefore be questioned whether verbal short-term memory is to
be conceptualized as a capacity extrinsic to the language system. On the
other hand, dissociations have been found between the comprehension
of sentences with reversible noun phrases and the ability to perform
simple comparative judgments (e.g., which is red, a poppy, or a head of
lettuce?) which involve the use of linguistic information in a subsequent
set of cognitive operations (McCarthy & Warrington, 1987). The two
aphasic patients who participated in this study displayed good comprehension of the individual words and relatively intact on-line processing
skills of verbal information. Their difficulties in performing the judgment tasks were therefore attributed to deficiencies in the capacity to
backtrack over spoken input. Auditory-verbal short-term memory is assumed to function as a backup resource which allows the individual to
"replay" the spoken input in subsequent attempts at constructing the
cognitive representation required by the demands of the task.

Impairments in this backup function of auditory-verbal short-term
memory may be detected on formal diagnostic testing by comparing the
performance of aphasic patients on the Token Test and on word-picture
matching tasks assessing auditory comprehension. The Token Test is
often used to assess auditory comprehension in patients with an aphasia.
The test was developed by De Renzi and Vignolo (1962) as a tool to tap
receptive disorders in aphasia. It consists of systematic arrangements of
20 tokens, varying in shape (squares and circles), size (large and small),
and color (red, yellow, blue, green, and white). The patient is asked to
identify the token indicated by the examiner. A more common way to
examine auditory comprehension abilities is to have patients match a
presented verbal stimulus with the corresponding picture in a choice set.
The distractors in the choice set are usually selected so that inferences
can be made about the functional locus of the processing deficit. Patients
with an aphasia of vascular etiology frequently show comparable levels

of performance in these two types of comprehension tests. However, marked differences in performance of some patients on the two tests can be found, with performance on the Token Test significantly more impaired.

HJ, a 50-year-old male biologist who sustained an infarct in the territory of the left middle cerebral artery in January 1985, had great difficulty with the instructions of the Token Test but performed the comprehension tasks of the Aachen Aphasia Test (AAT) (Huber, Poeck, Weniger, & Willmes, 1983; for a description of the test see Willmes, Poeck, Weniger, & Huber, 1983) with considerably fewer errors. His spontaneous speech was nonfluent and effortful, and contained numerous phonemic paraphasias; he was virtually unable to do confrontation naming, and his repetition was moderately impaired, with more omissions and semantically correct paraphrases as the length of the stimuli increased. His oral reading of real words was relatively preserved and was characterized by omissions and occasional phonemic substitutions. He could not read nonwords aloud, although he could distinguish them from real words quite reliably in lexical decision tasks. The patient appeared to be sensitive to the lexical status of phoneme strings. In writing to dictation, his errors consisted predominantly of omissions, the missing letters often being signalled by gaps between the written letters. Formal diagnostic testing was not possible until 2 months post-onset; the AAT was re-administered 19 months later. The patient achieved significantly better scores on all subtests except confrontation naming; his overall pattern of performance remained unchanged. His confrontation naming showed significant improvement when it was again assessed after 3 years. His poor performance on the Token Test persisted, whereas by this time he made only a few errors on the comprehension tasks of the AAT, which indicated that his lexical-semantic representations were relatively preserved.

The two tasks obviously entail different processing demands. Word-picture matching as required by the comprehension task involves two more or less sequentially organized processes: Access to the lexical-semantic representation of the presented verbal stimulus and then selection of a picture on the basis of the retrieved semantic information. Depending on the featural distinctions that have to be made in selecting the target picture, more precise semantic information needs to be retrieved. A correct solution is often possible with on-line retrieval of only fragmentary semantic information; with a certain amount of pragmatic intuition supported by the pictures in the given array, a reasonable guess can be made as to the target picture. The Token Test instructions are non-redundant and tied up with temporal constraints. If the on-line transcoding of a given instruction cannot be achieved within the time allotted by the processing system, the patient is forced to do some backtracking.

Unless the patient has access to a verbatim phonological record of the spoken instruction, backtracking is not possible.

One of HJ's problems lies in the impaired ability to retain access to the phonological form of spoken verbal input. This also becomes apparent in his repetition behavior. A comparably poor level of performance was observed on both the Token Test and the repetition subtest of the AAT. In repeating longer stimulus items, HJ frequently responded with a paraphrase of the auditorily presented word or sentence, suggesting that semantic information about a stimulus item was available. It might therefore be argued that the patient could have relied on lexical representations in accessing output phonology when the nonlexical route proved to be unsuccessful due to an inability to maintain a phonological record of the stimulus item. However, a pathological reduction in the activation of the phonological level of the production system appears to have made the lexical route less effective. Such an interpretation of the patient's repetition performance predicts that significantly lower test scores will be found in tasks that require spoken output than in tasks that do not. As can be seen in Table 12–1, this prediction is borne out by comparing the patient's test scores on confrontation naming and comprehension and repetition and comprehension. Also in agreement with the prediction is the patient's equally poor performance in repetition and confrontation naming.

Contrary to expectation, the patient did relatively well in reading aloud, and writing real words to dictation. In reading aloud, the ortho-

Table 12–1. Comparison of patient HJ's diagnostic test scores (Aachen Aphasia Test).

	Token Test	Repetition	Written Language	Confrontation Naming	Comprehension
Token Test		−3.04	−7.07*	−2.03	−13.36*
Repetition	34.79%		−4.03*	1.01	−10.32*
Written Language	11.41%	27.28%		5.04*	−6.29
Confrontation Naming	36.32%	43.54%	18.98%		−11.33*
Comprehension	2.68%	10.04%	17.66%	3.71%	

* significant difference (for an overall type I error of 10%, using the sequential multiple test procedure of Holm, 1979).
Note: The differences between the T-scores of the respective subtest scores are given on the upper half of the diagonal. On the lower half of the diagonal the probabilities are given for determining whether the T-score differences are diagnostically valid.

graphic form of the written words served as a reliable backup resource enabling HJ to reinforce activation of the nodes at the phonological output level. When writing to dictation a phonological trace of the stimulus word is again needed as a backup resource. But the transcoding process does not encompass the same temporal constraints as repetition. After spontaneously writing the initial two or three letters of the target word the patient added successive letters with much hesitation, and made errors predominantly at the end of words. It seems reasonable to assume that the patient's response behavior was guided by knowledge about possible orthographic word forms (letter combinations). To verify this assumption, the effects of word as well as letter transition frequencies would have to be examined.

Formal diagnostic testing of HJ revealed an impairment in the short-term retention of the phonological coding of speech input — in addition to difficulties in accessing the phonological output lexicon. In designing a treatment procedure for the patient's phonologically based word-finding difficulties, one cannot rely on short-term storage of phonological information. It is therefore rather unlikely that an approach aimed at activating the phonological forms of target words by aural stimulation would turn out to be successful. HJ does reasonably well in reading real words aloud and succeeds in writing the initial letters of target words. As has been demonstrated in a pilot study by Kremin et al. (1989), an improvement in the retrieval of the phonological form of target words can be achieved by training patients with considerable residual written language skills to use spelling information in retrieving word forms. Of particular relevance for a theory of rehabilitative interventions is whether the subsequently observed improvement of oral naming is the outcome of some restored access to output phonology from the semantic system. It might well reflect the acquired technique of producing an object name orally via its written form.

CONCLUDING COMMENTS

For the individual struck by an aphasia, the sudden loss of language represents not only a handicap in the use of language, it also places restrictions on numerous everyday activities. Most aphasic patients therefore will grasp the opportunities offered to reduce the impact of the language disorder. For both patients and therapists the goal of rehabilitative interventions lies in the improvement of impaired language functions and, consequently, spontaneous communicative skills. But there is a major difference in their prime concerns: Patients will content themselves with the feeling that treatment has worked; for the therapist the outcome of treatment raises the question of why the adopted approach worked or failed. The main concern of this chapter was to outline some of the issues that must be considered when determining the goals of treatment. Identifying the functional locus of a patient's linguistic processing deficits is just one side of the coin. In trying to set up a treatment program that promises some success, the other side of the coin, the neurological residuals, cannot be ignored. This has led us to the following schematic summary of rehabilitative interventions in aphasia.

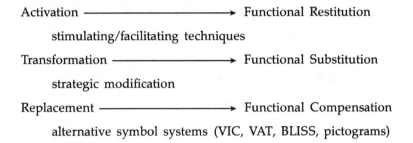

Activation ⟶ Functional Restitution

    stimulating/facilitating techniques

Transformation ⟶ Functional Substitution

    strategic modification

Replacement ⟶ Functional Compensation

    alternative symbol systems (VIC, VAT, BLISS, pictograms)

ACKNOWLEDGMENT

The authors wish to acknowledge the financial support of the Swiss Science Foundation (Grant No. 3.828-0.86).

REFERENCES

Allport, D. A. (1984). Auditory-verbal short term memory and aphasia. In H. Bouma & D. G. Bouwhuis (Eds.), *Attention and performance. X: Control of language processes* (pp. 313–325). Hillsdale, NJ: Lawrence Erlbaum.

Allport, D. A. (1985). Distributed memory, modular subsystems and dysphasia. In S. Newman & R. Epstein (Ed.), *Current perspectives in dysphasia* (pp. 32–60). Edinburgh: Churchill Livingstone.

Badecker, W., & Caramazza, A. (1985). On considerations of method and theory governing the use of clinical categories of neurolinguistics and cognitive neuropsychology: The case against agrammatism. *Cognition, 20,* 97–125.

Bertoni, B., Stoffel, A.-M., & Weniger, D. (1991). Communicating with pictographs: A graphic approach to the improvement of communicative interactions. *Aphasiology, 5,* 341–353.

Blumstein, S. E., Milberg, W., & Shrier, R. (1982). Semantic processing in aphasia: Evidence from an auditory lexical decision task. *Brain and Language, 17,* 301–315.

Bradley, D. C., Garrett, M. F., & Zurif, E. B. (1980). Syntactic deficits in Broca's aphasia. In D. Caplan (Ed.), *Biological studies of mental processes* (pp. 269–286). Cambridge, MA: M.I.T. Press.

Bruce, C., & Howard, D. (1987). Computer-generated phonemic cues: An effective aid for naming in aphasia. *British Journal of Disorders of Communication, 22,* 191–201.

Byng, S. (1988). Sentence processing deficits: Theory and therapy. *Cognitive Neuropsychology, 5,* 629–676.

Caramazza, A., & Berndt, R. S. (1985). A multicomponent deficit view of agrammatic Broca's aphasia. In M.-L. Kean (Ed.), *Agrammatism* (pp. 27–63). New York: Academic Press.

Caramazza, A., & Hillis, A. E. (1989). The disruption of sentence production: Some dissociations. *Brain and Language, 36,* 625–650.

Caramazza, A., & Hillis, A. E. (1990). Where do semantic errors come from? *Cortex, 26,* 95–122.

Coelho, C. A., & Duffy, R. J. (1987). The relationship of the acquisition of manual signs to severity of aphasia: A training study. *Brain and Language, 31,* 328–345.

Coelho, C. A., & Duffy, R. J. (1990). Sign acquisition in two aphasic subjects with limb apraxia. *Aphasiology, 4,* 1–8.

Cohen, R., Engel, D., Kelter, S., & List, G. (1979). Kurz- und langzeiteffekte vonbBenennhilfen bei aphatikern. In G. Peuser (Ed.), *Studien zur sprachtherapie* (pp. 350–360). Munich: Wilhelm Fink.

Cohen, R., Kelter, S., & Woll, G. (1980). Analytical competence and language impairment in aphasia. *Brain and Language, 10,* 331–347.

Damasio, A. R. (1990). Category-related recognition defects as a clue to the neural substrates of knowledge. *Trends in Neurosciences, 13,* 95–98.

de Lacy-Costello, A., & Warrington, E. (1989). Dynamic aphasia: The selective impairment of verbal planning. *Cortex, 25,* 103–114.

de Partz, M. P. (1986). Re-education of a deep dyslexic patient: Rationale for the method and results. *Cognitive Neuropsychology, 3,* 149–177.

De Renzi, E., & Vignolo, L. A. (1962). The Token Test: A sensitive test to detect receptive disturbances in aphasics. *Brain, 85,* 665–678.

Fillmore, C. J. (1971). Types of lexical information. In D. D. Steinberg & L. A. Jakobovits (Eds.), *Semantics: An interdisciplinary reader in philosophy, linguistics and psychology* (pp. 370–392). London: Cambridge University Press.

Friedrich, F., Glenn, C., & Marin, O. (1984). Interruption of phonological coding in conduction aphasia. *Brain and Language, 22,* 266–291.

Funnell, E., & Allport, A. (1989). Symbolically speaking: Communicating with blissymbols in aphasia. *Aphasiology, 3,* 279–300.

Gardner, H., Zurif, E. B., Berry, T., & Baker, E. (1976). Visual communication in aphasia. *Neuropsychologia, 14,* 275–292.

Garrett, M. F. (1976). Syntactic processes in sentence production. In R. Wales & E. Walker (Eds.), *New approaches to language mechanisms* (pp. 231–256). Amsterdam: North Holland.

Garrett, M. F. (1982). Production of speech: Observations from normal and pathological language use. In A. W. Ellis (Ed.), *Normality and pathology in cognitive functions* (pp. 19–78). London: Academic Press.

Glass, A. V., Gazzaniga, M. S., & Premack, D. (1973). Artificial language training in global aphasia. *Neuropsychologia, 11,* 95–103.

Gleason, J. B., Goodglass, H., Green, E., Ackerman, N., & Hyde, M. R. (1975). The retrieval of syntax in Broca's aphasia. *Brain and Language, 2,* 451–471.

Goodglass, H., Gleason, J. B., Bernholtz, N. A., & Hyde, M. R. (1972). Some linguistic structures in the speech of a Broca's aphasic. *Cortex, 8,* 191–212.

Grober, E., Perecman, E., Kellar, L., & Brown, J. (1980). Lexical knowledge in anterior and posterior aphasics. *Brain and Language, 10,* 318–330.

Gruber, J. S. (1965). *Studies in lexical relations.* Bloomington: Indiana Linguistics Club.

Heeschen, C. (1985). Agrammatism and paragrammatism: A fictitious opposition. In M. L. Kean (Ed.), *Agrammatism* (pp. 207–248). New York: Academic Press.

Hillis, A. E., & Caramazza, A. (1991). Mechanisms for accessing lexical representations for output: Evidence from a category-specific semantic deficit. *Brain and Language, 40,* 106–144.

Hillis, A. E., Rapp, B. C., Romani, C., & Caramazza, A. (1990). A selective impairment of semantics in lexical processing. *Cognitive Neuropsychology, 7,* 191–244.

Holm, S. (1979). A simple sequentially rejective multiple test procedure. *Scandinavian Journal of Statistics, 6,* 65–70.

Howard, D., & Franklin, S. (1990). *Dissociations in short-term memory.* Paper presented at the Attention and Performance Meeting.

Howard, D., & Orchard-Lisle, V. (1984). On the origin of semantic errors in naming: Evidence from the case of a global aphasic. *Cognitive Neuropsychology, 1,* 163–190.

Howard, D., & Patterson, K. (1989). Models of therapy. In X. Seron & G. Deloche (Eds.), *Cognitive approaches in neuropsychological rehabilitation* (pp. 39–64). London: Lawrence Erlbaum.

Howard, D., Patterson, K., Franklin, S., Orchard-Lisle, V., & Morton, J. (1985). The facilitation of picture naming in aphasia. *Cognitive Neuropsychology, 2,* 49–80.

Huber, W., Poeck, K., Weniger, D., & Willmes, K. (1983). *Der Aachener Aphasietest.* Göttingen: Verlag fr psychologie Dr. J. C. Hogrefe.

Jackendoff, R. (1972). *Semantic interpretation in generative grammar.* Cambridge, MA: M.I.T. Press.

Jackendoff, R. (1983). *Semantics and cognition.* Cambridge, MA: M.I.T. Press.

Jackson, H. (1878–79). On the affections of speech from disease of the brain. *Brain, 1,* 304–330.

Johannsen-Horbach, H., Cegla, B., Mager, U., & Schempp, B. (1985). Treatment of chronic global aphasia with a nonverbal communication system. *Brain and Language, 24,* 78–82.

Jones, E. V. (1986). Building the foundations for sentence production in a nonfluent aphasic. *British Journal of Disorders of Communication, 21,* 63–82.

Kay, J., & Ellis, A. (1987). A cognitive neuropsychological case study of anomia. *Brain, 110,* 613–629.

Kay, J., & Patterson, K. (1985). Routes to meaning in surface dyslexia. In K. Patterson, J. Marshall, & M. Coltheart (Eds.), *Surface dyslexia* (pp. 79–101). London: Lawrence Erlbaum.

Kean, M.-L. (1977). The linguistic interpretation of aphasia syndromes: Agrammatism in Broca's aphasia, an example. *Cognition, 5,* 9–46.

Kean, M.-L. (1979). Agrammatism: A phonological deficit? *Cognition, 7,* 69–83.

Kohn, S. E., & Goodglass, H. (1985). Picture naming in aphasia. *Brain and Language, 24,* 266–283.

Kolk, H., & Heeschen, C. (1990). Adaption symptoms and impairment symptoms in Broca's aphasia. *Aphasiology, 4,* 221–231.

Kremin, H., Larroque, C., Metz-Lutz, M. N., Perrier, D., Pichard, B., Quint, S., Cardebat, D., Deloche, G., Dordain, M., Ferrand, I., & Hannequin, D. (1989). The relation(s) between oral and written output for naming: Experimental evidence from aphasia rehabilitation. *Journal of Clinical and Experimental Neuropsychology, 11,* 355–356 (abstract).

Linebarger, M. C., Schwartz, M. F., & Saffran, E. M. (1983). Sensitivity to grammatical structure in so-called agrammatic aphasics. *Cognition, 13,* 361–392.

Luria, A. R. (1963). *Restoration of function after brain injury.* London: Pergamon Press.

Luria, A. R. (1970). *Traumatic aphasia.* The Hague: Mouton.

Luria, A. R., Naydin, V. L., Tsvetkova, L. S., & Vinarskaya, E. N. (1969). Restoration of higher cortical function following local brain damage. In P. J. Vinken & G. W. Bruyn (Eds), *Disorders of higher nervous activity* (pp. 368–433). Amsterdam: North-Holland.

Martin, N., & Saffran, E. M. (1990). Repetition and verbal STM in transcortical sensory aphasia: A case study. *Brain and Language, 39,* 254–288.

McCarthy, R. A., & Warrington, E. K. (1987). Understanding: A function of short-term memory? *Brain, 110,* 1565–1578.

Miceli, G., Silveri, M. C., Romani, C., & Caramazza, A. (1989). Variation on the pattern of omissions and substitutions of grammatical morphemes in the spontaneous speech of so-called agrammatic patients. *Brain and Language, 36,* 447–492.

Milberg, W., & Blumstein, S. E. (1981). Lexical decision and aphasia: Evidence for semantic processing. *Brain and Language, 14,* 371–385.

Patterson, K., & Coltheart, V. (1987). Phonological processes in reading: A tutorial review. In M. Coltheart (Ed.), *The psychology of language* (pp. 421–447). London: Lawrence Erlbaum.

Patterson, K., Purell, C., & Morton, J. (1983). Facilitation of word retrieval in aphasia. In C. Code & D. J. Muller (Eds.), *Aphasia therapy* (pp. 76–87). London: Arnold.

Pease, D. M., & Goodglass, H. (1978). The effects of cueing on picture naming in aphasia. *Cortex, 14,* 178–189.

Saffran, E. M. (1982). Neuropsychological approaches to the study of language. *British Journal of Psychology, 73,* 317–337.

Saffran, E. M., Schwartz, M. F., & Marin, O. S. M. (1980). The word order problem in agrammatism: II. Production. *Brain and Language, 10,* 263–280.

Sawyer-Woods, L. (1987). Symbolic function in a severe non-vebal aphasic. *Aphasiology, 1,* 287–290.

Seidenberg, M. S. (1988). Cognitive neuropsychology and language: The state of the art. *Cognitive Neuropsychology, 5,* 403–426.

Shallice, T. (1987). Impairments of semantic processing: Multiple dissociations. In M. Coltheart, R. Job, & G. Sartori (Eds.), *The cognitive neuropsychology of language* (pp. 111–127). London: Lawrence Erlbaum.

Shallice, T. (1988). *From neuropsychology to mental structure.* London: Cambridge University Press.

Shallice, T., & Warrington, E. K. (1977). Auditory-verbal short-term memory impairment and conduction aphasia. *Brain and Language, 4,* 479–491.

Singer, W. (1982). Recovery mechanisms in the mammalian brain. In J. G. Nicholls (Ed.), *Repair and regeneration of the nervous system* (pp. 203–226). Berlin: Springer Verlag.

Tissot, R. J., Mounin, G., & Lhermitte, F. (1973). *L'agrammatisme.* Brussels: Dessart.

von Stockert, T. R., & Bader, L. (1976). Some relations of grammar and lexicon in aphasia. *Cortex, 12,* 49–60.

Weigl, E. (1961). The phenomenon of temporary deblocking in aphasia. *Zeitschrift fur phonetik, sprachwissenschaft und kommunikationsforschung, 14,* 337–364.

Weniger, D., Springer, L., & Poeck, K. (1987). The efficacy of deficit-oriented therapy materials. *Aphasiology, 1,* 215–222.

Willmes, K., Poeck, K., Weniger, D., & Huber, W. (1983). Facet theory applied to the construction and validation of the Aachen Aphasia Test. *Brain and Language, 18,* 259–276.

Zurif, E. B., Caramazza, A., & Myerson, R. (1972). Grammatical judgements of agrammatic aphasics. *Neuropsychologia, 10,* 405–417.

Zurif, E. B., Caramazza, A., Myerson, R., & Galvin, J. (1974). Semantic feature representation for normal and aphasic language. *Brain and Language, 1,* 167–187.

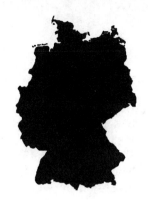

CHAPTER 13

Psychosocial Aspects on the Treatment of Adult Aphasics and Their Families: A Group Approach in Germany

HELGA JOHANNSEN-HORBACH
CONNY WENZ
School of Speech Therapy Freiburg
MATTHIAS FUNFGELD
Department of Psychiatry
University of Freiburg
MANFRED HERRMANN
Department of Rehabilitation Psychology
University of Freiburg
CLAUS-W. WALLESCH
Department of Neurology
University of Freiburg

Chronic aphasia results in considerable psychosocial changes and stress, both for the affected person and his or her relatives and for those close to them (Artes & Hoops, 1976; Bowling, 1977; Herrmann & Wallesch, 1989; Kinsella & Duffy, 1978, 1979). According to Matsumoto, Whisnant, Kurland, and Okasaki, (1973), fewer than 10% of aphasic stroke patients are professionally reintegrated, in comparison to one third of all stroke victims. Early retirement leads to loss of income and social status as well as to a restriction of social contacts. These changes affect both patients and their relatives. Within the family, social roles change and family members—in most instances wives—are faced with problems and tasks that were previously the aphasic person's responsibility (e.g., monetary matters). In addition, relatives encounter changes and impairments in the patient's mental and social capacities: Lack of endurance, concentration, and spontaneity; aggressiveness; resignation; irritability; cognitive impairment; depression; and sometimes confusion (for details, see Herrmann & Wallesch, 1989).

Wenz and Herrmann (1990) conducted a detailed investigation of emotional reactions and illness perception in 10 chronic aphasics and one relative of each patient. They found that the subjective impairment and the resulting emotional stress were independent. Whereas aphasic patients perceived little change with respect to interactions within the family and considered it a relief to be involved in a partnership, patients' relatives noted considerable changes within the family and complained about their own depressed mood. These findings strongly suggest that the psychosocial needs of aphasic individuals and their relatives differ considerably (Schulz, Tompkins, & Rau, 1988); thus, different psychotherapeutic strategies may be appropriate for each. Furthermore, the data of Schulz et al. (1988), and Tompkins, Schulz, and Rau (1988), indicate a variety of differences in the therapeutic needs of older compared with younger relatives.

PSYCHOTHERAPY FOR THE APHASIC AND HIS FAMILY

Divergent psychosocial requirements must be considered if the aphasic individual is treated within the family environment rather than in isolation. There appear to be different causes of emotional stress and different perceptions of the stability of the interaction within the family, as well as widely differing communication abilities. These factors render traditional family therapy approaches (Norlin, 1986; Rollin, 1984; Wahrborg, 1989) of questionable value for the treatment of psychosocial stress in families in which one member suffers from chronic aphasia. Herrmann (1989) suggested that a family system that includes an aphasic person is difficult to interpret in terms of traditional family therapy. The family therapy program outlined by Wahrborg (1989) for use in "aphasic families" is a communication-oriented treatment that integrates the family and focuses on communication within the family. Thus, the term "family communication training" might be very appropriate. However, we agree with Norlin (1986) that strategies taken from family therapy may be used for crisis intervention when aphasia is acute or when an acute change has taken place within the family (e.g., release from hospital).

On a more basic level, reports on the effect of family counseling (Derman & Manaster, 1967; Turnblom & Myers, 1952) and of integrating family members into therapy (Florance, 1979; Lesser, Bryan, Anderson, & Hilton, 1986) indicate that "family support" and behavioral changes on the part of the nonaphasic family members exert a positive influence on outcome. The possible advantages of such approaches must be weighed against the disadvantages of assigning the role of "co-therapist" to the spouse, thus altering the social equilibrium in the family even more in favor of its nonaphasic members.

Beyond attempts at recruiting family support to promote the goals of speech therapy, fundamental differences in the perception of emotional needs and the resultant stress (Wenz & Herrmann, 1990) indicate that some form of psychotherapy or professional counseling is required for both the chronic aphasic person and his or her partner. In consideration of these factors, we decided to offer psychosocially oriented group counseling to both patients and relatives, but separately. Figure 13–1 gives an overview of the divergent perceptions aphasics and their relatives have of the aphasic patient's illness.

Data from a study of illness perception and emotional reactions in chronic aphasics and their relatives indicated that relatives perceive their own depressive reaction as the most stressing factor (Wenz & Herrmann, 1990). The emotional burden of the relatives is greatly underrated by the aphasics, who view their family and partnership as the most consoling factor with respect to their own coping.

PSYCHOSOCIAL ASPECTS IN APHASIA REHABILITATION

Before outlining our therapeutic approach and its results, we will consider its status within a rehabilitation framework. With respect to the consequences of disease, the World Health Organization (1980) defined the three levels of impairment, disability, and handicap:

Impairment denotes a deviation from biomedical norms (e.g., anatomical, physiological, psychiatric, psychological). Impairments in aphasic patients include language, neuropsychological, and motor deficits.

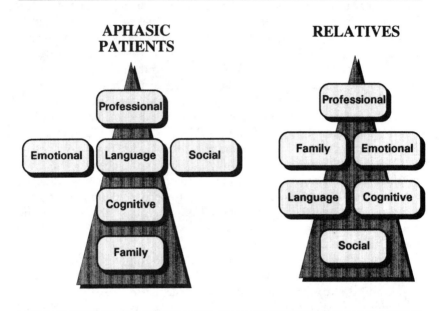

Figure 13–1. Hierarchy of perceived changes in various domains of functions.

Disabilities are secondary to impairments and include deficits of abilities and skills resulting from maladaptations and inadequate coping strategies that disturb social integrity and function. Such maladaptations may occur, for example, in the communicative strategies of aphasic patients.

Handicap denotes a social category as the third level of consequences of chronic disease, that is, the consequences of the impairment in a given social context. This level includes, for example, the social isolation of aphasic patients (and their families).

Based on this concept of level of deficits, the goals of a comprehensive medical-psychosocial rehabilitation would consist of:

1. training of residual capacities;
2. training of compensatory strategies; and
3. prevention of secondary and tertiary deficits (disabilities and handicaps) and promotion of social integration and emotional adaptation.

Therefore, aphasia rehabilitation would include language oriented, communication oriented, and psychosocially oriented approaches. Although all three levels are integral parts of our therapeutic strategy in the outpatient clinic of the Freiburg School of Speech Therapy, we will discuss only the psychosocially oriented aspects in the following sections.

A PSYCHOSOCIALLY ORIENTED GROUP APPROACH WITH CHRONIC APHASIC INDIVIDUALS

Most of the patients and their relatives who participate in psychosocially oriented groups have previously received individual speech and communication therapy for a long period of time (more than 1 year). They would have received therapy based on the neurolinguistic approach of the Aachen group (Springer & Weniger, 1980; Weniger, Huber, Stachowiak, & Poeck, 1980 and also described in Chapter 3) or communication oriented treatment, such as PACE (Davis & Wilcox, 1981, 1985). The strategies for group interactions are oriented along the lines of nondirective counseling (Rogers, 1942, 1959).

Our psychosocial group therapy approach for aphasics focuses on aspects of coping with the disease and its consequences at the levels of impairments, disabilities, and handicaps. We perceive coping as a process of both deficit perception and compensation, that includes individual psychosocial stresses and individual capacities to overcome deficits and burdens and to recruit social resources. The coping mechanisms depend on the individual's life situation.

In our opinion, age and age-related aspects of social structure are overwhelmingly important factors, which influence not only psychosocial status but also coping strategies and rehabilitation outcome (Tompkins et al., 1988). The intra-family interactions of older aphasics are well-established, and disintegration is unlikely. In most instances, both patient and spouse are able to accept the fact that advancing age may bring chronic impairment of one partner. In younger couples, on the other hand, the nonaffected member frequently perceives the illness of the other as a threat to his or her own expectations and may leave. Because of the different psychosocial situations and threats, we decided to offer two groups, one for younger and one for elderly aphasic patients.

The elderly group consisted of four males and three females who were 60 to 80 years old and who had suffered from aphasia for 2 to 5 years. Table 13–1 gives clinical and demographic data. The group protocol included three elements:

1. free interaction and exchange with psychosocial burdens and their emotional impact as the main topic;

Table 13-1. Profile of patients participating in the group of elderly aphasics.

Patient	Sex	Age	Years Post- onset	Profession	Life Situation	Clinical Diagnosis
1	M	80	4	civil servant	widowed	nonclassifiable (nonfluent)
2	M	73	2	civil servant	married	minimal aphasia
3	M	60	4	architect	married	severe Broca's
4	M	76	5	craftsman	married	severe Broca's
5	F	63	3	housewife	married	mild Broca's
6	F	68	3	housewife	widowed	Wernicke's
7	F	78	2	housewife	married	minimal deficit

2. elements from communication oriented therapy strategies such as PACE (Davis & Wilcox, 1981, 1985), pantomime, and topic-centered debates; and
3. tasks from a neuropsychological memory training program with verbal and visual material.

The group met once a week for 2 hours with a psychologist and a speech therapist, one of whom took notes. Over time, the free interaction gained weight and importance, and the patients increasingly included other topics, such as holiday events, experiences from the aphasics' self-help group, and everyday problems related to various impairments, such as arm paresis.

More than half of the patients raised the topic of an illness of their partner, which allowed them to express their own fears of being left alone or of dying. The group became an increasingly important social outlet for its members. Once the members of the elderly group got to know one another, communication problems ceased to be a relevant limitation to interaction. In this respect, the elderly group was quite different from the younger group, in which communication deficits posed a major obstacle to reaching the therapeutic goal. In the older group, therapeutic activities could be faded out; the group continued to meet with one therapist, who observed the group process.

The second group consisted of younger aphasics, five females and three males, who were 26 to 51 years old and who had suffered from aphasia for 2 to 11 years. Table 13-2 gives clinical and demographic data.

The younger group's protocol also included elements of free interaction. Because of the severe communication deficits of some group members (patients 4, 5, and 6), the communicative aim was oriented less to

Table 13–2. Profile of patients participating in the group of younger aphasics.

Patient	Sex	Age	Years Post-onset	Profession	Life Situation	Clinical Diagnosis
1	M	46	11	jeweler	divorced	Broca's
2	M	43	4	ambulance driver	with partner	Wernicke's
3	M	29	2	student	with partner	minimal deficit
4	F	29	5	ex-student	with partner	severe Broca's
5	F	51	5	housewife	married	severe Broca's
6	F	39	7	secretary	single	Broca's
7	F	26	2	ex-student	with partner	Broca's
8	F	36	2	educator	with partner	minimal deficit

discourse, and more to action. The two therapists played a more active role than in the older group. Group development could be subdivided into three stages.

The first phase contained role plays of everyday situations, such as shopping, dining out, business in a bank or insurance company office, or asking for information or help. The therapeutic goal at this stage was a more differentiated perception of the patient's own behavior and that of others as well as increasing awareness of situational obstacles. The group was encouraged to find a common position with respect to situational analysis and assessment. At this stage, the group was faced with the following difficulties:

1. *Communication impairment.* For example, key words were missing from statements, word-finding deficits resulted in utterance termination, or fluent aphasics could not communicate the intended message.
2. *Interactional impairment.* The central problem at this level was a lack of listener-oriented communication. That is, participants did not use non- or para-verbal communicative acts sufficiently to hold the attention of the listener.
3. *Psychological impairment.* This included intentional, attentional, emotional, and cognitive aspects of behavior. The patients tended to evade topics that were difficult to comment on or were controversial, or they terminated communication. Even patients suffering from minimal residual aphasia adopted this behavior as a strategy to avoid revealing their deficits.

These three levels of impairment tended to preclude the modification of behavior that should be based on experiences from role playing. Therefore, the next phase of group treatment focused on communication skills. The training was based on a simplified model of communication, consisting of a sender, a message, and a receiver. In the context of a group of aphasics of different degrees of impairment, the sender was required to use various verbal and nonverbal channels of communication, frequently in combination, in order to achieve comprehension. This skill was trained using elements of PACE (Davis & Wilcox, 1985), pantomime, and deliberate and conscious use of codified, symbolic and descriptive gesture (Herrmann, Reichle, Lucius-Hoene, Wallesch, & Johannsen-Horbach, 1988).

On the level of the message, the aphasics were required to analyze the elements that were crucial for understanding. Therapeutic tasks included formulating a telegram or selecting the critical elements from a complex story.

The aphasics analyzed the communication situation and concluded that the receiver played a crucially important role. The patients practiced holding the receiver's attention by, for example, maintaining eye contact and averting the loss of their conversational turn by using stereotyped phrases such as "hold on," "I need some more time," or "please, don't interrupt me."

The third phase aimed at applying these communicative skills in everyday life situations. Again, role-plays were used, now focusing on situations that had led to overload and termination in the first phase. They were performed with a normally speaking co-therapist, and the role-playing was videotaped. The videos were evaluated and analyzed by the group to identify crucial aspects, suboptimal communicative behavior, and ways of modification and improvement. The group developed individualized communication goals. For example:

1. A mildly impaired patient was to aim at better control of speed of productions by reducing speech rate during critical arguments;
2. A person with fluent aphasia was to develop a plan for an intended message before speaking; and,
3. One person with Broca's aphasia was instructed to keep eye contact to preclude interruption. Another was instructed to try to take the initiative in conversation.

Due to the severe illness of one member and the death of the spouse of another, the elderly group had to discontinue after 16 sessions, and later resumed with two new members. The younger group met 22 times. Only during the last sessions were the emotional and psychosocial aspects of coping, such as the impact of disease on individual life situations, discussed. However, these discussions were never as extensive as they were in the elderly group. We assume that social heterogeneity, a greater degree of social isolation in comparison to the elderly group and a less objective view of impairment and future prospects of some members (patients 5, 6, and 7) contributed to this delay in group interaction.

Our protocols of the group sessions do not allow statistical evaluation. However, a number of observations seem important. One positive aspect of group participation was that the protected atmosphere of the groups allowed the development and testing of new behavioral strategies. Both groups contributed to increases in patients' competence and performance and thus to a higher—or more realistic—degree of self-esteem. Our expectation that groups could be used to focus on individual psychosocial stresses and then to share these concerns with others was fulfilled only in the elderly group.

The difference in the respective group processes supports our initial decision to separate the groups according to age, and not according to aphasia type or severity. Most elderly patients were able to accept disability and could focus on its psychosocial consequences. Sharing these burdens with others had a stabilizing and relieving effect. Most younger patients, on the other hand, could accept neither their deficits nor the consequences of them. They were oriented more toward direct treatment of their deficits and only occasionally, and in the last sessions, raised the topic of psychosocial consequences on their own. We assume that the willingness to share psychosocial burdens with others in itself constitutes a stage in the process of overcoming these burdens. Therefore, it is an important aspect of compliance with rehabilitation and group therapy strategies.

We could not maintain, as was initially intended, the nondirective role of the therapist. Group communication requires that each member has a turn and that each member's comprehension is assured. At least in the initial phase, the therapist's guidance was required to accomplish this.

Especially in the younger group, avoidance strategies were a major problem for group interaction. The patients tended to avoid difficult or controversial topics. This led to incorrect perception of communicative competence (Helmick, Watamori, & Palmer, 1976) and contributed to social isolation. The topics of "(non-) acceptance" and "avoidance" in younger patients could perhaps better be addressed in individual psychotherapy than in a group. However, few strategies exist for psychotherapy with aphasic subjects.

A PSYCHOSOCIALLY ORIENTED GROUP APPROACH WITH RELATIVES OF CHRONIC APHASIC PATIENTS

As has been pointed out, aphasia in one member affects the whole family. The relatives, although not socially perceived as ill or disabled, suffer from a considerable degree of handicap as defined by the World Health Organization (1980). These handicaps are perceived and rated as severe. Therefore, we decided to offer a group for relatives.

The following approaches have been advanced for counseling of relatives of aphasic patients:

1. Family therapy (Derman & Manaster, 1967; Turnblom & Myers, 1952; Wahrborg, 1989);
2. Expert-directed counseling (Mykyta, Bowling, Nelson, & Lloyd, 1978); and,
3. "Non-directive" adaptation (Mulhall, 1978).

The aphasic's family is under severe stress, but its psychodynamic basis is usually not pathological. This, together with the imbalance in the means of communication, in our view rules out a family therapeutic approach in the strict sense. Expert counseling was intentionally kept separate from the group experience in order not to interfere with interaction on psychosocial aspects.

We chose the approach of an open, nondirective, client-centered group based on Rogers (1942, 1959). The therapist is cautioned to refrain from the role stereotypes of expert, leader, judge, caretaker, or therapist and from directing or guiding the group process. Instead, the therapist's role is to be empathic and accepting.

In September 1989, we invited 17 close relatives of chronic (more than 18 months post-onset) aphasics to an informal meeting. Interestingly, no relative under 40 years of age even responded to the invitation. Six spouses and one mother declined.

The group started with six and consolidated with three members. It met every fortnight for 1½ hours for 14 sessions. Table 13–3 gives demographic data for the group members and clinical data for the aphasic relatives.

Table 13–3. Profile of constant members of the relatives' group.

Member	Age (in years)	Occupation	Aphasic relative
Mrs. Sch.	55	former clerk	Mr. Sch., 61 yrs, former engineer, global aphasia for 28 months
Mrs. G.	62	former accountant	Mr. G., 78 yrs, former engineer, Wernicke's aphasia for 22 months
Mr. St.	68	former master baker	Mrs. St., 64 yrs, housewife, Wernicke's aphasia for 18 months

The therapeutic staff consisted of a psychologist trained in counseling and a speech therapist. Both were instructed to assume the role of passive hosts. The group progressed through three phases.

Contrary to our expectations, information concerning the illness, its prognosis, and therapy became the focus that dominated the first three sessions. Although this information had been supplied during the acute phase of the aphasic relatives' illness, the relatives seemed not to have had an opportunity to organize and accept it. Secondly, the relatives' illness constituted the only common ground for interaction in this phase. The group imposed the role of informed experts on the therapists, who were unable to remain passive during this stage.

The second stage, another three sessions, was characterized by increasing perplexity on the part of the relatives. They realized that they had no role model for dealing with the tearful outbursts of other participants, other than the social stereotype of ignoring them. When feelings overwhelmed one member, the others tended to change the subject. At this stage, the members questioned the purpose of the group and asked about the function of the psychologist. This gave the therapists an opportunity to present and discuss the group's concept and goals.

This discussion led to the third phase, comprising the remaining eight sessions. The group developed interaction strategies that allowed each member to give and receive attention for his or her or the others' needs. They learned to offer empathy and accept grief. Pauses, which had previously led to a change of topic, became acceptable, and their emotional content was shared. Only in this stage could the therapists remain passive and nondirective.

The group interaction in this phase focused on the following topics:

1. Problems with the patients' aggressiveness and changes of affect.
2. Not being able to leave the patient alone even for short periods of time.
3. Loss of social contacts, such as withdrawal of friends.
4. Own burdens and feelings.

In this phase, two of the members were able to alter their attitudes toward the aphasic patient and gain insight into their own feelings and requirements.

Mrs. Sch. learned to talk about her own stresses and felt relief at being able to shed tears. In the last sessions she was able to express her anger about the limitations the disability of her husband had brought for herself. Finally, she decided to seek psychotherapeutic aid.

Mr. St. maintained a "stiff upper lip" attitude ("one has to accept"), but became more flexible and open toward his own needs. He could reduce the fears that had not allowed him to leave his wife alone at all, and he looked for social contacts with other aphasic couples and with the self-help group.

Mrs. G. remained quite controlled ("you must not forget yourself"), and assumed the role of consoler and counselor in the group. She remained unable to express her own grief and fears. She terminated her participation when her husband died. We believe that she then assumed the socially acceptable role of the widow, which probably relieved her burdens.

This group demonstrates that an open, client-centered group for relatives of aphasics offers them an opportunity to express their own griefs, burdens, and fears. It also helps them to perceive their own feelings and needs, and thus may lead to relief and psychological stabilization. The experience may help members to progress from the exceptional state of emergency implied in being the "relative of someone severely disabled" to a state of individual normality. Our experience indicates that such a group requires a directive and therapist-guided initial phase.

THE RELATIVES' NEEDS

Before starting a second group of relatives, we decided to determine the relatives' psychosocial and therapeutic needs in more detail. We conducted a survey of seven chronic (more than 18 months duration) aphasics' relatives (six female, one male) concerning emotional stress resulting from disease symptoms and preferred partners to discuss these burdens. In parallel, the respective speech therapists were questioned about their assumptions concerning the relatives' responses. Both groups were asked to rank symptoms and preferred communication partners.

Figure 13–2 shows the rank order of symptoms of emotional stress. Whereas the relatives perceived aggressiveness, language deficit, depression, and changing moods as most stress producing, the therapists focused on motor and language impairment and their direct consequences. The strong impact of affective alterations was underestimated by the speech therapists.

The differences in perceptions were even greater with respect to ranking preferred communication partners with whom the relatives discussed their burdens (Figure 13–3). Whereas the therapists expected them to prefer the family doctor, the relatives expressed a wish for psychotherapy. None of them, however, had taken any steps to receive psychotherapy. Neither the self-help group nor relatives of other aphasics were considered particularly promising. This may explain why the relatives'

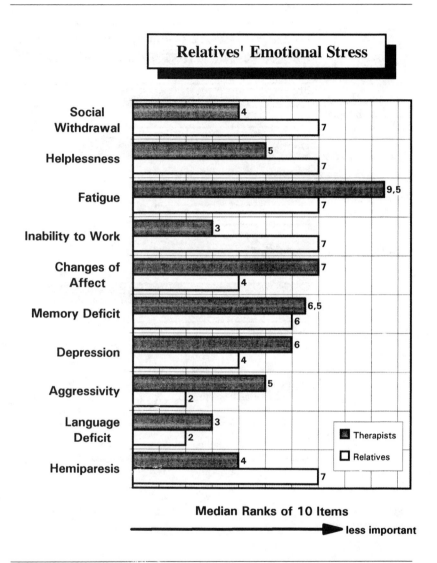

Figure 13-2. Relatives' emotional stress compared with therapists' assumptions.

group described above required a "warming-up" phase of six sessions. Furthermore, the relatives' statements clearly indicated that they wanted to keep discussion of their own burdens separate from the family.

When we asked the relatives what they thought would help them most, the majority responded, "If I could talk openly about my own problems."

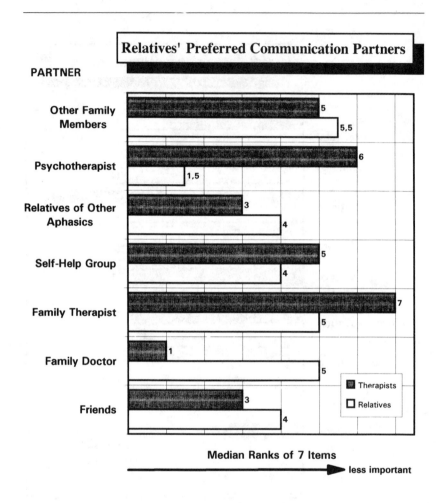

Figure 13–3. Relatives' preferred communication partners compared with therapists' assumptions.

In summary, the relatives perceived and suffered from psychosocial burdens. They also perceived a need for psychotherapy, but did not find ways or means to obtain it. Although they did not view interaction with other relatives of aphasics as promising, a relatives' group can contribute to clarifying their personal situation and stresses, and thus may help them to find adequate psychotherapy. However, psychosocially oriented individual psychotherapy techniques for relatives of aphasics have not yet been developed. We assume that the client-centered counseling approach of Rogers (1942, 1959) might be helpful for their particular life situation and its burdens. On the other hand, with more information and experience with respect to the therapeutic potential of a group setting, the relatives might decide to continue a therapeutic group. Family therapy might counteract the explicit wish of the relatives to keep their own emotional and psychosocial burdens apart from the family.

REFERENCES

Artes, R., & Hoops, R. (1976). Problems of aphasic and nonaphasic stroke patients as identified and evaluated by patients' wives. In Y. Lebrun & R. Hoops (Eds.), *Recovery in aphasia* (pp. 31–45). Amsterdam: Swets & Zeitlinger.

Bowling, J. H. (1977). Emotional problems of relatives of dysphasic patients. *Australian Journal of Communication Disorders, 5*, 29–41.

Davis, G. A., & Wilcox, J. (1981). Incorporating parameters of natural conversation in aphasia treatment. In R. Chapey (Ed.), *Language intervention strategies in adult aphasia* (pp. 169–193). Baltimore, MD: Williams & Wilkins.

Davis, G. A., & Wilcox, J. (1985). *Adult aphasia rehabilitation.* San Diego, CA: College-Hill Press.

Derman, S., & Manaster, A. (1967). Family counselling with relatives of aphasic patients at Schwab Rehabilitation Hospital. *ASHA, 9*, 175–177.

Florance, C. (1979). The aphasic's significant other: Training and counseling. In R. Brookshire (Ed.), *Clinical aphasiology conference proceedings.* Minneapolis: BRK Publishers.

Helmick, J. W., Watamori, T. S., & Palmer, J. M. (1976). Spouses' understanding of the communication disabilities of aphasic patients. *Journal of Speech and Hearing Disorders, 41*, 238–243.

Herrmann, M. (1989). On the possible value of family therapy in aphasia rehabilitation. *Aphasiology, 3*, 491–492.

Herrmann, M., Reichle, T., Lucius-Hoene, G., Wallesch, C. W., & Johannsen-Horbach, H. (1988). Nonverbal communication as a compensative strategy for severely nonfluent aphasics: A quantitative approach. *Brain and Language, 33*, 41–54.

Herrmann, M., & Wallesch, C. W. (1989). Psychosocial changes and psychosocial adjustment with chronic and severe nonfluent aphasia. *Aphasiology, 3*, 513–526.

Kinsella, G., & Duffy, F. D. (1978). The spouse of the aphasic patient. In Y. Lebrun & R. Hoops (Eds.), *The management of aphasia* (pp. 26–49). Amsterdam: Swets & Zeitlinger.

Kinsella, G., & Duffy, F. D. (1979). Psychosocial readjustment in the spouses of aphasic patients. *Scandinavian Journal of Rehabilitation Medicine, 11*, 129–132.

Lesser, R., Bryan, K., Anderson, J., & Hilton, R. (1986). Involving relatives in aphasia therapy: An application of language enrichment therapy. *International Journal of Rehabilitation Research, 9*, 259–267.

Matsumoto, N., Whisnant, J. P., Kurland, L. T., & Okasaki, H. (1973). Natural history of stroke in Rochester, Minnesota, 1955–1969. *Stroke, 4*, 20–29.

Mulhall, D. J. (1978). Dysphasic stroke patients and the influence of their relatives. *British Journal of Disorders in Communication, 13,* 127–134.

Mykyta, L. J., Bowling, J. H., Nelson, D. A., & Lloyd, E. J. (1976). Caring for the relatives of stroke patients. *Age and Aging, 5,* 87–90.

Norlin, P. F. (1986). Familiar faces, sudden strangers: Helping families cope with
the crisis of aphasia. In R. Chapey (Ed.), *Language intervention strategies in adult
aphasia* (2nd ed.). Baltimore, MD: Williams & Wilkins.

Rogers, C. R. (1942). *Counseling and psychotherapy.* Boston: Houghton Mifflin.

Rogers, C. R. (1959). A theory of therapy, personality and interpersonal relationships as developed in the client-centered framework. In S. Koch (Ed.), *Psychology: A study of a science* (Vol. 3). New York: McGraw-Hill.

Rollin, W. J. (1984). Family therapy and the aphasic adult. In J. Eisenson (Ed.),
Adult aphasia (2nd ed.). Englewood Cliffs, NJ: Prentice-Hall.

Schulz, R., Tompkins, C. A., & Rau, M. T. (1988). A longitudinal study of the psychosocial impact of stroke on primary support persons. *Psychology and Aging,
3,* 131–141.

Springer, L., & Weniger, D. (1980). Aphasietherapie aus logopadisch-linguisti-
scher Sicht. In G. Bohme (Ed.), *Therapie der sprach-sprech- und stimmstorungen*
(pp. 190–207). Stuttgart: Fischer.

Tompkins, C. A., Schulz, R., & Rau, M. T. (1988). Post-stroke depression in primary support persons: Predicting those at risk. *Journal of Consulting and Clinical Psychology, 56,* 502–508.

Turnblom, M., & Myers, J. S. (1952). Group discussion programs with the families of aphasic patients. *Journal of Speech and Hearing Disorders, 17,* 393–396.

Wahrborg, P. (1989). Aphasia and family therapy. *Aphasiology, 3,* 479–482.

Weniger, D., Huber, W., Stachowiak, F. J., & Poeck, K. (1980). Treatment of aphasia on a linguistic basis. In M. T. Sarno & O. Hook (Eds.), *Aphasia, assessment
and treatment.* Paris: Masson.

Wenz, C., & Herrmann, M. (1990). Emotionales erleben und subjektive krank-
heitswahrnehmung bei chronischer aphasie—ein vergleich zwischen patient-
en und deren familienangehorigen. *Psychotherapie, Psychosomatik, Medizinische
Psychologie, 40,* 488–495.

World Health Organization. (1980). *International classification of impairments, disabilities, and handicaps.* Geneva: WHO.

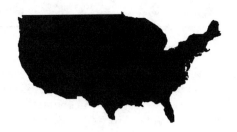

CHAPTER 14

Clinical Intervention for Aphasia in the United States of America

RICHARD K. PEACH

Departments of Otolaryngology,
Neurological Sciences and
Communication Disorders & Sciences
Rush University
Rush Presbyterian-St. Luke's Medical Center
Chicago, Illinois

This chapter provides an American perspective regarding the clinical management of aphasia. Similar to the charge given to all contributors to this volume, the editors have sought a practical overview of clinical aphasiology in the United States by asking me to provide a summary of my approach to aphasia rehabilitation. It should be stressed, therefore, that mine is not *the* American perspective on aphasia treatment, but simply one which has developed from the many influences that have been prominent in this country over approximately the past two decades and the personal experiences that have shaped my own philosophies with regard to clinical practice with this population.

To provide an historical context for what follows, it might be helpful to describe some of these personal experiences and how they relate to the contemporary practice of clinical aphasiology in America. My intent, of course, is not to provide a complete chronology of the clinical developments in the field during the period. Rather, I will highlight the particular achievements in clinical aphasiology to which I have received significant exposure and which, as a result, have provided an important background to my particular approach to this area. I will also assume that these experiences are similar in many respects to those of other practitioners who were trained in the clinical art of aphasia management during the same period in the United States.

Inasmuch as my formal training in clinical aphasiology began in 1975, I will focus on some important events in the early to late 1970's. At that time, not surprisingly, Dr. Hildred Schuell's stimulation approach (Schuell, Jenkins, & Jiminez-Pabone, 1964), which was developed over many years at the Minneapolis Veterans Administration Hospital, was the predominant approach to the treatment of aphasia, perhaps as it continues to be now. The conceptual bedrock of this approach emphasized a unidimensional character of aphasia, that is, all language modalities are impaired in approximately the same manner and to the same degree following aphasia (Duffy, 1986). Two of the most popular assessment instruments in use at that time, the *Minnesota Test for the Differential Diagnosis of Aphasia* (Schuell, 1965) and the *Porch Index of Communicative Abilities* (PICA) (Porch, 1967) reflected this orientation in their construction and schemes for classification of aphasic patients. However, the *Boston Diagnostic Aphasia Examination* (BDAE) (Goodglass & Kaplan, 1972) also had been published about this time, bringing with it an emphasis on aphasia syndromes associated with specific neuropathological profiles (e.g., Broca's aphasia, Wernicke aphasia, conduction aphasia). Most certainly, the approach was not a new one but, rather, brought existing principles of aphasia classification as practiced more frequently in other disciplines, such as neurology, into the mainstream of aphasia diagnosis. It has since become fairly common for clinicians to develop treatment plans based in large part on procedures adopted from the stimulation approach while describing their patients in ways that are consistent with the Boston system of aphasia classification.

Having attended Memphis State University, I had the opportunity to study with Dr. G. Albyn Davis. Several important research projects focusing on the speech acts of aphasic individuals, which would have a significant impact on the practice of clinical aphasiology, were in progress at Memphis State and the Memphis Veterans Administration Hospital during this period. Dr. Audrey Holland completed a major portion of the activities related to her development of the functional communication assessment instrument *Communicative Abilities in Daily Living (CADL)* (Holland, 1980) at these sites. Dr. M. Jeanne Wilcox, a doctoral student at that time, and Davis used speech act theory (Searle, 1969) as a framework for investigating language production in aphasic individuals and describing more adequately the communication abilities of these patients (Wilcox & Davis, 1977). A second study, conducted by these researchers and Dr. Laurence Leonard, also utilized speech act theory to describe the auditory comprehension of aphasic patients in more natural contexts than those found in situations involving standardized testing (Wilcox, Davis, & Leonard, 1978). These seminal studies provided the background for the development of a new treatment program called *Promoting Aphasics' Communicative Effectiveness* or *PACE* which, unlike most other treatment approaches, incorporated elements of natural face-to-face conversation (Davis, 1980; Davis, 1986; Davis & Wilcox, 1981, 1985; Wilcox & Davis, 1978, 1979). Until this time, formal assessment instruments that considered the pragmatic aspects of aphasic individuals' language were limited generally to Sarno's *Functional Communication Profile* (1969). The development of the CADL for assessment and the PACE program for treatment of aphasia signaled a renewed emphasis on the role of functional abilities in aphasia management. Since that time, each of these procedures has gained widespread acceptance and become an important part of many aphasia clinicians' armamentaria.

Several other significant events occurred during this period with regard to clinical aphasiology in the United States. Dr. Bruce Porch convened the Clinical Aphasiology Conference (CAC) for the first time in 1971 in Albuquerque, New Mexico; my first opportunity to participate in CAC was in 1978. Although originally conceived as a forum dedicated primarily to an exchange of ideas regarding the PICA and aphasia assessment, CAC has grown over these years, expanding its scope to include the full range of issues related to the clinical management of patients whose communication impairments result from language or other cognitive disorders secondary to brain damage (Wertz, 1991). Since its inception, the conference has had considerable influence on aphasia rehabilitation not only in the United States, but in many other countries as well. Support for this claim is found in the more than 75 data-based articles focusing on aphasia treatment which have been published in *Clinical Aphasiology* (Horner & Loverso, 1991). Included among these articles are descriptions and applications of such programs as Cuing Verb Treatments (Loverso, Prescott, Selinger, & Riley, 1989; Loverso, Prescott, Selinger, Wheeler, & Smith, 1985; Loverso, Selinger, & Prescott, 1979; Prescott, Selinger, & Loverso, 1982; Selinger, Prescott,

Loverso, & Fuller, 1987) and Response Elaboration Training (Kearns, 1985; Kearns & Potechin-Scher, 1989; Kearns & Yedor, 1991) among others. Now in its twenty-second year, CAC continues to provide the foremost colloquium in this country for the discussion of clinical research relating to aphasia.

Also during this period, Dr. Nancy Helm-Estabrooks and her colleagues at the Boston Veterans Administration Medical Center developed the first of several therapy programs designed specifically for certain subgroups of aphasic patients. These included Melodic Intonation Therapy (MIT) for severely nonfluent patients (Albert, Sparks, & Helm, 1973; Sparks, Helm, & Albert, 1974) and Visual Action Therapy (VAT) for global aphasia (Helm & Benson, 1978) to which I was exposed respectively during graduate training in 1976 and during a Veterans Administration traineeship in 1980. Since that time, the list of specific therapy programs has grown to include Voluntary Control of Involuntary Utterances (Helm & Barresi, 1980), the Helm Elicited Language Program for Syntax Stimulation (Helm-Estabrooks, Fitzpatrick, & Barresi, 1981), Back to the Drawing Board (Morgan & Helm-Estabrooks, 1987), Treatment of Aphasic Perseveration (Helm-Estabrooks, Emery, & Albert, 1987), and Treatment for Wernicke's Aphasia (Helm-Estabrooks & Albert, 1991). One of the important contributions these programs have made to clinical aphasiology in the United States is to focus attention on the efficacy of aphasia treatment programs for specific groups of patients (Peach, 1992).

The views of Dr. Gerald Canter, with whom I studied at Northwestern University in 1979, were another major influence, especially as they related to the articulatory behavior of aphasic adults. Between 1970 and 1977, Canter and two of his doctoral students at Northwestern, Judith Trost and Martha Burns, completed and published two studies identifying important distinguishing perceptual characteristics of apraxia of speech and phonemic paraphasia (Burns & Canter, 1977; Trost & Canter, 1974). Their findings were used to suggest that apraxia of speech is primarily the result of a disturbance in encoding phonological patterns into speech movements whereas phonemic paraphasia results from an impairment in the retrieval of phonological word patterns (Canter, Trost, & Burns, 1985). Given the terminological confusion at that time for surface articulatory disorders, the conclusions from these studies played a significant role in clarifying the nature and symptoms of these two disorders. In this way, the findings also made noteworthy contributions to the differential diagnosis and treatment of these disorders (Tonkovich & Peach, 1989).

There have been many other significant contributions in clinical aphasiology since these developments appeared during the 1980s. Although these contributions are too numerous to describe in detail, it seems appropriate to mention the evolution of computer applications as an important development in aphasia treatment during this time, especially given the current role of technology in rehabilitation. Although software programs for aphasia treatment have proliferated, there are several notable examples of programs in the United States which have been subjected to experimental analysis and, as a result, demonstrated to be effective. These programs include the reading, written confrontation naming, and spelling programs developed by Katz and his colleagues (Katz & Nagy, 1982, 1984, 1985; Katz & Wertz, 1992; Katz, Wertz, Davidoff, Shubitowski, & Devitt, 1988; Katz, Wertz, Lewis, Esparza, & Goldojarb, 1991). Also, computer-aided visual communication (C-ViC), a treatment program using an alternative visual symbol system for patients with no speech output, has been shown to be an effective tool for patients whose communication skills would otherwise be severely limited (Steele, Weinrich, Kleczewska, Carlson, & Wertz, 1987; Steele, Weinrich, Wertz, Kleczewska, & Carlson, 1989; Weinrich, Steele, Carlson, Kleczewska, Wertz, & Baker, 1989; Weinrich, Steele, Kleczewska, Carlson, Baker, & Wertz, 1989). These programs represent viable methods of using technology to facilitate the process of aphasia rehabilitation. There can be little doubt that the clinical management of aphasia in the future will continue to capitalize on these trends to maximize treatment outcomes.

Each of these developments influenced my practice in aphasia rehabilitation. Their effects will be noticeable as I describe my perspectives on aphasia treatment. The discussion will be organized in terms of three factors that I consider in choosing an aphasia treatment methodology: (a) the time since onset of the aphasia, (b) the nature or goals of the intervention, and (c) the type and severity of the aphasia. In practice, these factors more often than not interact to influence treatment decisions rather than presenting as mutually exclusive conditions. In this context, however, I will highlight some of the unique ways in which each of these factors may influence decisions in planning for intervention.

TIME SINCE ONSET OF APHASIA

Diverse sets of management issues confront clinicians providing aphasia treatment during the acute, subacute, and chronic phases of recovery. Treatment provided during these periods tends to be offered under different models of service delivery. Expectations vary when the service is provided in an acute inpatient health care institution (hospital), an inpatient rehabilitation facility, a long-term inpatient health care institution, an outpatient rehabilitation facility, in the patient's home, or in any of a variety of other service settings. Whether aphasia treatment is provided in one or another of these settings is dependent on, in most instances, the time that has elapsed since the onset of the patient's aphasia.

PHASES OF RECOVERY

Services provided during the acute period will usually be provided in an acute care hospital. Treatment will tend to be intensive, lasting approximately 1 to 3 weeks and consisting of more than one visit per day. Treatment sessions may be of shorter duration initially (15–20 minutes) and gradually increase in length based on the level of the patient's medical stability. As the patient approaches discharge, services may be provided on a schedule of one to two visits per day for a duration of 30–60 minutes per session. At approximately 3 to 4 weeks post-onset or at the time of discharge, the patient might be said to enter a subacute phase. Should the patient be transferred to an inpatient rehabilitation facility, the schedule attained at the end of the acute phase is likely to be maintained and integrated into a full regimen of therapeutic activities. Generally, the estimated length of stay for an uncomplicated rehabilitation stay might be 2 weeks to 2 months. Following this period, the patient enters a chronic phase of recovery at approximately 3 months post-onset where he or she may be discharged to the home to return to the hospital or rehabilitation unit for aphasia treatment on an outpatient basis or may be declared homebound and receive services in the home. Patients who are too sick to return home and require 24-hour skilled nursing may be discharged to a long-term inpatient health care facility (nursing home). In each of these chronic settings, aphasia treatment is likely to be provided perhaps two to three times per week for approximately 60 minutes per session. As treatment approaches termination, services may be reduced to one visit per week to facilitate maintenance of skills acquired previously, and upon dismissal, consist of follow-up visits once every few months as deemed appropriate.

TREATMENT CONSIDERATIONS

The nature of the aphasia treatment, be it primarily stimulatory, compensatory, or varying in degrees of both (see below), is affected in large measure by the patient's phase of recovery which, as approximated above, is related to the time post-onset of aphasia. During the acute phase, the severity of the patient's aphasia will be greatest and, depending on the degree to which the aphasia renders the patient unable to communicate even the most basic of needs, will necessitate that the first goals of treatment focus on establishing some basic means of communication, no matter how simple. Whether one considers the methods to accomplish this as stimulatory or compensatory might well rest on the choice of the medium through which this is accomplished. If the clinician attempts to establish reliable yes/no responding (Collins, 1990) or a basic vocabulary of functional items that are conveyed orally, the treatment would appear to be emphasizing stimulatory methods. Conversely, if the clinician attempts to achieve the same goals through gestural means such as head nodding, eye blinking, or pointing to pictures or specific icons, the treatment would be more compensatory in nature.

Although one of the goals of treatment during the acute phase may be to provide an immediate means of basic communication, the overwhelming focus generally is on remediation of language deficits via stimulation of disrupted cognitive processes to improve long-term outcomes. At times, it may be suggested that stimulation treatment be delayed during the acute period to observe the effects of spontaneous recovery before initiating language intervention. Such an approach is contradicted by clinical studies which indicate that patients who are treated during the acute and subacute phases of recovery have a better chance of improving than those who begin treatment later (Wertz, 1983). Hence, stimulation treatment during the acute phase should not be delayed, nor should it defer to strictly compensatory approaches while awaiting language outcomes at approximately 2 months post-onset before setting future goals for patient management.

During the subacute phase, aphasia treatment is most likely to consist of stimulation approaches which are geared toward long-term improvement of language. The clinical bias at this juncture is to provide a structured context for successful, graded language behaviors which in turn promote language utilization of an increasingly complex nature through the assumedly preferred auditory-verbal modalities. Put simply, the clinician is focused on language responses at successive levels that will ultimately build upon one another to help the patient understand and speak better.

During this period, few clinicians elect to focus their efforts on purely compensatory approaches to the treatment of their aphasic patients. Compensatory approaches are designed to ameliorate language performance in deficient areas which are not expected to recover even in the presence of language stimulation or facilitation. They are the methods of choice, therefore, when there is limited, if any, potential for language recovery in the areas of deficit. However, reliable prediction of language outcome remains elusive due to many factors, not the least of which is patient heterogeneity. Beyond the most obvious of prognostic factors such as the severity of aphasia, it is frequently difficult to know which of similar patients will or will not demonstrate good improvement. Until such factors are more completely understood with regard to the way they influence aphasia treatment and language outcome, clinicians will continue to use the reasonable approach of applying stimulation methods in aphasia management during the subacute period when measurable progress can be observed. This will be the case (a) so long as clinicians honor the rights of patients to have the opportunity for rehabilitation, regardless of their potential for recovery, or (b) until more powerful methods of predicting language outcome are developed.

Naeser and her colleagues at the Boston Veterans Administration Medical Center have reported findings which are beginning to provide these predictive methods. Using scaling techniques developed to assess the amount of infarction in different neuroanatomical areas identified by CT scans at 2 to 3 months post-onset (Naeser, Gaddie, Palumbo, & Stiassny-Eder, 1990; Naeser, Helm-Estabrooks, Haas, Auerbach, & Srinivasan, 1987; Naeser, Palumbo, Helm-Estabrooks, Stiassny-Eder, & Albert, 1989), these investigators have identified lesion profiles during the subacute phase that are highly suggestive of the type of outcome a patient will demonstrate in the areas of auditory language comprehension and spontaneous speech production. The neuroanatomical areas associated with these language outcomes include Wernicke's area and the temporal isthmus for recovery of auditory language comprehension and the medial subcallosal fasciculus and middle one third of the periventricular white matter for recovery of spontaneous speech production. Naeser (1991) and colleagues have extended these profiles to predict which patients will respond positively or negatively to specific verbal or nonverbal treatment programs such as Melodic Intonation Therapy and Computer-aided Visual Communication Therapy (C-ViC). The thrust of this work is that clinicians now have data to make treatment decisions regarding the selection of verbal (stimulatory) versus nonverbal (compensatory) treatment programs during the subacute phase that will be consistent with predicted long-term outcomes. As a result, efficiency and accountability of aphasia treatment can be expected to improve for patients who demonstrate severe deficits in auditory comprehension and spontaneous speech production. Although CT scan approaches to predicting outcome are not yet completely accurate, they do provide one of the most powerful, contemporary methods for treatment planning, especially as it relates to the quandaries of selecting stimulatory or compensatory treatment programs during this phase of recovery.

Long-term language deficits are most apparent during the chronic phase of recovery (beyond 3 months post-onset). Treatment during the early portions of this period continues to be primarily stimulatory based on continued spontaneous recovery to approximately 6 months post-onset (Darley, 1982; Rosenbek, LaPointe, & Wertz, 1989) and the desire to take advantage of cerebral reorganization and its positive effects on language functioning during this time. Beyond the latter portions of the first year post-onset, aphasia treatment will likely have taken on a decidedly compensatory approach. These approaches may take a variety of forms which may be categorized generally as those that involve (a) training of more efficient and/or effective strategies and (b) substitution of nonverbal communication modes for impaired verbal modes. Examples of techniques that emphasize training strategies include matrix training for increasing phrase length (Loverso & Milione, 1992), nonconfrontational naming activities such as practical lexical accessing and priming to decrease naming impairments (Holland, 1991), and increasing use of contingent queries for improving auditory comprehension (Rosenbek et al., 1989). Techniques that emphasize substitution of nonverbal communication modes include PACE therapy (Davis & Wilcox, 1985), drawing therapy (Lyon & Sims, 1989), gestural treatment (Skelly, 1979), communication boards (Collins, 1990), and C-ViC (Steele et al., 1989). These and other approaches will be described further in the next section.

THE NATURE OF TREATMENT

Once the clinician has considered relevant factors such as time post-onset to determine the degree to which treatment will be primarily stimulatory or compensatory, aphasia intervention may be implemented using approaches that satisfy these general objectives. In this section, some viewpoints are described with regard to each general rubric.

STIMULATION TECHNIQUES

Stimulation techniques utilize structured methods which are carefully controlled for levels of difficulty to provide a context that will facilitate successful language responses and shape succeeding language behaviors of increasing complexity. Schuell (Jenkins, Jiminez-Pabon, Shaw, & Sefer, 1975) described treatment planning for these techniques in the following way:

> It is always necessary to begin at the level where language breaks down for each patient, and to proceed systematically from easier to more difficult tasks. A good method may fail if materials are too easy or too difficult at a given time. The patient should build from success to success at gradually increasing levels of complexity. (p. 307)

Given the basic role of auditory-verbal association in language processing, stimulation treatment begins with intensive auditory stimulation, as advocated by Schuell, and comprises the primary modality through which treatment is provided to all aphasic patients regardless of the type or severity of the aphasia. Auditory input is often enhanced by pairing each stimulus simultaneously with its counterpart in another modality, (e.g., pictorial, gestural, graphic).

In designing the task continuum for treatment, a number of factors which are considered to increase complexity for the various language activities are manipulated both within and between treatment levels. These factors include the type of task, the size of the response field, the frequency of occurrence of lexical items, the number of modalities through which information is presented, the number and types of cues provided to the patient, the semantic relatedness of the stimuli, the processing demands imposed within the task, the length of the stimuli, and the number of different syntactic or semantic representations associated with the stimuli. All factors will not always apply simultaneously in the commission of a given task. Others will cluster together because of the characteristics of a task. These factors are discussed in the context of the tasks that might be used to treat specific areas of deficit within each of the broad categories of language impairment following aphasia.

At each level of treatment within or between tasks, baseline measures are collected to establish stability in the patient's performance before initiating treatment. This information is used subsequently to assess the efficacy of treatment for particular behaviors. I adopt a fairly standard criterion for moving from one level of treatment to the next. That criterion is usually 85 to 90% accuracy over two consecutive sessions for any given task unless specific circumstances dictate otherwise. I also attempt to select comparable sets of stimuli from a larger corpus of items and rotate the specific stimuli within a task from session to session to minimize the effects of improvement due to simple learning. Treatment probes are incorporated to assess the generalization of treatment effects to untreated stimuli or behaviors.

Due to the restrictions imposed by the space limitations of this volume, I will confine my remarks to approaches for the treatment of auditory comprehension and verbal expressive disturbances. Although treatments for disturbances of naming, reading and writing are integral components of aphasia treatment, they will not be covered here. The reader is referred to the works of Gonzales-Rothi, Raymer, Maher, Greenwald, and Morris (1991) and Rosenbek et al. (1989) for treatment of naming disturbances; Gonzales-Rothi and Moss (1992), Rosenbek et al. (1989), Webb (1990), and Webb and Love (1986) for treatment of reading disturbances; and Hillis (1992), McNeil and Tseng (1990), and Rosenbek et al. (1989) for treatment of writing disturbances. Also, because computerized treatment "appears more appropriate for improving reading and writing than for treating auditory comprehension and oral expressive language" (Rosenbek et al., 1989, p. 269), the reader is referred to Katz (1986; also see above referenced works) for a description of procedures that can be used to treat reading and writing disturbances via this medium.

Auditory Comprehension

Auditory comprehension tasks are included in the treatment plan for all of my aphasic patients. This applies naturally for patients who demonstrate observable auditory language comprehension deficits. But it also includes patients for whom auditory comprehension appears to be relatively preserved or even clinically intact on formal test batteries or in conversation. Clinical investigations designed specifically to probe the auditory processing of sentences or narratives that vary along such dimensions as syntactic complexity, semantic reversibility, or contextual support have consistently demonstrated that even mildly aphasic patients have difficulties with these and other materials (Peach, Canter, & Gallaher, 1988; Pierce & Grogan, 1992). Therefore, using tasks that are sensitive to the wide range of comprehension impairments which may be found following aphasia, evidence can be found to support the inclusion of auditory comprehension treatment in all aphasic cases.

For auditory comprehension, I give first consideration to the different types of tasks used to stimulate these processes: Matching pictures, recognizing words, sequencing items, answering questions, and following directions. Depending on the degree of comprehension impairment, treatment may focus exclusively on this modality using a full range of tasks such as those listed above or may be limited to only tasks that are commensurate with the patient's area(s) of deficit. For the most severe comprehension deficits, picture matching, accompanied by the clinician's production of the name of the items to be matched, may provide the most basic level of auditory stimulation. Even in cases where the patient has no understanding of the auditory stimulus accompanying the pictures, it is assumed that the response elicited by the matching task evokes auditory representations of the visual stimuli which may underlie subsequent association of meaning with the name of the pictures. Complexity may be increased within this task by (a) increasing the size of the response field (i.e., beginning with matching one picture to its counterpart from among 2 or 3 choices and increasing to matching from among 10 choices); (b) moving from pairing real objects to realistic pictures of objects to line drawings of the objects; (c) matching objects to pictures and pictures to objects, a technique that is incorporated in Visual Action Therapy (Helm-Estabrooks & Albert, 1991; Helm-Estabrooks,

Fitzpatrick, & Barresi, 1982); and (d) using sets of pictures that represent nouns with decreasing frequency of occurrence in language usage.

Word recognition by object, picture, or body part identification is also used with patients whose auditory comprehension is severely impaired. Task complexity can be increased in several ways. The first method would encompass varying objects or pictures and the response fields to the appropriate extent as in the matching tasks described above. Another is achieved by providing the stimuli through multiple modalities and then withdrawing one input at a time until the patient receives the stimulus through the auditory modality only. In a related vein, cues provided through multiple modalities can also be used to control task complexity. For example, the name of an object might be presented initially with a verbal description and gesture of the function of that object. These cues may then be withdrawn one at a time until the patient meets criterion when provided the name of the picture only. Of course, multiple levels within this one task can be constructed by combining both of these approaches (i.e., providing multimodal stimuli and cues and systematically withdrawing each to attain an auditory-only condition for picture identification). Then, the semantic relatedness of the stimuli within the response field can be used to increase complexity by moving from pictures that are classified in different semantic categories in the above levels to pictures that are from the same semantic category or categories. Once it has been established that the patient can recognize single words to criterion levels in a response field as large as 10 items and perhaps from among semantically related items, 1 use one or both of two methods to increase the depth of lexical processing for such items and, as a result, the strength of their verbal associations. The first method consists of imposing a delay between the presentation of the stimulus and the patient's response. The delay might be 3 seconds initially and then be lengthened systematically to perhaps 10 seconds or more to increase complexity within this task. The second method would consist of identifying sequences of two or three stimuli. After achieving criterion levels of performance on this task, varying lengths of delay may again be imposed to increase stimulus processing.

In addition to word recognition tasks, patients receive concurrent auditory comprehension treatment by responding to simple questions. These questions are limited to yes/no responses so as not to allow response contamination as a result of expressive disturbances. The form of the questions usually requires affirmation or denial of some information that has been presented. The information may be personal ("Do you have red hair?"), relate to recent events ("Did you eat lunch?") or the environment ("Is the door closed?"), or be based on general knowledge ("Do you use a comb to brush your teeth?"). The complexity of the questions is increased by the number of critical units of information that are required for full comprehension. So, complexity is increased by moving from questions with one critical unit ("Do you shave?") to two units ("Do you shave your arms?") to three or more critical units ("Do you shave your beard with cologne?"). The reliability of the responses can be increased by incorporating contrasting information into sequences of paired questions ("Do you shave your arms?" and "Do you shave your beard?").

Patients are also asked to follow directions that require a demonstration of some response using parts of the body or objects which have been placed in front of them. The complexity of the directions increases according to the number of critical elements in the sentence that are necessary for comprehension, similar to that described for answering questions. At a basic level, the directions could be composed of a single action ("Smile" or "Wave"). Patients will demonstrate more success, however, on directions containing an action and some body part or object ("Close your eyes" or "Touch the book") because of the greater redundancy or predictability in such stimuli, especially when there is a limited array of objects in front of them. Treatment using these tasks, therefore, starts with directions of at least two critical elements and progresses by increasing the number of actions and/or objects on which the actions are to be performed in each direction (e.g., "Pick up the comb and the pencil" or "Pick up the comb and move the pencil").

Once a patient successfully comprehends sentences with as many as three or more critical elements, complexity can be increased within this level by utilizing sentences that contain different syntactic constructions or semantically reversible constituents. When varying syntactic structure, the approach is similar to that used in Part V of the Token Test (De Renzi & Vignolo, 1962) which assesses the patient's appreciation of grammatical relations. For example, one set of materials I have used (Ross & Spencer, 1980) incorporates sentences that contain temporal ("Touch the cup after I raise my hand"), spatial ("Put the spoon under the book"), conditional ("If your name is John, hold up two fingers; if not, put up four"), and comparative ("Is a briefcase bigger than a suitcase?") relations. As can be seen from the examples, a variety of tasks can be used for these purposes, including picture or body part manipulation and yes/no questions. Patients who do well with these types of sentences may still demonstrate marked difficulties with sentences that contain semantically reversible constituents (e.g., "Patti is chasing Kevin") (Carramaza & Zurif, 1976; Peach et al., 1988; Schwartz, Saffran, & Marin, 1980). If such difficulties are detected during assessment of auditory comprehension, then these types of sentences are included in the treatment. Byng (1988) has suggested an approach to treating these sentence processing deficits which relies on visual cues to assist the patient in mapping the appropriate thematic roles associated with these reversible items onto their corresponding grammatical structures.

Recent work has also suggested that sentence complexity may vary as a result of the number of syntactic subcategorizations or predicate-argument structures taken by a verb in a sentence (Caplan, Baker, & Dehaut, 1985; Shapiro & Levine, 1989, 1990). Syntactic subcategorization refers to the way in which different verbs select for different phrases or clauses called complements. For example, the verb *fix* in the sentence *Jimmy fixed the sink* subcategorizes for the noun phrase *the sink*. The verb *send* also subcategorizes for a noun phrase, as in the sentence *Karen sent the jacket*, but may also select for a prepositional phrase, as in the sentence *Karen sent the jacket to the cleaners*. Verbs such as *send* are considered, therefore, to be more complex than verbs such as *fix* because of the number of syntactic subcategorizations taken by each respectively. Sentences containing such verbs would also be considered to vary commensurately in their complexity.

Predicate-argument structure refers to the thematic roles that are associated with the actions described by the verb in a sentence. Again, the verb *fix* takes the arguments Agent and Theme in the sentence *Jimmy fixed the sink*, but the verb *send* can take as many arguments as Agent, Theme, and Goal in the sentence *Karen sent the jacket to the cleaners*. Once again, verbs such as *send* would be considered to have a more complex structure than those including *fix* because of the greater number of arguments for which they select.

Although much of the work investigating the role of these factors in auditory language comprehension following aphasia is still exploratory, these issues may have an impact on treatment planning. At a minimum, sentences controlled initially by verbs that select for the fewest syntactic subcategorizations or the simplest argument structure may be conceptually easier for aphasic patients. These sentences also tend to be shorter in most instances because of the interaction between these factors and sentence length (i.e., sentences including simpler verbs will take fewer complements or arguments which influences their length). Sentences might be ordered subsequently according to verb complexity as an additional means of increasing complexity for stimuli of this length.

Auditory comprehension stimulation beyond the sentence level consists of presenting narratives controlled for length (total number of sentences in the narrative) and assessing the patient's comprehension by his responses to yes/no questions concerning the stimuli. Recent work has suggested also that narratives containing semantically reversible sentences may be more difficult for these patients to comprehend than narratives containing semantically constrained sentences (Alexander & Peach, in press). In addition, semantic reversibility was found to exert a greater effect on narrative comprehension following aphasia than the length of the narratives or their syntactic complexity.

Treatment at this level is directed toward patients who have made significant recovery from a more severe form of their aphasia or whose aphasia has been relatively mild since onset. However, in most instances, a plan for patients at this level of auditory comprehension performance will be concerned primarily with improving production rather than comprehension disturbances. Some reasons for this would include the perception (by the patient if not also clinician and family) of functional comprehension abilities and the salience of remaining expressive difficulties. In addition, the factors that influence the comprehension of narratives in different environments cannot be controlled adequately in a purely clinical setting. As a result, the task becomes decidedly artificial, especially as the patient demonstrates improved comprehension of narratives in contextual settings, whether they are in the clinic or not. In some instances, treatment may focus exclusively on factors such as those described above that are related to narrative comprehension when patients have specific complaints in this area. When it does, the nature of the treatment tends to be more strategic than stimulatory. Greater gains are more often made by teaching the patient effective means for coping with inputs of this length or with these characteristics rather than by attempting to improve processing capacities by repeatedly exposing the patient to stimuli of this sort. This will be discussed further under compensatory approaches for comprehension impairment.

Verbal Expression

Aphasic patients who receive treatment for verbal expressive disorders may present a range of abilities that varies from complete mutism to fluent production of speech in adequate amounts that contains minor grammatical problems, impairments in word-retrieval or word-substitution, or discourse failures. The particular profile the patient presents at the time of treatment is dependent, of course, on such factors as the time post-onset of aphasia and the type and severity of the aphasia. In this section, I describe treatment for verbal expressive disorders within a framework which is organized by the aphasic patient's level of speech fluency, beginning with severe nonfluency and continuing with increasing levels of speech fluency. For each task described, patient responses that do not meet specified levels of accuracy are shaped to criterion by varying degrees of cuing until successful production of the target is (ideally) achieved.

The first consideration in treating a patient with a severe verbal expressive impairment is whether the deficits are due to aphasia, apraxia of speech, or both. When the condition is the result of a single cerebrovascular event, it is highly probable that the deficits are the result of *both* aphasia and apraxia of speech. This suggestion is based on epidemiologic findings which show that thrombotic infarctions are six times more likely than embolic infarctions (Kurtzke & Kurland, 1983). Because the intracranial involvement resulting from thrombosis is more generalized than that due to embolism, the neurological damage presumably will consist of a more extensive opercular syndrome, therefore increasing the likelihood that the condition is the result of linguistic *and* motor programming deficits (Tonkovich & Peach, 1989). Treatment planning may be directed, therefore, toward the amelioration of deficits in each of these areas.

In the patient who is totally mute, the inability to produce volitional laryngeal sounds may be due to apraxia of speech. Treatment at this most basic level would attempt to establish control for phonation. One approach would consist of using reflexive coughing or throat-clearing to establish voluntary phonation, then shaping these behaviors to incorporate humming and production of vowels (Aronson, 1990). Once the patient is able to initiate phonation at this level, treatment would increase to the production of words and phrases.

Initial training at the word and phrase level in severely nonfluent patients utilizes Hughlings Jackson's (1864) notion of propositional versus automatic speech production. Patients who are unable to use words voluntarily for meaningful, intentional communication frequently retain the ability to produce more automatic verbalizations such as counting, reciting the days of the week and months of the year, memorized sequences including prayers or songs, social expressions, and emotional speech (Davis, 1983). As a result, these stimuli provide natural targets for successful responses at a very early stage of treatment which serves the dual purpose of (a) stimulating verbal expression in the context of very limited abilities and (b) reinforcing productive client behaviors that will facilitate treatment at later, more complex levels of response.

When a high degree of success has been achieved in the production of automatic verbal sequences, treatment begins to focus on the production of words for more propositional purposes. The first tasks I present for these purposes utilize a sentence completion format. These tasks facilitate the transition between automatic and propositional production because the stimuli and responses they elicit communicate meaningful and voluntary information while retaining varying degrees of verbal automaticity due to the redundancy and predictability of the responses. In sentences requiring the patient to provide a noun or a verb, predictability (from highest to lowest) can be varied using the following items: (a) sentences constructed from idioms (e.g., "He's a chip off the old _____"), nursery rhymes (e.g., "Humpty Dumpty sat on a _____"), or other rote-learned items; (b) sentences which constrain the missing noun or verb by the remaining information (e.g., "You tell time with a _____," "Comb your _____," "Soap is for _____"); (c) paired-associates (e.g., "Bacon and _____"); and (d) open-ended sentences (e.g., "Put the suitcase in the _____," "Tonight we are going to begin _____").

As the patient improves in his or her ability to produce single words under these conditions, other tasks that stimulate single word production may be gradually introduced. These tasks include word repetition with or without a visual stimulus such as a picture or an object, word reading, answering questions that contain the target response (e.g., "What do you write with — a pen or a book?"), responsive naming ("What do you drive?"), recall of one or more items in a category (word fluency), and confrontation naming. Clinicians may opt at this stage to accept responses that contain apractic errors if the primary focus of the intervention is stimulation of word production. Subsequently, treatment may incorporate methods for improving articulatory precision for single words before increasing the length of the target response. In either case, the stimuli used for the various reading and naming tasks at this level should be well within the patient's capabilities so as not to conceal the patient's true productive capacities by failures in reading or word retrieval.

Some severely impaired nonfluent patients do not recover to a level where they demonstrate productive usage of single words in tasks like those above. Instead, their speech output is restricted to single word stereotypies. The treatment program Voluntary Control of Involuntary Utterances (VCIU) (Helm & Barresi, 1980) can be used with these patients to bring these stereotypies into more productive usage. In this program, words that are involuntarily and inappropriately produced in the contexts of testing and treatment are identified and used as later targets in treatment. The words are trained in a sequence including oral reading, confrontation naming, and, finally, conversational usage until a vocabulary of between 200–300 words is established.

Once the patient is successful in using single words with a high degree of accuracy under controlled circumstances, subsequent treatment can be directed toward improving volitional production of linguistic units of increasing length. At this level, treatment may promote reacquisition of syntactic form, articulatory precision, or both.

I have used a variety of methods to improve syntactic form. Subject-plus-verb and verb-plus-object constructions can be trained using such techniques as matrices or cuing verb treatments (Loverso & Milione, 1992). In matrix training, patients are trained to produce two-word constructions composed of words from the above grammatical categories. Once the patient is successful in producing trained combinations to a criterion level, generalization of these language productions to untrained combinations of these types is evaluated. Cuing verb treatments (CVT) uses wh-question cuing strategies to train subject-plus-verb constructions (Loverso, Prescott, & Selinger, 1988). In this treatment approach, "verbs are presented as pivots and wh-questions provide strategic cues to elicit thematic associations in a actor-action-recipient framework" (Loverso & Milione, 1992, p. 47). The final levels of CVT also incorporate training for subject-plus-verb-plus object constructions.

Kearns (1985) has described response elaboration training (RET) which is also useful for improving phrase length in chronic nonfluent patients. Unlike the other approaches described here, RET relies on patient-initiated utterances rather than demanding specific target responses selected by the clinician. RET uses a "forward chaining technique to lengthen patient-initiated utterances" (p. 198). The patient's one- to two-word responses to pictures are expanded and modeled by the clinician. The patient is then prompted for additional information which again is expanded and modeled by the clinician. The clinician then combines the patient responses and requests a repetition of this model. The patient is thereafter reinforced for expanded utterances.

Alternatively, patients may be asked simply to read aloud or repeat whole phrase- or sentence-length stimuli with or without accompanying pictures to stimulate increased phrase lengths. To facilitate the transition from simple repetition to more propositional language usage, patients may be asked to provide responses where the target is embedded in the verbal stimuli and elicited by intervening questions (e.g., "I'm going to buy baseball tickets tomorrow. What am I going to buy?"). This approach has been formalized in the Helm Elicited Language Program for Syntax Stimulation (HELPSS) (Helm-Estabrooks et al., 1981; Helm-Estabrooks & Ramsberger, 1986). HELPSS targets 11 sentence types which are hierarchically ordered in terms of their difficulty as demonstrated by previous research. A short story accompanied by a simple line drawing is substituted for single sentences. Two task levels differ only·on the basis of whether or not intervening questions are presented as described above.

Patients can also be asked to respond to a question containing incorrect information by transforming the question to a statement in its corrected form (e.g., "Do you write with a shoe? No, I write with a pen"). Subsequently, patients can respond to questions asking for different types of information including, for example, the function of objects ("What do you do with a toothbrush?"), routines ("How do you get to this hospital?," "How do you make a sandwich?"), or other items of general knowledge ("What do you do at the beach?").

Another approach consists of having patients construct sentences when given a specific noun, verb, or functor. Variations include constructing sentences when provided interrogative pronouns or modal verbs (to stimulate formulation of questions), two or more words (to be included in the same sentence), phrases, or parts of sentences. Patients may also be given whole sentences followed by questions that are designed to stimulate formulation of different syntactic constructions such as passive sentences (e.g., "The woman is making the bed. What is happening to the bed?"), relative clauses (e.g., "The man stood beside the train. The train was leaving. Combine these sentences to tell me what is happening") and adverbial clauses (e.g., "Mr. McCarthy was upset. He heard about the news. Using both of these sentences, when was Mr. McCarthy upset?") (Shewan & Bandur, 1986).

Subsequent tasks designed to stimulate complex sentence production may be structured to be more open-ended. For example, patients may be asked to provide descriptions of pictured activities or objects. Describing occupations, animals, and places would be variations on the same task. Complex responses can also be elicited to wh-questions (e.g., "Why is gasoline" taxed? What is a stroke?"), requests for the similarities and differences between two objects (e.g., "What are the similarities and differences between soccer and football?"), explanations of idiomatic expressions (e.g., "What does 'Don't count your chickens before they hatch' mean?"), and word definitions, as well as a variety of similar types of tasks (see, for example, Brubaker, 1978, or Ross & Spencer, 1980).

Verbal expressive tasks eliciting utterance lengths in excess of those produced in the above tasks will target discourse abilities in narrative or conversational contexts. Examples would include story retellings and open-ended conversation on unrestricted topics, respectively. Story retellings provide the preferred approach because the patient's performance can be assessed relative to a given model. Using the model proposed by Ulatowska and Chapman (1989), the target for intervention is defined by the integrity of the superstructure of the patient's discourse. According to Chapman and Ulatowska (1992), superstructure "defines the form of the discourse in terms of the elements . . . (which) include abstract, complicating action, resolution, evaluation, and coda" (p. 66). It is evaluated by assessing the setting, complicating action, and resolution of the patient's story retellings. For patients whose superstructure is deficient, treatment is focused on assisting the patient in structuring information according to the above story components. Chapman and Ulatowska propose using an outline of the stimulus story to cue these major components. Conversely, if superstructure is intact, these authors recommend treatment tasks that focus on elaborating, adding, or changing information rather than continued story retellings.

COMPENSATORY TECHNIQUES

Often, factors including the time post-onset, the severity of aphasia, and/ or the outcome achieved from an extended course of aphasia treatment will interact to result in a poor prognosis for attaining measurable increases in auditory comprehension or verbal expression. In these cases, language stimulation may no longer appear to be the treatment approach of choice. Whether due to the above considerations or a management decision that emphasizes improving the patient's functional communicative skills concurrent with language facilitation, aphasia treatment may utilize compensatory approaches to treat language behaviors. Broadly defined, compensatory approaches include techniques that exploit the patient's residual linguistic and nonlinguistic cognitive skills to increase successful communication. In contrast to the narrow view of aphasia treatment as consisting of language stimulation only, the demonstrated effectiveness of compensatory techniques provides at least one reason that all aphasic patients are entitled to the opportunity for aphasia rehabilitation, even when the outlook for language recovery may be considered bleak.

With regard to improving an aphasic patient's auditory verbal comprehension, one approach consists of training the patient to follow a comprehension breakdown with a contingent query (Davis & Wilcox, 1985; Rosenbek, et al., 1989). Contingent queries consist of requests for clarification of the input or additional information and may be either (a) nonvocal, consisting of any facial or other behavior that indicates a need for more information; (b) vocal, consisting of some vocal behavior which indicates a need for more information; or (c) verbal, consisting of an appropriate linguistic response. In addition, a contingent query may simply consist of the patient's asking a speaker to slow down the rate of speech. By utilizing contingent queries, aphasic patients use natural processes found in the discourse of nonaphasic speakers to manipulate auditory input according to their needs. As a result, comprehension frequently improves due to the increased opportunities patients have to understand the message.

Several compensatory approaches have been utilized to improve patients' expressive abilities, including gestural programs, drawing, and computer applications. Probably the best known of the gestural programs is Amer-Ind Code (Rao, 1986; Skelly, 1979). Amer-Ind Code is adapted from American Indian sign, a gestural system based on the concepts underlying words rather than on the words themselves (Skelly, Schinsky, Smith, Donaldson, & Griffin, 1975). According to Rao and Horner (1980), Amer-Ind is concrete, pictographic, highly transmissible, easily learned, agrammatic, and generative. The system can be applied in aphasia rehabilitation as an alternative means of communication, as a facilitator of verbalization, especially in patients with apraxia of speech, and as a deblocker of other language modalities (Rao, 1986). Although a few reports exist demonstrating the usefulness of Amer-Ind Code as an alternative means of communication (Rao et al., 1980; Tonkovich & Loverso, 1982), the greatest utility of the technique appears to be as a facilitator of verbalization, although reports of its effectiveness vary (Hanlon, Brown, & Gerstman, 1990; Hoodin & Thompson, 1983; Kearns, Simmons, & Sisterhen, 1982; Rao & Horner, 1978; Raymer & Thompson, 1991; Skelly, Schinsky, Smith, Donaldson, & Griffin, 1974). Rosenbek et al. (1989) describe a treatment program for gestural reorganization which utilizes Amer-Ind Code as the primary system of gestures and has as its end goal verbalization without gestural accompaniment. Visual Action Therapy (VAT) (Helm-Estabrooks & Albert, 1991; Helm-Estabrooks et al., 1982; Helm-Estabrooks, Ramsberger, Brownell, & Albert, 1989; Ramsberger & Helm-Estabrooks, 1989) also utilizes gestures to reduce apraxia and improve the patient's verbal expression or ability to use symbolic gestures as a means of communication. Three programs constitute the approach, including proximal limb, distal limb, and buccofacial VAT. A hierarchical procedure is used in each program to "move the patient along a performance continuum from the basic task of matching pictures and objects to the communicative task of representing hidden items with self-initiated gestures" (Helm-Estabrooks & Albert, 1991, p. 178). The method has been shown to produce improvements not only in the area of pantomime, as indicated by formal assessments, but also in the areas of auditory and reading comprehension, verbal repetition, and graphic copying.

Other gestural approaches include pantomime; limited manual sign systems for hospitals and nursing homes such as manual shorthand, manual self-care signals, or a hand-talking chart, gestures for yes and no; eye-blink encoding; and pointing (Silverman, 1989). Silverman (1989) offers a number of suggestions for the selective use of each of these approaches. For example, pantomime may be appropriate for the aphasic patient who cannot use Amer-Ind Code. Limited manual sign systems may be used initially on an interim basis until other communication systems can be developed but ultimately may provide the only means of communication in the most severely impaired patients (e.g., see Coelho, 1990, 1991). Pointing is desirable for the patient who is going to use a communication board.

Silverman (1989) also describes gestural communication strategies assisted by nonelectronic or electronic means. Strategies using nonelectronic assistance include transmission of messages by communication boards, manipulation of symbol sequences, and drawing. Communication boards vary in type and complexity and are generally used in aphasia rehabilitation with severely expressively impaired patients (Bellaire, Georges, & Thompson, 1991). One of the most notable applications of manual symbol systems following aphasia was the visual communication (VIC) system reported by Gardner, Zurif, Berry, and Baker (1976). Drawing has received considerable attention both as a communicative medium and as a means to deblock verbal and written communication. In response, several programs for training picture drawing for these purposes have been described in recent reports (Helm-Estabrooks & Albert, 1991; Lyon & Helm-Estabrooks, 1987; Lyon & Sims, 1989; Morgan & Helm-Estabrooks, 1987).

With regard to gestural-assisted strategies using electronic means, computer-aided visual communication (C-ViC) (Steele et al., 1987; Steele et al., 1989; Weinrich, Steele, Carlson et al., 1989; Weinrich, Steele, Kleczewska et al., 1989) provides one of the most promising approaches to establishing alternative communication in severely impaired patients. Using procedures similar to those of visual communication (ViC) (Gardner et al., 1976) but in a microcomputer environment, C-ViC is an iconographic system in which patients construct communications by selecting symbols from six "card decks" and arranging them according to certain syntactic conventions. The card decks contain interjections, animate nouns, verbs, prepositions, modifiers, and common nouns. Formal procedures have been developed that extend training from introductory phases which teach the patient to follow simple commands to later phases designed to transfer C-ViC communication skills to use in a home setting (Baker & Nicholas, 1992).

As has been reported with other gestural strategies, we have also noted verbal facilitation in patients using C-ViC. Some have produced successful naming not seen in the same patients in other communicative contexts (e.g., conversation or formal testing). While the ultimate goal of C-ViC is not verbalization without computer assistance (as might be the case with some of the foregoing gestural strategies), these observations suggest that C-ViC is a powerful verbal reorganizer that enhances language production in patients using the system. Further investigation of this point is needed to fully understand its long-term effects for language recovery. Nonetheless, for the severely impaired aphasic patient, a patient for whom successful treatment approaches are too often lacking, C-ViC offers an important tool for communication.

The last approach which will be considered here is Promoting Aphasics' Communicative Effectiveness or PACE treatment (Davis, 1980; Davis, 1986; Davis & Wilcox, 1981, 1985; Wilcox & Davis, 1978). Because PACE procedures allow patients to freely choose the channel(s) through which they will communicate, the technique provides opportunities for patients to use a verbal strategy or any of the gestural or gestural-assisted strategies described above, with or without verbal accompaniment, to convey messages. In this way, the approach emulates natural conversation by allowing participants to exchange information through multiple modalities. In addition to free selection, some of the other characteristics of natural conversation that provide guiding principles for PACE treatment include: (a) clinician and patient participate equally as senders and receivers of messages; (b) the interaction incorporates the exchange of new information between clinician and patient; and (c) the clinician's feedback is based on the patient's success in communicating a message (Davis & Wilcox, 1985). PACE treatment utilizes a multidimensional scoring system to better capture the full range of behaviors that may be observed in this interactive approach. Generalization of language gains observed following PACE treatment has been demonstrated on formal language assessment instruments. Given its emphasis on the pragmatic aspects of language, PACE is well suited as a means to incorporate compensatory strategies into communication treatment. An additional strength of the approach, however, lies in its use as a framework for incorporating traditional language stimulation techniques into a communicatively dynamic context.

In the United States, the model for clinical aphasiology has evolved in recent years from one that is medically oriented, stressing identification and remediation of pathologic conditions, to one that is more socially based and includes such concepts as disability and handicap (Holland & Wertz, 1988). Aphasia rehabilitation considered in the latter terms emphasizes compensatory gains that result in more functional communication rather than simply changes in language structure, for example, due to a given treatment (Peach, 1992). With their emphasis on communication in natural settings, many of the techniques that have been described in this section may be more suitably applied to intervention in this contemporary environment.

THE TYPE AND SEVERITY OF APHASIA

It has been common practice in the literature to describe various approaches to aphasia intervention in terms of either the type (LaPointe, 1990; Perkins, 1983; Rosenbek et al., 1989) or severity (Holland, 1984) of the aphasia. In practice, however, type and severity of aphasia are so often nested within one another that it becomes impractical to discuss these parameters independently. In this final section, many of the approaches which have been described will be discussed briefly in terms of their application to specific types of aphasia with their associated levels of severity of impairment. Recent trends have placed increased importance on identifying the particular treatments that are most effective for specific groups of aphasic patients (Nicholas & Helm-Estabrooks, 1990; Peach, 1992). In keeping with these trends, emphasis will also be placed on additional programs that have been found to be effective with certain groups of aphasic patients.

NONFLUENT APHASIA

The nonfluent aphasias which will be discussed here include Broca's, transcortical motor, mixed transcortical (isolation syndrome), and global aphasia. Although the defining characteristic for grouping these patients is expressive in nature, each of these groups will be considered in terms of treatments for both expressive *and* receptive language disturbances.

In describing treatment for acute Broca's aphasia, I assume a profile of limited phrase length accompanied by mild or mild-to-moderate auditory comprehension deficits. The syndrome is frequently accompanied by apraxia of speech so that treatment for this population often emphasizes motor speech programming as well as syntactic facilitation (Tonkovich & Peach, 1989). Depending on the level of severity, treatment incorporates many of the stimulation techniques described earlier to increase phrase lengths from production of single words to more syntactically complete utterances. For improving articulatory precision, programs such as the eight-step continuum (Rosenbek, Lemme, Ahern, Harris, & Wertz, 1973), speech sound sequencing (Dabul & Bollier, 1976), the content network for verbal dyspraxia (Shewan, 1980), and Melodic Intonation Therapy (MIT) (Helm-Estabrooks & Albert, 1991) are useful. MIT is, of course, the treatment approach that theoretically exploits the intact right hemisphere of the severely nonfluent aphasic patient for verbal improvements by using intoned phrases of increasing complexity. Intoning is gradually faded so that phrases are subsequently produced with exaggerated prosody and, finally, with normal prosody. Naeser, Frumkin, Helm-Estabrooks, Fitzpatrick, and Palumbo (1991) have identified language and CT scan criteria in patients which predict a particularly good response to MIT. The language criteria include three out of the following four observations: (a) poorly articulated, nonfluent, or severely restricted verbal output; (b) at least moderately preserved auditory comprehension; (c) poor repetition; and (d) poorly articulated speech. With regard to CT scan findings, patients who have lesions that comprise less than half of the medial subcallosal fasciculus and the middle one third of the periventricular white matter or who have patchy lesions including more than half of these areas, and have a lesion in less than half of Wernicke's area and the temporal isthmus, are the best candidates for MIT. Auditory comprehension treatment for Broca's aphasic patients targets sentences of moderate complexity or greater (i.e., three or more critical units representing a variety of grammatical relations) or the parsing impairments that produce difficulty for these patients in assigning thematic roles to sentence constituents (Byng, 1992).

Patients with transcortical motor aphasia (TMA) also demonstrate reduced phrase lengths and relatively preserved auditory comprehension. As with the other transcortical aphasias, repetition is fairly intact. Unlike Broca's aphasia, nonfluency in TMA is related more to deficits in verbal initiation rather than grammatical or motor speech programming deficits. Treatment approaches have included methods that use deblocking procedures to improve the volitional initiation of motor responses, self-generation of category names and complete sentences, and traditional language training using stimulation techniques (Gonzales-Rothi, 1990). Pharmacotherapy using the dopamine agonist bromocriptine to increase speech initiation has been attempted with TMA patients with mixed results (Albert, Bachman, Morgan, & Helm-Estabrooks, 1988; MacLennan, Nicholas, Morley, & Brookshire, 1991). I have observed mild improvements on post-testing in such a patient when relying on tasks that require sentence production (e.g., providing the function of objects, constructing a sentence when given two words) and naming (e.g., sentence completion, responsive naming, category recall, and antonym production) accompanied by complex auditory processing. Because repetition generally is preserved in TMA, some consideration may be given to using such tasks to improve verbal output, especially if the approach is to use an intact function to facilitate an impaired one. However, such use of repetition tasks generally has received little support except in the initial stages of treatment because of the limited results that it provides (Alexander & Schmitt, 1980).

Patients with mixed transcortical aphasia demonstrate the verbal deficits described above but with accompanying deficits in auditory comprehension. Gonzales-Rothi (1990) has suggested that treatments similar to those used in transcortical motor aphasia be applied for the expressive disturbances in mixed transcortical aphasia. Auditory comprehension stimulation will also be included at a level commensurate with the more severe receptive impairments observed in these patients.

The verbal recovery in chronic global aphasia is generally poor (Kertesz & McCabe, 1977; Lomas & Kertesz, 1978). As a result, treatment for these patients is largely compensatory except, perhaps, in the earliest stages following onset of the aphasia. VCIU (Helm & Barresi, 1980) is specifically designed to bring the limited spontaneous utterances of severely impaired patients under productive control. Any of the compensatory approaches described earlier may also be appropriate for treatment of the global aphasic patient. These approaches include, among others, gestural programs such as Amer-Ind or VAT, drawing programs

such as Back to the Drawing Board (Helm-Estabrooks & Albert, 1991) or
that of Lyon and Sims (1989), computer applications such as C-ViC, and
communication boards. Or, the clinician may use the integrative framework found in the PACE treatment program to incorporate any of these
or the patient's other natural attempts into a communication system.

FLUENT APHASIA

The fluent aphasias to be discussed here include Wernicke's, transcortical sensory, conduction, and anomic aphasia. Approaches for the more
severely aphasic Wernicke's and transcortical aphasic groups emphasize
auditory-verbal processing, whereas programs for conduction and anomic aphasia focus more on remediation of expressive deficits.

Treatment for Wernicke's aphasia is directed toward reducing the severe auditory comprehension deficits found in this syndrome and serves
as a prerequisite to improving expressive functioning as well. The stimulation procedures outlined earlier, beginning at the most basic levels of
picture matching, provide a continuum for treating the comprehension
disturbances in Wernicke's aphasia. If the patient is capable of understanding selected printed words, the program entitled Treatment for
Wernicke's Aphasia (Helm-Estabrooks & Albert, 1991) may be useful for
improving word recognition. Task complexity increases in a manner
commensurate with the patient's level of severity. From a more functional standpoint, training may emphasize the use of contingent queries to
provide additional exposure to speech input, thereby enhancing the
chances for successful comprehension. Educating families and significant others to simplify their input, and accompany their speech with additional cues such as pointing or gestures, is another important component to the treatment program for these patients.

As in Wernicke's aphasia, the major goal of treatment for transcortical
sensory aphasia (TSA) is improved auditory-verbal comprehension.
Gonzales-Rothi (1990), citing previous work, proposes that the receptive deficits in TSA may be due to (a) disconnection between the cognitive system and the input and output lexicons, (b) impairment of the
cognitive system itself, or (c) evolution from Wernicke's aphasia. She
suggests that treatment for impairments following the initial two conditions should focus, respectively, on pairing auditory input with another
modality and reconstructing semantic relationships. Treatment for the
latter condition might simply utilize methods that are most appropriate
for Wernicke's aphasia.

Conduction aphasia is characterized by generally preserved auditory
comprehension and a disproportionate impairment in repetition relative
to spontaneous speech. Treatment programs for this syndrome frequent-

ly emphasize repetition training to provide a transition to spontaneous speech production. The approach does little, however, to circumvent the impaired mechanisms responsible for the repetition deficit. Oral reading has also been used, but with minimal generalization to other forms of language expression (Beard & Prescott, 1991; Sullivan, Fisher, & Marshall, 1986). Caramazza, Basili, Koller, and Berndt (1981) and Shallice and Warrington (1977) proposed that the repetition deficit in conduction aphasia is the result of auditory-verbal short-term memory deficits. Based on this hypothesis, I have used a treatment approach that utilizes tasks of auditory and oral word sequencing to improve auditory verbal span (Peach, 1987). The results of this approach, using a multiple baseline design, showed generalization to the repetition of novel stimuli. In addition, improvements also were noted in spontaneous speech as evidenced by significantly reduced paraphasic errors on post-testing. Although several varieties of repetition deficit appear to exist, this treatment approach has been successful in improving repetition in patients whose deficit is related to auditory-verbal short-term memory deficits and, therefore, may be useful in treating the expressive impairments in conduction aphasia.

Anomic aphasia is characterized primarily by lexical retrieval deficits. Recent work has demonstrated, however, that these patients also have difficulty with parsing semantically reversible sentences presented either auditorily or visually (Peach et al., 1988). Other clinical observations have supported at least mild or mild-to-moderate auditory comprehension deficits for sentences of three or more critical units containing varying grammatical relations. So, while emphasis in the treatment programs of these patients is given to improving word retrieval abilities through a variety of confrontational and nonconfrontational naming tasks (e.g., recall of category members, word associations, antonym/synonym production, descriptions of busy pictures), auditory comprehension tasks targeting the affected syntactic processes may also be included. Generalization of the naming improvements achieved through these means to functional forms of expression may be fostered through tasks such as picture description, monologues, story retellings, and role-playing (Linebaugh, 1990).

These overviews are by no means intended to provide an in-depth discussion of treatment for each of the aphasias. The reader should consult the works contained in Holland (1984), LaPointe (1990), Perkins (1983), and Rosenbek et al. (1989) for additional American perspectives on treatment of each of these types of aphasia. The discussion in this section does provide the reader with some indication of the way that the severity and type of aphasia interact with the nature of the selected approaches in treatment planning for aphasia in the United States.

CONCLUSION

The current state of aphasia rehabilitation in the United States is the product of significant contributions from practitioners all over the world. To attempt to summarize this literature, or for that matter, just the literature that emanates from the United States, would be a formidable, if not unrealistic task due to the sheer number of resources. The purpose of this book, therefore, is to provide at least an initial comparison of how the art is practiced in different countries by asking contributors from a host of different countries to provide an overview of their own accounts of how one goes about treating the communication deficits associated with aphasia.

As described at the beginning of this chapter, my perspectives on aphasia treatment are very much the result of the influences to which I have been exposed and, therefore, are not necessarily the same as many of my colleagues. I have not attempted to cover all of the relevant literature because, as stated above, it would be difficult to accomplish that goal. More importantly, surveying all of the literature is not necessarily the best way to provide my own perspective. However, because all of my training occurred in this country, I feel comfortable in saying that there probably would be more agreement than disagreement among practitioners in this country with regard to the representativeness of this approach for aphasia rehabilitation in the United States. I hope, therefore, that this chapter is helpful in providing a useful and instructive counterpoint as to how clinicians treat their aphasic patients in different parts of the world.

REFERENCES

Albert, M. L., Bachman, D., Morgan, A., & Helm-Estabrooks, N. (1988). Pharmacotherapy of aphasia. *Neurology, 38,* 877–879.

Albert, M., Sparks, R., & Helm, N. (1973). Melodic Intonation Therapy for aphasia. *Archives of Neurology, 29,* 130–131.

Alexander, L., & Peach, R. K. (1992). Syntactic and semantic factors influencing narrative comprehension in aphasia [Abstract]. *Asha, 34*(10), 202.

Alexander, M. P., & Schmitt, M. A. (1980). The aphasia syndrome of stroke in the left anterior cerebral artery territory. *Archives of Neurology, 37,* 97–100.

Aronson, A. E. (1990). *Clinical voice disorders: An interdisciplinary approach* (3rd ed.). New York: Thieme.

Baker, E., & Nicholas, M. (1992). *C-ViC training manual.* Unpublished manuscript.

Beard, L. C., & Prescott, T. E. (1991). Replication of a treatment protocol for repetition deficit in conduction aphasia. *Clinical Aphasiology, 19,* 197–208.

Bellaire, K. J., Georges, J. B., & Thompson, C. K. (1991). Establishing functional communication board use for nonverbal aphasic subjects. *Clinical Aphasiology, 18*, 219–227.

Brubaker, S. H. (1978). *Workbook for aphasia.* Detroit, MI: Wayne State University Press.

Burns, M. S., & Canter, G. J. (1977). Phonemic behavior of aphasic patients with posterior cerebral lesions. *Brain and Language, 4*, 492–507.

Byng, S. (1988). Sentence processing deficits: Theory and therapy. *Cognitive Neuropsychology, 5*, 629–676.

Byng, S. (1992). Testing the tried: Replicating sentence-processing therapy for agrammatic Broca's aphasia. *Clinics in Communication Disorders, 2*(1), 34–42.

Canter, G. J., Trost, J. E., & Burns, M. S. (1985). Contrasting speech patterns in apraxia of speech and phonemic paraphasia. *Brain and Language, 24*, 204–222.

Caplan, D., Baker, C., & Dehaut, F. (1985). Syntactic determinants of sentence comprehension in aphasia. *Cognition, 21*, 117–175.

Caramazza, A., Basili, A. G., Koller, J. J., & Berndt, R. S. (1981). An investigation of repetition and language processing in a case of conduction aphasia. *Brain and Language, 14*, 235–271.

Caramazza, A., & Zurif, E. B. (1976). Dissociation of algorithmic and heuristic processes in language comprehension: Evidence from aphasia. *Brain and Language, 3*, 572–582.

Chapman, S. D., & Ulatowska, H. K. (1992). Methodology for discourse management in the treatment of aphasia. *Clinics in Communication Disorders, 2*(1), 64–81.

Coelho, C. A. (1990). Acquisition and generalization of simple manual sign grammars by aphasic subjects. *Journal of Communication Disorders, 23*, 383–400.

Coelho, C. A. (1991). Manual sign acquisition and use in two aphasic subjects. *Clinical Aphasiology, 19*, 209–218.

Collins, M. J. (1990). Global aphasia. In L. L. Lapointe (Ed.), *Aphasia and related neurogenic language disorders* (pp. 113–129). New York: Thieme.

Dabul, B., & Bollier, B. (1976). Therapeutic approaches to apraxia. *Journal of Speech and Hearing Disorders, 41*, 268–276.

Darley, F. L. (1982). *Aphasia.* Philadelphia: W. B. Saunders.

Davis, G. A. (1980). A critical look at PACE therapy. *Clinical Aphasiology, 10*, 248–257.

Davis, G. A. (1983). *A survey of adult aphasia.* Englewood Cliffs, NJ: Prentice-Hall.

Davis, G. A. (1986). Pragmatics and treatment. In R. Chapey (Ed.), *Language intervention strategies in adult aphasia* (2nd ed., pp. 251–265). Baltimore, MD: Williams & Wilkins.

Davis, G. A., & Wilcox, J. (1981). Incorporating parameters of natural conversation in aphasia. In R. Chapey (Ed.), *Language intervention strategies in adult aphasia* (pp. 169–194). Baltimore, MD: Williams & Wilkins.

Davis, G. A., & Wilcox, M. J. (1985). *Adult aphasia rehabilitation: Applied pragmatics.* San Diego, CA: College-Hill Press.

De Renzi, E., & Vignolo, L. A. (1962). The Token Test: A sensitive test to detect receptive disturbances in aphasics. *Brain, 85*, 665–678.

Duffy, J. R. (1986). Schuell's stimulation approach to rehabilitation. In R. Chapey

(Ed.), *Language intervention strategies in adult aphasia* (2nd ed., pp. 187–214). Baltimore, MD: Williams & Wilkins.

Gardner, H., Zurif, E. B., Berry, T., & Baker, E. (1976). Visual communication in aphasia. *Neuropsychologia, 14*, 275–292.

Gonzales-Rothi, L. J. (1990). Transcortical aphasias. In L. L. LaPointe (Ed.), *Aphasia and related neurogenic communication disorders* (pp. 78–95). New York: Thieme.

Gonzales-Rothi, L. J., & Moss, S. (1992). Alexia without agraphia: Potential for model assisted therapy. *Clinics in Communication Disorders, 2*(1), 11–18.

Gonzales-Rothi, L. J., Raymer, A. M., Maher, L., Greenwald, M., & Morris, M. (1991). Assessment of naming failures in neurological communication disorders. *Clinics in Communication Disorders, 1*(1), 7–20.

Goodglass, H., & Kaplan, E. (1972). *The assessment of aphasia and related disorders.* Philadelphia: Lea & Febiger.

Hanlon, R. E., Brown, J. W., & Gerstman, L. J. (1990). Enhancement of naming in nonfluent aphasia through gesture. *Brain and Language, 38*, 298–314.

Helm, N. A., & Barresi, B. (1980). Voluntary control of involuntary utterances: A treatment approach for severe aphasia. *Clinical Aphasiology, 10*, 308–315.

Helm, N. A., & Benson, D. F. (1978, October). *Visual Action Therapy for global aphasia.* Paper presented at the annual meeting of the Academy of Aphasia, Chicago, IL.

Helm-Estabrooks, N., & Albert, M. L. (1991). *Manual of aphasia therapy.* Austin, TX: Pro-Ed.

Helm-Estabrooks, N., Emery, P., & Albert, M. L. (1987). Treatment of Aphasic Perseveration (TAP) program. *Archives of Neurology, 44*, 1253–1255.

Helm-Estabrooks, N., Fitzpatrick, P. M., & Barresi, B. (1981). Responses of an agrammatic patient to a syntax stimulation program for aphasia. *Journal of Speech and Hearing Disorders, 46*, 422–427.

Helm-Estabrooks, N., Fitzpatrick, P. M., & Barresi, B. (1982). Visual action therapy for global aphasia. *Journal of Speech and Hearing Disorders, 47*, 385–389.

Helm-Estabrooks, N., & Ramsberger, G. (1986). Treatment of agrammatism in long-term Broca's aphasia. *British Journal of Disorders of Communication, 21*, 39–45.

Helm-Estabrooks, N., Ramsberger, G., Brownell, H., & Albert, M. (1989). Distal versus proximal movement in limb apraxia. *Journal of Clinical and Experimental Neuropsychology, 7*, 608.

Hillis, A. E. (1992). Facilitating written production. *Clinics in Communication Disorders, 2*(1), 19–33.

Holland, A. L. (1980). *Communicative abilities in daily living.* Baltimore: University Park Press.

Holland, A. L. (Ed.). (1984). *Language disorders in adults: Recent advances.* San Diego, CA: College-Hill Press.

Holland, A. L. (1991, April). *New approaches to working with naming disorders.* Symposium conducted at the annual meeting of the Georgia Speech-Language-Hearing Association, Jekyll Island.

Holland, A. L., & Wertz, R. T. (1988). Measuring aphasia treatment effects: Large-group, small-group, and single-subject studies. In F. Plum (Ed.), *Language, communication, and the brain* (pp. 267–273). New York: Raven Press.

Hoodin, R. B., & Thompson, C. K. (1983). Facilitation of verbal labeling in adult aphasia by gestural, verbal or verbal plus gestural training. *Clinical Aphasiology, 13,* 62–64.

Horner, J., & Loverso, F. L. (1991). Models of aphasia treatment in *Clinical Aphasiology 1972–1988. Clinical Aphasiology, 20,* 61–75.

Jackson, J. H. (1864). Loss of speech: Its association with valvular disease of the heart and with hemiplegia on the right side. *Brain, 38,* 28–42.

Jenkins, J. J., Jimenez-Pabon, E., Shaw, R. E., & Sefer, J. W. (1975). *Schuell's aphasia in adults: Diagnosis, prognosis, and treatment* (2nd ed.). Hagerstown, MD: Harper & Row.

Katz, R. C. (1986). *Aphasia treatment and microcomputers.* San Diego, CA: College-Hill Press.

Katz, R. C., & Nagy, V. T. (1982). A computerized treatment system for chronic aphasic patients. *Clinical Aphasiology, 12,* 153–160.

Katz, R. C., & Nagy, V. T. (1984). An intelligent computer-based spelling task for chronic aphasic patients. *Clinical Aphasiology, 14,* 65–72.

Katz, R. C., & Nagy, V. T. (1985). A self-modifying computerized reading programs for severely-impaired aphasic patients. *Clinical Aphasiology, 15,* 184–188.

Katz, R. C., & Wertz, R. T. (1992). Computerized hierarchical reading treatment in aphasia. *Aphasiology, 6*(2), 165–177.

Katz, R. C., Wertz, R. T., Davidoff, M., Schubitowski, Y. D., & Devitt, E. W. (1988). A computer program to improve written confrontation naming in aphasia. *Clinical Aphasiology, 18,* 321–337.

Katz, R. C., Wertz, R. T., Lewis, S. M., Esparza, C., & Goldojarb, M. (1991). A comparison of computerized reading treatment, computer stimulation, and no treatment for aphasia. *Clinical Aphasiology, 19,* 243–254.

Kearns, K. P. (1985). Response elaboration training for patient initiated utterances. *Clinical Aphasiology, 15,* 196–204.

Kearns, K. P., & Potechin-Scher, G. (1989). The generalization of response elaboration training effects. *Clinical Aphasiology, 18,* 223–245.

Kearns, K., Simmons, N. N., & Sisterhen, C. (1982). Gestural sign (Amer-Ind) as a facilitator of verbalization in patients with aphasia. *Clinical Aphasiology, 12,* 183–191.

Kearns, K. P., & Yedor, K. (1991). An alternating treatments comparison of loose training and a convergent treatment strategy. *Clinical Aphasiology, 20,* 223–238.

Kertesz, A., & McCabe, P. (1977). Recovery patterns and prognosis in aphasia. *Brain, 100,* 1–18.

Kurtzke, J. F., & Kurland, L. T. (1983). The epidemiology of neurologic disease. In A. B. Baker & L. H. Baker (Eds.), *Clinical neurology.* Philadelphia: Harper & Row.

LaPointe, L. L. (Ed.). (1990). *Aphasia and related neurogenic language disorders.* New York: Thieme.

Linebaugh, C. W. (1990). Lexical retrieval problems: Anomia. In L. L. LaPointe (Ed.), *Aphasia and related neurogenic language disorders* (pp. 96–112). New York: Thieme.

Lomas, J., & Kertesz, A. (1978). Patterns of spontaneous recovery in aphasic groups: A study of adult stroke patients. *Brain and Language, 5,* 388–401.

Loverso, F. L., & Milione, J. (1992). Training and generalization of expressive syntax in nonfluent aphasia. *Clinics in Communication Disorders, 2*(1), 43–53.

Loverso, F .L., Prescott, T. E., & Selinger, M. (1988). Cuing verbs: A treatment strategy for aphasic adults (CVT). *Journal of Rehabilitation Research and Development, 25,* 47–60.

Loverso, F. L., Prescott, T. E., Selinger, M., & Riley, L. (1989). Comparison of two modes of aphasia treatment: Clinician & computer-clinician assisted. *Clinical Aphasiology, 18,* 297–319.

Loverso, F. L., Prescott, T. E., Selinger, M., Wheeler, K. M., & Smith, R. (1985). The application of microcomputers for the treatment of aphasic adults. *Clinical Aphasiology, 15,* 189–195.

Loverso, F. L., Selinger, M., & Prescott, T. E. (1979). Application of verbing strategies to aphasia treatment. *Clinical Aphasiology, 9,* 229–238.

Lyon, J. G, & Helm-Estabrooks, N. (1987). Drawing: Its communicative significance for expressively restricted aphasic adults. *Topics in Language Disorders, 8*(1), 61–71.

Lyon, J. G., & Sims, E. (1989). Drawing: Its use as a communicative aid with aphasic and normal adults. *Clinical Aphasiology, 18,* 339–355.

MacLennan, D. L., Nicholas, L. E., Morley, G. K., & Brookshire, R. H. (1991). The effects of bromocriptine on speech and language function in a man with transcortical motor aphasia. *Clinical Aphasiology, 20,* 145–155.

McNeil, M. R., & Tseng, C. H. (1990). Acquired neurogenic dysgraphias. In L. L. LaPointe (Ed.), *Aphasia and related neurogenic language disorders* (pp. 147–176). New York: Thieme.

Morgan, A. L. R., & Helm-Estabrooks, N. (1987). Back to the Drawing Board: A treatment program for nonverbal aphasic patients. *Clinical Aphasiology, 17,* 64–72.

Naeser, M. A. (1991, November). *How to analyze CT scans to predict potential for recovery and good response to specific verbal and nonverbal treatment programs in aphasia.* Symposium conducted at the annual scientific meeting of the Academy of Neurologic Communication Disorders and Sciences, Atlanta.

Naeser, M. A., Frumkin, N. L., Helm-Estabrooks, N., Fitzpatrick, P. M., & Palumbo, C. L. (1991). *Predicting successful treatment with Melodic Intonation Therapy (MIT) using CT scan.* Manuscript submitted for publication.

Naeser, M. A., Gaddie, A., Palumbo, C. L., & Stiassny-Eder, D. (1990). Late recovery of auditory comprehension in global aphasia: Improved recovery observed with subcortical temporal isthmus lesion versus Wernicke's cortical area lesion. *Archives of Neurology, 47,* 425–432.

Naeser, M. A., Helm-Estabrooks, N., Haas, G., Auerbach, S., & Srinivasan, M. (1987). Relationship between lesion extent in "Wernicke's Area" on CT scan and predicting recovery of comprehension in Wernicke's Aphasia. *Archives of Neurology, 44,* 73–82.

Naeser, M. A., Palumbo, C. L., Helm-Estabrooks, N., Stiassny-Eder, D., & Albert, M. L. (1989). Severe non-fluency in aphasia: Role of the medial subcallosal fasciculus plus other white matter pathways in recovery of spontaneous speech. *Brain, 112,* 1–38.

Nicholas, M., & Helm-Estabrooks, N. (1990). Aphasia. *Seminars in Speech and Language, 11*(3), 135–144.

Peach, R. K. (1987). A short-term memory treatment approach to the repetition deficit in conduction aphasia. *Clinical Aphasiology, 17,* 35–45.

Peach, R. K. (1992). Efficacy of aphasia treatment: What are the real issues? *Clinics in Communication Disorders, 2*(1), 7–10.

Peach, R. K., Canter, G. J., & Gallaher, A. J. (1988). Comprehension of sentence structure in anomic and conduction aphasia. *Brain and Language, 35,* 119–137.

Perkins, W. H. (Ed.). (1983). *Language handicaps in adults.* New York: Thieme-Stratton.

Pierce, R. S., & Grogan, S. (1992). Improving listening comprehension of narratives. *Clinics in Communication Disorders, 2*(1), 54–63.

Porch, B. E. (1967). *Porch index of communicative ability.* Palo Alto, CA: Consulting Psychologists Press.

Prescott, T. E., Selinger, M., & Loverso, F. L. (1982). An analysis of learning, generalization and maintenance of verbs by an aphasic patient. *Clinical Aphasiology, 12,* 178–182.

Ramsberger, G., & Helm-Estabrooks, N. (1989). Visual Action Therapy for bucco-facial apraxia. *Clinical Aphasiology, 18,* 395–406.

Rao, P. R. (1986). The use of Amer-Ind code with aphasic adults. In R. Chapey (Ed.), *Language intervention strategies in adult aphasia* (2nd ed., pp. 360–367). Baltimore, MD: Williams & Wilkins.

Rao, P. R., Basili, A. G., Koller, J., Fullerton, B., Diener, S., & Burton, P. (1980). The use of Amer-Ind code by severe aphasic adults. In M. S. Burns and J. R. Andrews (Eds.), *Neuropathologies of speech and language: Diagnosis and treatment* (pp. 18–35). Evanston, IL: Institute for Continuing Professional Education.

Rao, P. R., & Horner, J. (1978). Gesture as a deblocking modality in a severe aphasic patient. *Clinical Aphasiology, 8,* 180–187.

Rao, P. R., & Horner, J. (1980). Nonverbal strategies for functional communication in aphasic persons. In M. S. Burns & J. R. Andrews (Eds.), *Neuropathologies of speech and language: Diagnosis and treatment* (pp. 108–133). Evanston, IL: Institute for Continuing Professional Education.

Raymer, A. M., & Thompson, C. K. (1991). Effects of verbal plus gestural treatment in a patient with severe apraxia of speech. *Clinical Aphasiology, 20,* 285–295.

Rosenbek, J. C., LaPointe, L. L., & Wertz, R. T. (1989). *Aphasia: A clinical approach.* Austin, TX: Pro-Ed.

Rosenbek, J. C., Lemme, M. L., Ahern, M. B., Harris, E. H., & Wertz, R. T. (1973). A treatment for apraxia of speech in adults. *Journal of Speech and Hearing Disorders, 38,* 462–472.

Ross, D., & Spencer, S. (1980). *Aphasia rehabilitation: An auditory and verbal task hierarchy.* Springfield, IL: Charles C. Thomas.

Sarno, M. T. (1969). *The functional communication profile: Manual of directions* (Rehabilitation Monograph 42). New York: New York University Medical Center, Institute of Rehabilitation Medicine.

Schuell, H. (1965). *The Minnesota test for differential diagnosis of aphasia.* Minneapolis: University of Minnesota Press.

Schuell, H. M., Jenkins, J. J., & Jimenez-Pabon, E. (1964). *Aphasia in adults: Diagnosis, prognosis, and treatment.* New York: Harper & Row.

Schwartz, M. F., Saffran, E. M., & Marin, O. S. M. (1980). The word order problem in agrammatism. I. Comprehension. *Brain and Language, 10,* 249–262.

Searle, J. (1969). *Speech acts: An essay in the philosophy of language.* London: Cambridge University Press.

Selinger, M., Prescott, T. E., Loverso, F., & Fuller, K. (1987). Below the 50th percentile: Application of the verb as core model. *Clinical Aphasiology, 17,* 55–63.

Shallice, T., & Warrington, E. K. (1977). Auditory-verbal short term memory impairment and conduction aphasia. *Brain and Language, 4,* 479–491.

Shapiro, L. P., & Levine, B. A. (1989). Real-time sentence processing in aphasia. *Clinical Aphasiology, 18,* 281–296.

Shapiro, L. P., & Levine, B. A. (1990). Verb processing during sentence comprehension in aphasia. *Brain and Language, 38,* 21–47.

Shewan, C. M. (1980). Verbal dyspraxia and its treatment. *Human Communication, 5,* 3–12.

Shewan, C. M., & Bandur, D. L. (1986). *Treatment of aphasia: A language oriented approach.* San Diego, CA: College-Hill Press.

Silverman, F. H. (1989). *Communication for the speechless* (2nd ed.). Englewood Cliffs, NJ: Prentice-Hall.

Skelly, M. (1979). *Amer-Ind gestural code based on universal American Indian hand talk.* New York: Elsevier.

Skelly, M., Schinsky, L., Smith, R., Donaldson, R., & Griffin, P. (1974). American Indian Sign (Amer-Ind) as a facilitator of verbalization for the oral-verbal apraxic. *Journal of Speech and Hearing Disorders, 39,* 445–456.

Skelly, M., Schinsky, L., Smith, R., Donaldson, R., & Griffin, P. (1975). American Indian Sign: Gestural communication for the speechless. *Archives of Physical Medicine and Rehabilitation, 56,* 156–160.

Sparks, R., Helm, N., & Albert, M. (1974). Aphasia rehabilitation resulting from Melodic Intonation Therapy. *Cortex, 10,* 303–316.

Steele, R. D., Weinrich, M., Kleczewska, M. K., Carlson, G. S., & Wertz, R. T. (1987). Evaluating performance of severely aphasic patients on a computer-aided visual communication system. *Clinical Aphasiology, 17,* 46–54.

Steele, R. D., Weinrich, M., Wertz, R. T., Kleczewska, M. K., & Carlson, G. S. (1989). Computer-based visual communication in aphasia. *Neuropsychologia, 27,* 409–426.

Sullivan, M. P., Fisher, B., & Marshall, R. C. (1986). Treating the repetition deficit in conduction aphasia. *Clinical Aphasiology, 16,* 172–180.

Tonkovich, J. D., & Loverso, F. L. (1982). A training matrix approach for gestural acquisition by the agrammatic patient. *Clinical Aphasiology, 12,* 283–288.

Tonkovich, J., & Peach, R. (1989). What to treat: Apraxia of speech, aphasia, or both. In P. Square-Storer (Ed.), *Acquired apraxia of speech in aphasic adults: Theoretical and clinical issues* (pp. 115–144). London: Taylor & Francis.

Trost, J. E., & Canter, G. J. (1974). Apraxia of speech in patients with Broca's aphasia: A study of phonemic production accuracy and error patterns. *Brain and Language, 1,* 63–79.

Ulatowska, H. K., & Chapman, S. B. (1989). Discourse considerations for aphasia management. *Seminars in Speech and Language, 10,* 298–314.

Webb, W. G. (1990). Acquired alexias. In L. L. LaPointe (Ed.), *Aphasia and related neurogenic language disorders* (pp. 130–146). New York: Thieme.

Webb, W. G., & Love, R. J. (1986). Therapy for retraining reading. In R. Chapey (Ed.), *Language intervention strategies in adult aphasia* (2nd ed., pp. 394–401). Baltimore, MD: Williams & Wilkins.

Weinrich, M., Steele, R., Carlson, G. S., Kleczewska, M., Wertz, R. T., & Baker, E. H. (1989). Processing of visual syntax in a globally aphasic patient. *Brain and Language, 36,* 391–405.

Weinrich, M., Steele, R., Kleczewska, M., Carlson, G. S., Baker, E. H.,& Wertz, R. T. (1989). Representation of "verbs" in a computerized visual communication system. *Aphasiology, 3,* 501–512.

Wertz, R. T. (1983). Language intervention context and setting for the aphasic adult: When? In J. Miller, D. E. Yoder, and R. Schiefelbusch (Eds.), *Contemporary issues in language intervention* (ASHA Reports 12, pp. 196–220). Rockville, MD: American Speech-Language-Hearing Association.

Wertz, R. T. (1991). Glasnost in aphasiology: On opening up systems. *Clinical Aphasiology, 20,* 1–8.

Wilcox, M. J., & Davis, G. A. (1977). Speech act analysis of aphasic communication in individual and group settings. *Clinical Aphasiology, 7,* 166–174.

Wilcox, M. J., & Davis, G. A. (1978). *Procedures for promoting communicative effectiveness in an aphasic adult.* Symposium conducted at the annual meeting of the American Speech and Hearing Association, San Francisco.

Wilcox, M. J., & Davis, G. A. (1979, November). *Promoting aphasic communicative effectiveness.* Paper presented to the American Speech-Language-Hearing Association, Atlanta, GA.

Wilcox, M. J., Davis, G. A., & Leonard, L. (1978). Aphasics' comprehension of contextually conveyed meaning. *Brain and Language, 6,* 362–377.

Index